a LANGE

Pulmonary Pathophysiology

A CLINICAL APPROACH

3rd edition

Edited by

Juzar Ali, MD
Professor of Medicine
Louisiana State University Health Sciences Center
School of Medicine
Section of Pulmonary/Critical Care Medicine
New Orleans, Louisiana

Warren R. Summer, MD
Professor of Medicine
Louisiana State University Health Sciences Center
School of Medicine
Section of Pulmonary/Critical Care Medicine
New Orleans, Louisiana

Michael G. Levitzky, PhD
Professor of Physiology, Anesthesiology, and Cardiopulmonary Science
Louisiana State University Health Sciences Center
Department of Physiology
New Orleans, Louisiana

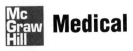 **Medical**

New York Chicago San Francisco Lisbon London Madrid Mexico City
Milan New Delhi San Juan Seoul Singapore Sydney Toronto

This book was set in Adobe Garamond by Newgen North America.
The editors were Michael Weitz and Peter J. Boyle.
The production supervisor was Catherine H. Saggese.
Project management was provided by Newgen North America.
RR Donnelley was printer and binder.

This book is printed on acid-free paper.

McGraw-Hill books are available at special quantity discounts to use as premiums and sales promotions, or for use in corporate training programs. To contact a representative please e-mail us at bulksales@mcgraw-hill.com.

Contents

Contributors

Juzar Ali, MD
Professor of Medicine, Louisiana State University Health Sciences Center, School of Medicine, Section of Pulmonary/Critical Care Medicine, New Orleans, Louisiana

LaSandra Barton, MD
Assistant Professor, Louisiana State University Health Sciences Center, School of Medicine, Section of Pulmonary/Critical Care Medicine, New Orleans, Louisiana

Peter DeBlieux, MD
Professor of Medicine, Louisiana State University Health Sciences Center, School of Medicine, Section of Pulmonary/Critical Care Medicine, New Orleans, Louisiana

Bennett P. deBoisblanc, MD
Professor of Medicine and Physiology, Louisiana State University Health Sciences Center, School of Medicine, Section of Pulmonary/Critical Care Medicine, New Orleans, Louisiana

Susan Gunn, MD
Assistant Professor, Louisiana State University Health Sciences Center, School of Medicine, Section of Pulmonary/Critical Care Medicine, New Orleans, Louisiana

Suma Jain, MD
Assistant Professor, Ochsner Medical Center, Pulmonary Department, Jefferson, Louisiana

Stephen P. Kantrow, MD
Associate Professor of Medicine, Louisiana State University Health Sciences Center, School of Medicine, Section of Pulmonary/Critical Care Medicine, New Orleans, Louisiana

Jason M. Konter, MD
Senior Fellow, Department of Medicine, Section of Pulmonary Medicine, Boston University Medical School, Boston, Massachusetts

Michael G. Levitzky, PhD
Professor of Physiology, Anesthesiology, and Cardiopulmonary Science, Louisiana State University Health Sciences Center, Department of Physiology, New Orleans, Louisiana

Carol M. Mason, MD
Professor of Medicine, Louisiana State University Health Sciences Center, School of Medicine, Section of Pulmonary/Critical Care Medicine, New Orleans, Louisiana

Kendra J. McAnally , MD
Louisiana State University Health Sciences Center, School of Medicine, Section of Pulmonary/Critical Care Medicine, New Orleans, Louisiana

Richard Morrison, MD
Louisiana State University Health Sciences Center, Department of Medicine, Section of Pulmonary/Critical Care Medicine, New Orleans, Louisiana

Jennifer Ramsey, MD
Assistant Professor of Medicine, Louisiana State University Health Sciences Center, Department of Medicine, Section of Pulmonary/Critical Care Medicine, New Orleans, Louisiana

Kevin Reed, MD
Associate Professor of Medicine, Louisiana State University Health Sciences Center, School of Medicine, Section of Pulmonary/Critical Care Medicine, New Orleans, Louisiana

Leonardo Seoane, MD
Program Director of Internal Medicine,
Staff Physician, Section of Pulmonary
and Critical Care Medicine, Ochsner
Clinic Foundation, New Orleans,
Louisiana

Judd Shellito, MD
Professor of Medicine and Microbiology,
Immunology, and Parasitology,
Louisiana State University Health
Sciences Center, School of Medicine,
Section of Pulmonary/Critical Care
Medicine, New Orleans, Louisiana

Michael Stumpf, MD
Department of Medicine, Earl
K. Long Hospital, Baton Rouge,
Louisiana

Ross S. Summer, MD
Associate Professor, Pulmonary
Center, Boston University, Boston,
Massachusetts

Warren R. Summer, MD
Professor of Medicine, Louisiana State
University Health Sciences Center,
School of Medicine, Section of
Pulmonary/Critical Care Medicine,
New Orleans, Louisiana

David Taylor, MD
Clinical Associate Professor of
Medicine, Louisiana State University
Health Sciences Center, School of
Medicine, Section of Pulmonary/
Critical Care Medicine, New Orleans,
Louisiana

Dwayne A. Thomas, MD
Professor of Medicine, Louisiana State
University Health Sciences Center,
School of Medicine, Section of
Pulmonary/Critical Care Medicine,
New Orleans, Louisiana

David A. Welsh, MD
Associate Professor of Medicine,
Louisiana State University Health
Sciences Center, School of Medicine,
Section of Pulmonary/Critical Care
Medicine, New Orleans, Louisiana

Preface

The third edition of *Pulmonary Pathophysiology* elaborates on the clinical implications of the subjects discussed, with the pathogenesis and the pathophysiological aspects of each topic made more concise. More tables and charts have been incorporated and certain redundancies eliminated. Algorithms and Key Concepts summarizing each chapter have been maintained. Some chapters have been reorganized or rewritten.

We wish to acknowledge the assistance and cooperation of the staff of McGraw-Hill and Newgen North America in preparing this edition.

Juzar Ali
New Orleans, Louisiana   *Warren R. Summer*
August, 2009   *Michael G. Levitzky*

SECTION 1
Basic Evaluation: Symptoms/Problem Based

Dyspnea

Richard Morrison & Warren R. Summer

OBJECTIVES

- ▶ *Define dyspnea and its pathophysiologic relationship to various disease processes.*
- ▶ *Identify types of respiratory disease by the recognition of spirometric patterns.*
- ▶ *Identify appropriate tests used in the systematic evaluation of dyspnea.*

GENERAL CONSIDERATIONS

Dyspnea is a sensation of breathlessness or subjective "shortness of breath." It defies strict definition with many individual descriptions and varies widely among patients for comparable objective dysfunction. The American Thoracic Society (ATS) has defined dyspnea as "a term used to characterize a subjective experience of breathing discomfort that is comprised of quantitatively distinct sensations that vary in intensity." The sensation of breathlessness can be experienced by healthy subjects with exercise or at high altitudes and those with diseases that affect the respiratory, cardiac, endocrine, renal, neurologic, hematologic, or rheumatologic systems. It is a frequent clinical complaint. Occasionally, a source cannot be clearly identified, and dyspnea is attributed to psychophysiologic disturbances.

ETIOLOGY & PATHOGENESIS

Dyspnea in patients with chronic obstructive pulmonary disease (COPD) is due to narrowing of the airways, increased airway resistance, and reduction of lung elastic recoil. Very often, concominant hyperinflation is seen, which alters respiratory muscle mechanics, thereby increasing the sensation of dyspnea. Infiltration of the lung parenchyma in diffuse lung disease such as pulmonary fibrosis can also result in similar ventilatory impediment due to increased elastic work of breathing. This is also seen in conditions causing acute respiratory distress syndrome (ARDS) and pulmonary edema with congestive heart failure (Table 1–1). Excessive secretions and inability to clear such secretions can compromise airways and increase airway resistance. Chest wall mechanics can also be compromised by pleural disease and cause dyspnea. Some patients with chronic lung disease have increased minute ventilation at rest and on exertion due to increased dead space (wasted ventilation), increased carbon dioxide production, and enhanced drive to breathe.

The sensation of dyspnea increases when the demand to breathe is disproportionate to the requirement. Increased work of breathing resulting from an imbalance between afferent inputs and respiratory muscle output due to poor nutrition and muscle strength can contribute to the sensation of dyspnea. Common to the processes causing metabolic acidosis, such as aspirin, methanol ingestion, increased lactic acidosis due to poor tissue perfusion, overproduction of ketones secondary to metabolism of fatty acids (eg, diabetic ketoacidosis, alcoholism, or starvation), renal failure (decreased excretion of hydrogen ions), or bicarbonate loss (eg, diarrhea, renal dysfunction, or pancreatic disease), is an increase in hydrogen ions, which stimulate arterial receptors, especially those in the carotid bodies. This respiratory compensation is often appreciated or perceived as dyspnea.

PATHOPHYSIOLOGY & MECHANISM OF DYSPNEA

Breathing is an unconscious act; we are only aware of our breathing effort when something is wrong. Many respiratory conditions can present acutely with the sensation of dyspnea. Dyspnea is not a single sensation and the mechanism of dyspnea is not well understood. Similar to pain, dyspnea appears to be multidimensional encompassing unpleasantness and emotional impact. Dyspnea has two dimensions, sensory and affective, and both can be independently identified in the laboratory and in clinical situations. Also, it is a perception or subjective experience and it must be explained by human experiments. New brain imaging studies indicate that the sensation of different respiratory efforts is perceived in several areas of the brain stem and sensory cortex with dyspnea resulting when the degree of stimulation in respiratory-related neurons is perceived as being excessive. Stimulation may arise from different situations (eg, exercise, hypoxia, or breath-holding), medical conditions (eg, increased airway resistance, decreased compliance, or increased work of breathing), physical discomfort (pain), metabolic changes (acidosis), emotional discomfort, excitement, and depression. Receptors in the heart may also give rise to perceptions of

Table 1–1. Pathophysiologic correlates of disease causing dyspnea

Structural or mechanical interference with ventilation

Obstruction of flow
  Emphysema
  Asthma
  Chronic bronchitis
  Tracheal (after prolonged mechanical ventilation, vocal cord dysfunction)
  Endobronchial disease, primary lung carcinoma, foreign body

Restriction to lung or chest wall expansion

Intrinsic: diseases involving lung parenchyma
  Interstitial fibrosis
  Acute respiratory distress syndrome
  Congestive heart failure
Extrinsic: processes not involving lung parenchyma
  Kyphoscoliosis
  Obesity
  Ascites
  Pregnancy
  Pleural fibrosis

Increases in dead space ventilation

Emphysema: obstruction of airflow
Pulmonary embolus: interruption of blood flow

Respiratory muscle weakness

Poliomyelitis
Neuromuscular disease
Systemic diseases
Guillain-Barré syndrome

Increases in respiratory drive

Hypoxemia: secondary to any cause
  Exercise
  Metabolic acidosis: diabetic ketoacidosis and renal failure
  Significant decreases in hemoglobin or cardiac output

Psychological disturbances

Anxiety/panic attacks
Depression and somatization disorders

Source: Adapted with permission from Stulbarg MS, Adams L. Dyspnea. In: Murray JF, Nadel JA, eds. *Textbook of Respiratory Medicine*. Vol. 1, 3rd ed. Philadelphia, PA: WB Saunders; 2000:511–528.

dyspnea (orthopnea) since awareness of breathing may occur with apparently normal lungs and gas exchange.

The increased afferent stimulation of the respiratory complex from a variety of receptors (chemoreceptors, proprioreceptors, or emotions) results in increasing efferent neural drive to the respiratory muscles. Additional stimuli of other afferent pathways can contribute (eg, bronchospasm, inflammation, pulmonary hypertension, or lung edema). This information is simultaneously relayed to sensory areas within the cortex.

The sense of respiratory effort intensifies with increases in central efferent respiratory motor activity. This sense of effort is proportional to the ratio of the pressures generated by the respiratory muscles to the maximum pressure-generating capacity of these muscles. Mechanical support during exercise therefore reduces the sensation of dyspnea. Externally supported increases in minute ventilation (by a mechanical device) are associated with little or no dyspnea.

The final perception of dyspnea may best relate to total neural traffic. Both the "sense of effort" (augmented requirements to overcome mechanical constraints or muscle weakness) and the "urge to breathe" (hypoxia, hypercapnia, airway compression, and anxiety) contribute to the global perception of dyspnea. There is polymorphism in neurotraffic with some (patients) producing greater neurotraffic for similar experience. This may explain individual "panic attacks" in certain patients. The addition of oral or parenteral opioids reduces dyspnea in patients with severe disease whereas the use of antidepressants may reduce dyspnea in some patients.

Dyspnea is worse when unexpected or perceived to be dangerous. Adaptation or acclimatization seems to occur with hypoxemia, exercise conditioning, and some mechanical constraints.

Thus, dyspnea increases when ventilatory impedance increases as during an acute asthma attack, when ventilatory demand increases as during exercise, when respiratory muscle function is abnormal as in hyperinflation states, and when perception of dyspnea is increased as during an anxiety attack. The correlation between dyspnea and objective measures of lung and cardiac function is weak.

DIAGNOSTIC & CLINICAL CONSIDERATIONS

An understanding of basic respiratory physiology enables the clinician to categorize and evaluate dyspnea. Basic concepts such as increased respiratory drive, respiratory muscle weakness, dead space ventilation, and mechanical impairment of ventilation, all contribute to an understanding of the underlying causes and mechanisms of dyspnea. It is possible to narrow the differential diagnosis and evaluation of dyspnea by asking whether the symptoms are acute or chronic (see Figures 1–1 and 1–2). Acute changes are more likely to be seen in congestive heart failure, myocardial infarction, exacerbations of COPD, asthma attacks, pulmonary embolism, and pneumonia. Dyspnea is usually recognized as chronic when it is present for at least 4–8 weeks. Common causes and observed frequencies for chronic dyspnea are listed in Table 1–2.

Evaluation of the History

A comprehensive history is required and will help to define the timing, precipitating or aggravating factors, related conditions, severity of symptoms, their relationship to activity, and any identifiable alleviating factors. Patients with certain diseases tend to describe the shortness of breath in similar terms (Table 1–3),

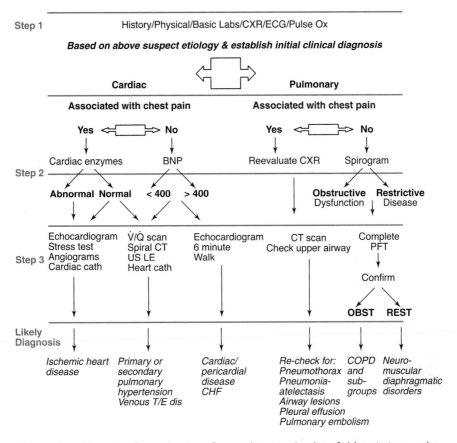

Figure 1–1. Algorithm for evaluation of acute dyspnea. See list of abbreviations at the end of the book.

but the reliability of specific descriptions is suspect. Nocturnal dyspnea may be related to several disease processes, such as asthma, congestive heart failure, gastroesophageal reflux, or nasal congestion. In the supine position, dyspnea may be related to something that upwardly displaces the abdominal contents, such as pregnancy, ascites, diaphragmatic paralysis, or redistribution of intravascular volume to the central circulation that is not compensated due to a failing heart. If symptoms are intermittent, the clinician should consider reversible diseases such as asthma (bronchoconstriction), heart failure, or recurrent pulmonary emboli. Progressive symptoms usually signal more chronic diseases, such as interstitial pulmonary fibrosis, sarcoidosis, COPD, amylotrophic lateral sclerosis, or cancer.

Dyspnea that has its onset in conjunction with physical activity is generally of physiologic origin. For example, dyspnea may be due to deconditioning, anemia (decreased oxygen delivery), or exercise-induced asthma. If the patient complains of shortness of breath that is independent of physical activity, the

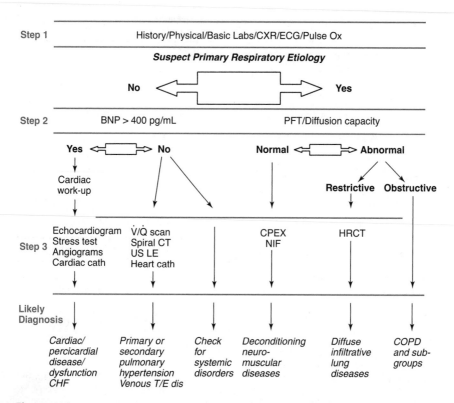

Figure 1–2. Algorithm for evaluation of a patient reporting chronic dyspnea. See list of abbreviations at the end of the book.

Table 1–2. Frequency (%) of respiratory conditions presenting to an emergency department with a chief complaint of breathlessness

Asthma	20–30
Cardiac	15
COPD	5–15
Interstitial lung disease	5–15
Deconditioning and obesity	5–15
Psychophysiologic	5–25
Unexplained upper airway	5–7
Pulmonary vascular	5
Neuromuscular	5
Endocrine (hyperthyroid) and GI	5

Note: COPD, chronic obstructive pulmonary disease; GI, gastrointestinal.

Table 1–3. Often-used patient descriptions of dyspnea as reported in asthma

My breathing is heavy
I feel a hunger for more air
I feel out of breath
I have an uncomfortable awareness of my breathing
I am gasping for breath
My chest feels tight
I can't take a deep breath
My breathing is rapid
I can't get enough air
I feel I am smothering or suffocating

Table 1–4. American Thoracic Society shortness of breath scale

Description	Grade	Degree
Not troubled by shortness of breath when hurrying on the level or walking up a slight hill	0	None
Troubled by shortness of breath when hurrying on the level or walking up a slight hill	1	Mild
Walks slower than people of the same age on the level because of breathlessness or has to stop for breath when walking at own pace	2	Moderate
Stops for breath after walking 100 yards or after a few minutes on the level	3	Severe
Too breathless to leave the house, or breathless on dressing or undressing	4	Very severe

Note: This scale has been used in this or a similar form for many years, especially for epidemiologic studies.

Source: Adapted with permission from Stulbarg MS, Adams L. Dyspnea. In: Murray JF, Nadel JA, eds. *Textbook of Respiratory Medicine.* Vol. 1, 3rd ed. Philadelphia, PA: WB Saunders; 2000:511–528.

clinician should consider psychological problems. If the dyspnea is clearly out of proportion to objective findings, it may be related to personal gain or litigation (malingering).

There are several specific questions related to the dyspnea experience, which can help the clinician identify the true cause of the patient's dyspnea and overall impact on quality of life (Table 1-4). Patients do not always associate external factors with breathlessness and may need further prompting through focused questioning regarding such precipitating factors as foods, medications, cleaners, perfumes, and cigarettes. Correlation with exposure to animals, plants, or the workplace environment may also be a significant clue to the origin of the dyspnea.

Physical Examination

The patient's respiratory rate should be noted along with body habitus (eg, the barrel chest of COPD or obesity) and use of accessory muscles of respiration. The sensation of dyspnea is analogous to pain and as a result may play a protective role as does pain by causing an individual to reduce his or her level of activity when distressed. Dyspnea is multifactorial in its perception; the patient's degree of physical fitness, weight, level of awareness, levels of hemoglobin, blood pH, oxygen tension, and the psychological state influence the sensation of dyspnea. But dyspnea is often difficult to quantify. Objective signs of breathlessness are the use of accessory muscles of respiration, tachypnea, flaring of the nasal alae, and cyanosis. These objective factors are easier to quantify. Several scales to grade degrees of dyspnea have been developed and are individually reproducible on repeated testing.

The Borg scale for assessing dyspnea (Table 1–5) uses verbal descriptions ("slight," "moderate," and "severe") to rate the intensity of symptoms, usually during a particular activity. Numerical equivalents are assigned to each choice so that various levels of activity can be scored and levels of dyspnea graded for individuals and compared to assess improvement after therapy. Another popular dyspnea scale is the ATS shortness of breath scale (Table 1–4). Both scales are relatively simple to understand and are widely used for clinically assessing dyspnea. It must be kept in mind that they are insensitive to significant differences in functional impairment over time.

Table 1–5. Modified Borg category scale

Rating	Intensity of sensation
0	Nothing at all
0.5	Very, very slight (just noticeable)
1	Very slight
2	Slight
3	Moderate
4	Somewhat severe
5	Severe
6	Very severe
7	Very severe
8	Very severe
9	Very, very severe (almost maximal)
10	Maximal

Source: Adapted with permission from Stulbarg MS, Adams L. Dyspnea. In: Murray JF, Nadel JA, eds. *Textbook of Respiratory Medicine*. Vol. 1, 3rd ed. Philadelphia, PA: WB Saunders; 2000:511–528.

Breath sounds also give important clues to the underlying cause: crackles (heart failure), wheezing (asthma or COPD), decreased or absent breath sounds (emphysema, pneumothorax, or pleural effusion). A right ventricular heave and a loud second pulmonic (P_2) sound (ie, an accentuated component of the second heart sound representing closure of the pulmonic valve) suggest pulmonary hypertension. Jugular venous distention and pedal edema are clues to the diagnosis of heart failure. Dry (velcro) crackles, clubbing, and cyanosis are signs of significant interstitial lung disease.

Laboratory Evaluation

Other helpful and objective data obtained during this phase of the evaluation include the results of blood chemistries, hemoglobin, chest x-ray, pulmonary function tests (PFTs), and an electrocardiogram, especially if the patient is over 40 years of age and has symptoms referable to the cardiac system. The chest x-ray may reveal the presence of pneumonia, infiltrates, masses, effusions, hyperinflated lungs, or unexpected cardiomegaly.

Dyspnea caused by respiratory dysfunction can be divided into several physiologic categories through careful evaluation of pulmonary function as we discuss in the next section of this chapter.

Arterial blood gases may be very helpful in understanding the underlying mechanism for dyspnea (Figure 1–3). Maintaining appropriate ventilation–perfusion relationships within the lung is critical to good gas exchange. Normal alveolar ventilation occurs at a rate of approximately 4–6 L/min, similar to the rate of pulmonary blood flow, making the ratio of ventilation to perfusion or $\dot{V}/\dot{Q}$ approximately 0.8–1.2. Therefore, if it is severe enough, any disease process that disturbs this fundamental relationship will alter gas exchange. Airflow obstruction moves the $\dot{V}/\dot{Q}$ toward, but rarely to, zero. Hypoxemia usually has to be severe before it is perceived as dyspnea. Increases in dead space or wasted ventilation move the $\dot{V}/\dot{Q}$ toward infinity and can be demonstrated in emphysema. Dead space or wasted ventilation must be massive and will usually cause other problems with mechanics or respiratory acidosis to produce dyspnea. Dyspnea may be experienced with reduced minute ventilation as a function of respiratory muscle weakness and is seen in patients with a history of polio, severe hypothyroidism, and Guillain-Barré syndrome.

Another disease process that alters gas exchange producing hypoxemia is pulmonary embolism in which blood flow is interrupted and $\dot{V}/\dot{Q}$ moves toward infinity. Dyspnea is reported in 80%–90% of patients with pulmonary embolism. Acute hypoxia is present in 85%–90% of patients with significant emboli.

Lung and chest wall mechanics may also be adversely affected by hyperinflation with flattening of the diaphragm and airway narrowing (eg, as in asthma, emphysema). In addition, patients with a pneumothorax, pleural effusion, pleural fibrosis, and thoracic cage deformities have altered mechanics.

Psychosomatic disorders are diagnoses of exclusion, and a thorough work-up should be completed prior to labeling any patient as having such a disorder.

Objective measures such as respiratory rate, oxygen tension, or PFTs do not correlate with the subjective experience of dyspnea.

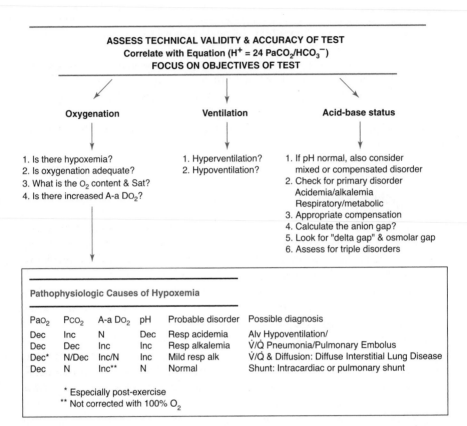

ASSESS TECHNICAL VALIDITY & ACCURACY OF TEST
Correlate with Equation (H^+ = 24 $PaCO_2$/HCO_3^-)
FOCUS ON OBJECTIVES OF TEST

Oxygenation

1. Is there hypoxemia?
2. Is oxygenation adequate?
3. What is the O_2 content & Sat?
4. Is there increased A-a DO_2?

Ventilation

1. Hyperventilation?
2. Hypoventilation?

Acid-base status

1. If pH normal, also consider
   mixed or compensated disorder
2. Check for primary disorder
   Acidemia/alkalemia
   Respiratory/metabolic
3. Appropriate compensation
4. Calculate the anion gap?
5. Look for "delta gap" & osmolar gap
6. Assess for triple disorders

Pathophysiologic Causes of Hypoxemia

PaO_2	PCO_2	A-a DO_2	pH	Probable disorder	Possible diagnosis
Dec	Inc	N	Dec	Resp acidemia	Alv Hypoventilation/
Dec	Dec	Inc	Inc	Resp alkalemia	V̇/Q̇ Pneumonia/Pulmonary Embolus
Dec*	N/Dec	Inc/N	Inc	Mild resp alk	V̇/Q̇ & Diffusion: Diffuse Interstitial Lung Disease
Dec	N	Inc**	N	Normal	Shunt: Intracardiac or pulmonary shunt

* Especially post-exercise
** Not corrected with 100% O_2

COMPENSATION EQUATIONS

Primary Disorder	pH Change	Appropriate Secondary Changes
Respiratory acidosis & Alkalosis $PaCO_2$ change (Acute) $PaCO_2$ change (Chronic)	Δ pH = 0.008 x Δ in PCO_2 Δ pH = 0.003 x Δ in PCO_2	Δ HCO_3 minimal Δ HCO_3 = 0.4 x Δ PCO_2
Metabolic Acidosis Drop in HCO_3	Variable	Δ $PaCO_2$ = 1.2 xΔ HCO_3
Metabolic Alkalosis Rise in HCO_3	Variable	Δ $PaCO_2$ = 0.6 xΔ HCO_3

Figure 1-3. Algorithm and synopsis for interpretation of arterial blood gases. See list of abbreviations at the end of the book.

Pulmonary Function Tests

The nature and severity of many respiratory diseases can be reliably and effectively evaluated using PFTs. The tests are noninvasive and reproducible and can be completed in a relatively short time. Airflow, lung volumes, and diffusion capacity are routinely measured and provide a quantitative measure of lung function (Figure 1–4).

The forced vital capacity (FVC) and forced expiratory volume in the first second (FEV_1) are primary values and form the basis of the spirometric evaluation. This test enables the clinician to recognize expiratory obstructive airway diseases, suspect restrictive lung disease, define disease severity, and serially follow disease progression or response to therapy. Spirometry may help assess preoperative risk and predict post–lung resection symptoms.

Common obstructive airway diseases include asthma, chronic bronchitis, and emphysema and are defined by increased resistance to airflow. Reduction in airflow may also be caused by tracheal stenosis, large airway tumors, toxic insults, hypersensitivity, and inflammatory diseases. Obstruction is defined as a decrease in the FEV_1:FVC ratio to below 70%, primarily through a decrease in the FEV_1. Patients usually do not report symptoms until the FEV_1 is <60% predicted. Severe obstruction is considered to be present when the FEV_1 is below 50% of predicted, although symptoms only loosely correlate with objective measurements.

There are several conditions in which obstruction may not be accompanied by a low FEV_1:FVC ratio. These conditions include central airway obstruction, acute air trapping with increased residual volume (RV), and premature termination of the forced expiratory maneuver (expiratory time less than 6 seconds).

Reduced lung or expansion can be divided into two categories: intrinsic (those that involve the pulmonary parenchyma, eg, interstitial fibrosis, ARDS, and congestive heart failure) and extrinsic (eg, kyphoscoliosis, obesity, tense ascites, and pregnancy). These diseases change lung volume measurements. The lungs consist of four standard compartments, or volumes, that vary with diaphragm position (Figure 1–5). The tidal volume (TV) is the volume of air that enters and leaves the lungs with each breath and is approximately 500 mL in a 70-kg adult. The inspiratory reserve volume (IRV) is the maximum volume of air that can be inhaled to reach the total lung capacity (TLC) over and above the TV. It is influenced by muscle strength, elastic recoil of the chest wall and lungs, and the appropriate starting point (ie, the end of a normal tidal breath). A normal IRV in a 70-kg adult is approximately 2.5 L. The expiratory reserve volume (ERV) is the maximum volume of air that can be exhaled from end-expiration (ie, the end of a normal tidal breath), and is approximately 1.5 L in a 70-kg subject. It is reduced in pregnancy, obesity, and neuromuscular disease. The volume of air that remains in the lung after maximal expiration is the RV, also about 1.5 L (Figure 1–5).

Four additional volumes, referred to as capacities, are made up of two or more volumes. The TLC is the volume of air in the lungs after maximal inspiration and is the sum of all lung volumes. The vital capacity (VC) is the volume of gas that can be exhaled after maximal inhalation (from TLC). It is the sum of IRV, TV, and ERV. The funcitonal residual capacity FRC is the volume of air remaining in the lungs at the end of a normal expiration and is the sum of RV and ERV (Figure 1–5). The inspiratory capacity (IC) is the total volume of air that can be inhaled from the FRC (end of normal quiet breathing). It is the sum of TV and IRV (Figure

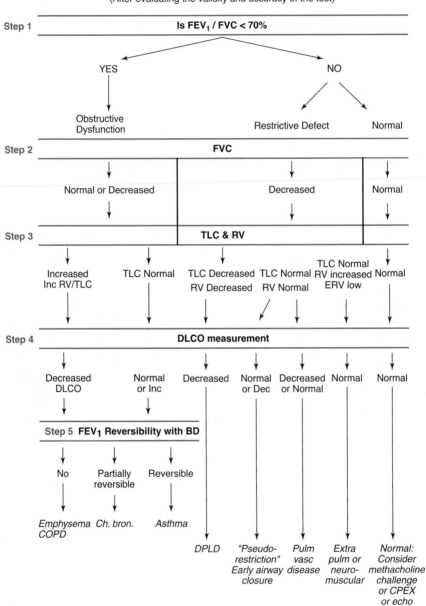

Figure 1-4. Algorithm for interpretation of pulmonary function tests. See list of abbreviations at the end of the book.

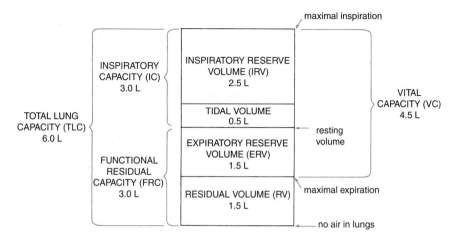

Figure 1–5. Standard lung volumes and capacities for a 70-kg adult male. (Reproduced with permission from Levitzky MG. *Pulmonary Physiology*, 7th ed. New York, NY: McGraw-Hill/ Lange; 2007:55–65.)

1–5). IC may increase after bronchodilator use as the only indication of an effective response. When reduced, this function may correlate with dyspnea and the ratio of IC/TLC correlates with survival in a COPD patient. The measurement of lung volumes helps to clarify and further define specific diseases. A TLC that is >120% predicted defines hyperinflation, whereas a reduction below 80% predicted defines restriction.

Diffusion occurs when there is net movement of a gas from an area of high partial pressure to one of lower partial pressure. Each gas moves according to its own partial pressure gradient, which is dependent on temperature. The transfer of a gas across a membrane is proportional to the area of the membrane and concentration gradient (Fick's law). Other less significant but nevertheless important factors in diffusion include membrane thickness and hemoglobin (Hgb) level. Therefore, disease processes that affect any of these factors will adversely affect diffusion capacity (DLCO) (Table 1–6). There are also conditions in which an increase in DLCO may be seen, including early congestive heart failure, asthma with acute bronchospasm, and pulmonary hemorrhage. Measurement of diffusing capacity may vary up to 20% over time, making small changes difficult to interpret.

Patterns associated with normal, obstructive, restrictive, fixed, and variable upper and lower airway obstructions can help in identifying different mechanisms of airway obstruction. Familiarity with the shape of flow-volume loops allows for the rapid recognition of spirometric abnormalities and the various patterns of airway obstruction (Figures 1–6 and 1–7). Consistency of PFTs is best achieved in the same laboratory. Table 1–7 lists several pulmonary function patterns commonly seen in patients with respiratory dysfunction and forms the basis for understanding and interpreting PFTs.

Table 1–6. Conditions that lead to reductions in diffusion capacity

Alveolar capillary membrane
Quantitative loss
Decreased lung volume (pulmonary resection)
Decreased surface area or lung volume (emphysema, atelectasis, compression)
Qualitative change
Membrane thickening
Circulatory factors
Hgb concentration (anemia)
Pulmonary blood volume reduction
Ventilation-perfusion changes
Nonperfusion of ventilated alveoli (pulmonary embolus)
Miscellaneous factors
Changes in CO_2 back-pressure (elevated carboxyhemoglobin)

Table 1–7. Common pulmonary function testing patterns found in respiratory dysfunction

Disorder	FEV_1	FVC	FEV_1/FVC	TLC	RV	FRC	DLCO
Asthma	↓	↓	↓	N or ↑	↑	N or ↑	N
COPD	↓	N or ↓	↓	N or ↑	↑	N or ↑	N or ↓
Fibrosis	↓	↓	N or ↑	↓	↓	↓	↓
Muscle weakness	↓	↓	N or ↑	↓	N or ↑	N	N
Kyphoscoliosis	↓	↓	N or ↑	↓	N or ↓	↓	N

Note: COPD, chronic obstructive pulmonary disease; DLCO, diffusion capacity; FEV, forced expiratory volume; FVC, forced vital capacity; N, normal; RV, residual volume; TLC, total lung capacity.

Other Tests in the Evaluation of Dyspnea

The first objective measure of suspected lung disease should be PFTs. They will usually give concrete clues to the underlying abnormality. However, many patients will need additional testing. The appropriate selection of tests will depend on the patient's history. For example, if the PFT results are normal and the patient has symptoms of intermittent shortness of breath, asthma or cardiovascular disease may be present. If asthma is suspected, bronchoprovocation testing may be indicated. This method uses nonspecific mediators of bronchoconstriction (methacholine) to determine whether airway hyperreactivity is present. If the concentration of methacholine required to produce a 20% or greater fall in the FEV_1 (PC_{20}) is very low (<1 µg/mL), the likelihood of moderate to severe asthma is high. If there is no response to a concentration of >16 µg/mL, asthma is very unlikely. Patients

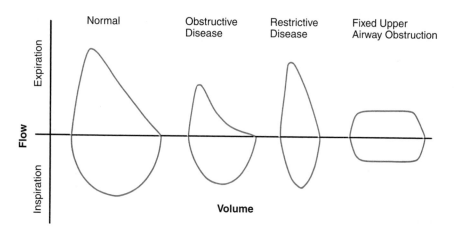

Figure 1–6. Flow-volume curves. The shape of the flow-volume curves allows rapid qualitative assessment of pulmonary function. The flow is plotted on the *y* axis, and the volume is plotted on the *x* axis. (Reproduced with permission from Schwartzstein RM, Weinberger SE. Use and interpretation of pulmonary function tests. *Resident Staff Phys.* 1986;32:43.)

with methacholine PC_{20} responses at 4–16 μg/mL have increased airways reactivity, but the test is of borderline significance for diagnosing asthma. Mild asthmatics usually have a PC_{20} between 1 and 4 μg/mL.

A chest x-ray will help in identifying the presence of hyperinflation and changes in the pleura or lung parenchyma. High-resolution computed tomography (HRCT) scanning may be useful in identifying subtle inflammatory lung diseases and differentiating various causes of interstitial pneumonitis. Electrocardiograms are recommended if the patient has symptoms referable to the cardiac system, especially if the patient is older than 40 years of age. Exercise testing may provide a more precise assessment of the patient's functional capacity or impairment than PFTs, and may uncover unsuspected cardiovascular disease. Diseases that affect the heart, lungs, and circulation will invariably cause an abnormal response to exercise. Although the test results do not lead to a specific diagnosis, they can help to categorize the disease state. Cardiopulmonary exercise testing helps to evaluate unexplained dyspnea, determine factors (cardiac or pulmonary) that limit activity, measure the degree of ventilatory limitation, and follow the natural course of several diseases. Treadmill and cycle ergometry are the two main exercise modes in cardiopulmonary exercise testing. If the history or physical exam points primarily toward underlying cardiac disease, echocardiograms should be performed early and cardiac catheterization may be indicated. Ventilation-perfusion scanning is the most sensitive screening test in the evaluation of pulmonary vascular disease. Contrast spiral CT and pulmonary angiography are very specific to pulmonary emboli. When any of these three studies are normal, significant emboli can be excluded. In patients with an elevated hemidiaphragm, fluoroscopy may be diagnostic of paralysis if paradoxical movement of the elevated diaphragm is present.

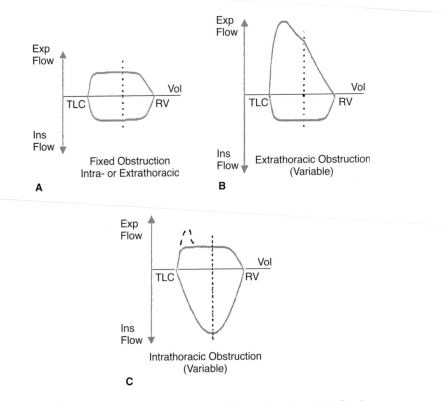

Figure 1–7. Maximal inspiratory and expiratory flow-volume curves in fixed obstruction (**A**), extrathoracic variable obstruction (**B**), and intrathoracic variable obstruction (**C**). The dashed line represents a flow transient that is occasionally observed just before the plateau in intrathoracic obstruction. (Reproduced with permission from Kryger M, Bode F, Antic R, et al. Diagnosis of obstruction of the upper and central airways. *Am J Med*. 1976;61:85.)

MANAGEMENT PRINCIPLES

The management of a dyspneic patient should be based on the principles of altering the underlying pathophysiology while attempting to correct the underlying cause. As the work-up of dyspnea proceeds (see Figures 1–1 and 1–2), management and treatment goals should include disease-focused general education, and attempts to (1) improve pulmonary mechanics, (2) diminish ventilatory demand, (3) improve respiratory muscle function, and (4) alter the perception of dyspnea.

Airway obstruction can be reduced by general measures such as smoking cessation and pharmacologic therapy with bronchodilators. These may be supplemented with long-term inhaled corticosteroids in the treatment of asthma and COPD. Airway resistance can be further reduced by aerosol treatment and pulmonary toilet that help in the clearance of secretions. Where there is a definite cause of altered mechanics, such as a significant pleural effusion, removal of pleural fluid will help in relieving the symptoms of dyspnea.

A comprehensive program of breathing exercises, exercise training, and pulmonary rehabilitation, along with psychosocial support, can reduce ventilatory demand. These programs should focus on general body strengthening, endurance, efficiency for activities of daily living, perception of shortness of breath, and improving quality of life. Supplemental oxygen therapy may also reduce ventilatory drive and pulmonary vascular resistance and has been shown to increase survival in severely hypoxemic patients with COPD. Oxygen delivered in a customized controlled dose-regulated manner through nasal prongs, masks, or transtracheal catheters ensures compliance. Palliative oxygen may relieve dyspnea in cancer or congestive heart failure patients but this is controversial. Ventilatory demand can also be diminished if minute ventilation and the sensation of breathlessness are reduced by the administration of opiates such as oral codeine or morphine. The use of these agents must be done cautiously while keeping in mind their long-term side effects and short-term intolerance.

Attempts to improve respiratory muscle strength may not always be successful. Nutritional supplements to enhance muscle strength and endurance may help in relieving the sensation of dyspnea in selected cases. Although not totally substantiated, mechanical devices such as respiratory muscle trainers are sometimes used to help in decreasing the sense of ventilatory load and "urge to breathe." Ventilatory demand may be diminished by reduction in dead space ventilation and dietary carbohydrates.

Home noninvasive positive pressure ventilatory devices such as continuous positive airway pressure and bilevel positive airway pressure machines used for variable periods have been demonstrated to improve exercise tolerance and quality of life when combined with pulmonary rehabilitation and other physical training exercise programs in selected cases of advanced COPD. Instructions regarding head elevation and forward leaning positional maneuvers may help in improving diaphragmatic muscle efficiency and function.

CLINICAL SCENARIOS

Case 1

The patient is a 66-year-old man found to be unresponsive to verbal stimuli by his wife. He has a long-standing history of COPD. His past medical history also includes pneumonia and mild hypertension. His medications include theophylline 300 mg bid, metaproterenol 2 puffs qid, haloperidol 10 mg hs, and temazepam 30 mg as needed for sleep.

Physical Examination: On physical examination, the patient is comatose and cachectic with a mild odor of alcohol on his breath. His vital signs are pulse 116 beats/min and regular, respiratory rate 36 breaths/min, systolic blood pressure 96 mm Hg, and temperature 37.0°C (98.6°F). Other pertinent aspects of his physical examination reveal the following: mild conjunctival injection with the nasal mucosa slightly edematous. *Lungs*: increased resonance and reduced tactile fremitus with prolonged expiratory phase is noted. Scattered inspiratory rhonchi are present. *Heart*: the point of maximum impulse is not palpable. S_1 and S_2 are present without murmurs, rubs, or clicks. *Abdomen*: there are no scars and bowel sounds are present but diminished. No bruits are noted. The liver span is 8 cm to percussion and no masses or organomegaly is noted. Extremities reveal no cyanosis, clubbing, or edema with normal and symmetrical pulses. His neurologic examination is nonfocal with pinpoint pupils. Movement is minimal but symmetric to deep pain. Deep tendon reflexes are 11 and symmetric.

Lab data reveal white blood cell count is 9200 with a normal differential. Electrolyte levels are as follows: sodium 134 mEq, potassium 3.5 mEq, chloride 98 mEq, and HCO_2 29. The arterial blood gas measurements on 2 L of oxygen reveal a pH of 7.07, P_{CO_2} 113 mm Hg, P_{O_2} 64 mm Hg, and 90% saturation. The electrocardiogram reveals sinus tachycardia, right atrial enlargement, and an incomplete right bundle-branch block. The chest x-ray reveals hyperinflation, a small heart, flattened diaphragms, and radiolucent lung fields. The theophylline level is 4.4 mg/mL. A 50% dextrose solution along with naloxone is administered without a change in the neurologic status. The patient requires intubation and mechanical ventilatory support.

Discussion: The patient's history is compatible with a diagnosis of CO_2 narcosis induced by sedatives and alcohol. The relevant factors include his history of COPD, his medications (haloperidol and temazepam), alcohol on his breath, pinpoint pupils, a chest x-ray compatible with hyperinflation, and an elevated P_{CO_2} of 113 mm Hg (normal values are between 35 and 45 mm Hg) on the initial arterial blood gas measurement. Although the patient is comatose, a cerebrovascular accident is unlikely because he does not have any focal findings on examination. Although the patient has a history of mild hypertension, he was actually hypotensive at the time of presentation. There is no evidence of infection or septic foci. If severe enough, any obstructive disease can result in the retention of CO_2 secondary to hypoventilation, whether the obstruction is the result of a loss of elasticity and early airway closure, as seen in emphysema, or the result of bronchospasm and airway inflammation, as seen in asthma. In the acute phase, both these disease processes require the use of steroids and bronchodilators. If the patient had a superimposed infection, antibiotic therapy would also be required. Therapy would be directed at supporting alveolar ventilation either by a noninvasive or an invasive technique.

CLINICAL PEARLS

- Change in mental status with central nervous system (CNS) derangement may reflect CO_2 narcosis in a patient prone to hypercarbia.
- Factors contributing to CO_2 narcosis include sedation and alcohol intake.

Case 2

A 52-year-old obese man with a body mass index (BMI) of 34, a smoker, presents with a 11-month history of progressive shortness of breath. On careful questioning, the patient recalls having a "cold" the previous winter and states that the shortness of breath started after that. The symptoms are accompanied by a dry, nonproductive cough but no fever or other constitutional symptoms. He denies any exposure to inhalants or environmental toxins.

Physical Examination: On physical examination, the patient's vital signs are normal. Auscultation of the chest reveals "velcro" rales throughout both lungs with no wheezing. Findings upon cardiac examination are normal. The extremities reveal obvious clubbing but no cyanosis or edema. Laboratory values are normal with the exception of a hematocrit of 47%. Room air arterial blood gas measurements are as follows: pH 7.46, P_{CO_2} 36 mm Hg, P_{O_2} 69 mm Hg, and 92% saturation. A chest x-ray reveals bilateral interstitial markings with small lung volumes.

Discussion: Pulmonary function testing will allow the clinician to categorize and define the severity of the patient's respiratory abnormality. PFTs in this case would likely show a restrictive ventilatory defect with a significant reduction in the D$_{LCO}$. These findings along with the patient's prolonged history of progressive shortness of breath and chest x-ray changes are compatible with a diagnosis of idiopathic pulmonary fibrosis (IPF) (see Chapter 7). A high-resolution computed tomography (CT) scan would be helpful in defining the extent and type of parenchymal changes such as honeycombing and/or ground glass pattern, without gaining additional information regarding the physiologic changes that are present. The evaluation of dyspnea should include the consideration of chronic thromboembolic disease, but without any potential risk factors for thromboembolic disease, the diagnosis would be unlikely. A scan would be indicated in a patient in whom a diagnosis of pulmonary embolism is suspected.

CLINICAL PEARLS

- The combination of dyspnea, cough, clubbing, and "velcro" rales should raise the suspicion of idiopathic pulmonary fibrosis.
- Other causes of dyspnea with a restrictive defect but without any reduction in diffusion capacity include obesity and diaphragmatic and neuromuscular disorders.

KEY CONCEPTS

Increased respiratory drive, respiratory muscle weakness, dead space ventilation, central perception of shortness of breath, and mechanical impairment of ventilation may all play a role in the underlying causes and mechanisms of dyspnea.

Pulmonary function testing helps in distinguishing the various pulmonary and extra pulmonary causes of dyspnea.

Management and treatment of dyspnea is based on altering the pathophysiological derangements that contribute to dyspnea, such as reducing ventilatory demand and airflow impedance while correcting the underlying cause.

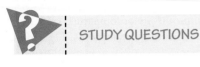

STUDY QUESTIONS

1-1.   Spirometry is a useful tool in helping to distinguish various types of lung disorders. Airway obstruction is defined by which of the following?

    a. normal FEV_i:FVC ratio

    b. an FEV_1 of 45% of the predicted value

    c. a supranormal FEV_i:FVC ratio

    d. an FEV_i:FVC ratio of <70%

    e. an FVC of less than 75% of the predicted value

1-2.   Which of the following are pathophysiologic causes of dyspnea?

    a. resistance to lung or chest wall expansion

    b. respiratory muscle weakness

    c. airflow obstruction

    d. increased in respiratory drive

    e. all of the above

1-3.   Airway obstruction is defined as a decrease in the FEV1:FVC ratio secondary to a decrease in FEV_1. Which of the following examples of airway obstruction may NOT be accompanied by a decrease in the FEV_i:FVC ratio?

    a. central airway obstruction

    b. acute air trapping

    c. premature termination of the forced expiratory maneuver (expiratory time less than 6 seconds)

    d. all of the above

    e. a and c only

SUGGESTED READINGS

American Thoracic Society. Dyspnea: mechanisms, assessment and management: a consensus statement. *Am J Respir Crit Care Med.* 1999;159:321–340.

Levitzky MG. *Pulmonary Physiology,* 7th ed. New York, NY: McGraw-Hill/Lange; 2007:chapters 2, 3, 6.

Stulbarg MS, Adams L. Dyspnea. In: Murray JF, Nadel JA, eds. *Textbook of Respiratory Medicine.* Vol. 1, 3rd ed. Philadelphia, PA: WB Saunders; 2000:541–549.

Cough

Juzar Ali

OBJECTIVES

▶ *Outline the common causes of cough and discuss the underlying mechanism and pathogenesis.*

▶ *Develop a clinically based algorithm for the diagnosis and management of chronic cough relative to disease-specific pathophysiology.*

GENERAL CONSIDERATIONS

Cough is not common in healthy persons. It plays a major role in maintaining the defense of the airways and in clearing mucus and foreign particles. Cough can also spread disease, signify an underlying serious pathologic condition, affect the quality of life, and interfere with a person's daily routine or occupation. Chronic cough, defined as cough persistent for three or more weeks, is one of the most troubling symptoms for which a patient seeks medical attention and is a common problem seen in both pulmonary and general medical practice. Referrals of patients with chronic cough account for up to 30% of the outpatient practice of a pulmonologist in the United States.

ETIOLOGY & PATHOGENESIS

Acute cough is generally a manifestation of an acute inflammatory or infectious process and may not require any specific investigation. Although it is usually self-limiting, it can be protracted after an acute viral respiratory tract illness and may linger for several weeks. In smokers, bronchial secretions induced by smoking may cause cough. Although most smokers have cough, they often do not complain of it. Almost every pulmonary disorder, either directly or indirectly, can cause cough. Chronic cough may be associated with altered mucus expectoration as in chronic bronchitis or with increased reactivity of airways as in asthma. It can be present with aspiration, as in esophageal dysfunction or neurologic disorders, or associated with signs of local compression, as in lung/bronchogenic cancer, mediastinal tumors, thyroid or vascular enlargement. It is also seen

21

with pulmonary edema or pulmonary fibrosis. It has been observed that in more than 90% of immunocompetent patients complaining of cough with a nonlocalizing chest radiograph, the cause is upper airway cough syndrome (UACS), previously called postnasal drip. Other causes in this category include gastroesophageal reflux disease (GERD), asthma, or chronic bronchitis. Therefore, in nonsmoking patients and in those not taking any medication that can cause cough, such as an angiotensin-converting enzyme (ACE) inhibitor, chronic cough is most likely due to one of these conditions.

Mechanism

Cough is a complex event that protects against thermal, chemical, or mechanical insult or injury. It is a normal response to inhalational exposure to particulate matter or chemicals and after aspiration. However, it may be the only sign of a number of diseases and disorders, including inflammatory processes, mechanical changes, or chronic inhalation of irritants. The mucus normally produced by the secretory cells of the airways entraps irritant particles and chemical and endogenous debris, with the clearance mechanism being initiated by mucociliary action. A cough dramatically enhances this process by narrowing the airway and increasing the velocity of airflow, resulting in more turbulence and clearance of pollutants in larger airways. Vagal receptors and recurrent laryngeal nerve receptors can induce coughing when stimulated by airways secretion, foreign bodies, or tumors. Sensory nerve receptors such as rapidly adapting receptors (RARs), slowly adapting receptors (SARs), and C-fiber receptors form the conducting pathway in the response of external stimuli causing cough. These stimuli may be external, such as external cigarette smoke, mechanical stimuli, acidic or alkaline, hypo- or hypertonic solutions, or intrinsic, such as bronchoconstriction, pulmonary congestion, atelecasis, or pulmonary/interstitial fibrosis. An abnormal increase in the sensitivity of these cough receptors can cause a lower threshold for coughing, such as seen with cough induced by ACE inhibitors. Diabetic patients with autonomic neuropathy also have an increased cough reflex threshold.

The components of the cough reflex have been well described. They are the (1) receptors, (2) afferent pathways, (3) cough center, (4) efferent pathway, and (5) effectors. The irritant receptors, such as those sending afferent myelinated fibers via the vagus nerve, are primarily in the large airway and on the luminal side of the tracheobronchial tree. Stimulation of the mechanical and chemoreceptors produces cough, airway constriction, and increased mucus secretion. These receptors are also abundant at the bifurcations of bronchi, especially at the carina. The cough reflex (Table 2–1) is initiated by stimulation of sensory nerves beneath and between the epithelium of the larynx and tracheobronchial tree. Involuntary coughing appears to be entirely vagally mediated and can be initiated by irritation of any structure innervated by the vagus nerve or its branches. These structures include the oropharynx, the larynx, the lower respiratory tract, and the esophagus. Afferent impulses travel to the cough center in the brain via various neural pathways. Efferent signals are then transmitted to the glottis, diaphragm, intercostals, and abdominal muscles. This culminates in (1) an inspiratory phase, (2) closure

Table 2–1. Components of cough reflex

Receptors	Afferent pathways	Cough center	Efferent pathways	Effectors
Larynx Trachea Bronchi Ear canal Pleura Stomach	Branches of vagus nerve		Vagus nerve	Muscles of larynx, trachea, and bronchi
		Diffusely located in medulla near respiratory center; under control of higher brain centers	Phrenic nerve Intercostal and lumbar nerves	Diaphragm, intercostal, abdominal, and lumbar muscles
Nose Paranasal sinuses	Trigeminal nerve			
Pharynx	Glossopharyngeal nerve		Trigeminal, facial, hypoglossal, and accessory nerves	Upper airways and accessory respiratory muscles
Pericardium Diaphragm	Phrenic nerve			

Source: Reproduced with permission from Braman SS, Corrao WM: Cough: Differential diagnosis and treatment. *Clin Chest Med.* 1987;8:178.

of the glottis, (3) diaphragmatic relaxation, (4) active contraction of the expiratory muscles with intrapleural pressures rising up to 200 mm Hg, and (5) rapid opening of the glottis. The physiologic process of coughing, specifically that which originates from the lower airways (Figure 2–1), starts with rapid inspiration, usually but not necessarily followed by glottal closure for about 200 ms, a rise in pleural and abdominal pressure to 50–100 mm Hg by expiratory muscle contraction, followed by an explosive exhalation. When the glottis suddenly opens, the high pressure gradient between the pleura and the airway produces an explosive release of air accompanied by a sound produced by turbulence. Although expiratory volume is no greater than during forced exhalation, narrowing of the airways caused by the large transpulmonary pressure gradient leads to a high flow velocity. The cough event lasts about 0.5 s, during which up to a liter of air may be expelled. This expulsion is followed by glottic closure and then respiratory muscle relaxation. At times, there is a series of coughs during a single exhalation phase, diminishing in intensity as the residual volume is approached. During cough, dynamic compression of airways occurs initially in segmental or lobar bronchi immediately above the equal pressure point. Maximum flow is determined by the resistance of upstream intrapulmonary airways, by the elastic recoil of the lungs, and by the collapsibility of the airways.

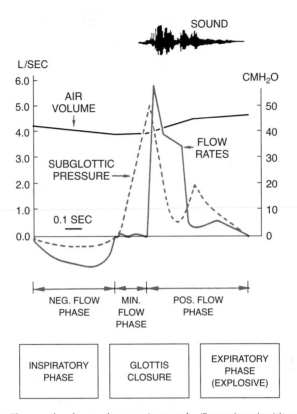

Figure 2–1. Flow and volume changes in cough. (Reproduced with permission from Bianco S, Robuschi M: Mechanics of cough. In: Braga PC, Allegra L, eds. *Cough.* New York, Raven Press, 1989, pp 29–36.)

Measurement of the effectiveness of coughing is difficult. Furthermore, patients with severe chronic lung disease may generate low linear velocities and thus have ineffectual cough. In chronic bronchitis, cough may account for 50% clearance, thus compensating for any defective mucociliary transport. Clinical studies show that coughing is highly effective in central airways clearance but not in the peripheral airways.

As a defense mechanism, cough helps prevent any foreign material from entering the lower respiratory tract and also clears excessive secretions. The effectiveness of cough depends on the viscosity of the secretions and the linear velocity of air moving through the lumen. Once there is material of sufficient thickness for expulsion from the airways, the effectiveness of cough depends on the high flow rate of air and the small cross-sectional area of the airway in order to achieve a high linear velocity. Therefore, any condition associated with a diminished expiratory flow rate or reduced ability to dynamically compress airways may lead to an ineffective cough. Since expiratory flow rates are directly related to lung volume, failure to take an initial breath and reluctance to give a forceful expiratory effort often lead to an ineffective cough velocity. Unconscious patients who have central nervous system depression may also have decreased cough due to central depression of cough reflexes. Pulmonary disorders may have cough impairment associated with decreased expiratory flow rates or production of overwhelming amounts of secretions. In asthma, both these conditions may cause cough ineffectiveness. Inflammation, edema, smooth muscle contraction, narrowing of airways, increased resistance to inspiratory and expiratory flow rates, and tenacious viscous secretions may partly occlude the lumen. This occlusion, combined with respiratory muscle fatigue, may diminish flow rates.

PATHOPHYSIOLOGY

Causes of chronic cough include a number of clinical conditions, some of which are mentioned in the following section. The disease-specific pathogenesis and pathophysiology are discussed.

Asthma & Cough-Variant Asthma

One of the three most common causes of chronic cough in a nonsmoker is asthma and/or cough-variant asthma. Cough due to asthma is usually accompanied by wheezing and chest tightness. These accompanying symptoms may be absent in cough-variant asthma. Typically, the onset of cough in cough-variant asthma occurs for a few months following an upper respiratory tract infection and persists for several months. These patients may progress to asthma in 30% of cases. This cough is worse at night, and it may also increase after exercise. Overt wheezing is generally undetectable and spirometric test results are normal. Allergy testing may show a positive reaction to ragweed. Exercise testing or methacholine challenge reveals a decrease in flow rates with protracted cough consistent with airway hyperreactivity and asthma. Sputum eosinophilia is frequent with increased submucosal and bronchoalveolar lavage eosinophilia. Exhaled nitric oxide concentration is raised in these conditions. Management of asthma relieves the cough, and response to corticosteroids is generally good. There is no significant correlation between cough sensitivity and bronchial hyperreactivity, even in inflammation or asthma. Asthma stimulates cough through induction of airways secretion, bronchial hyperreactivity, and eosinophilic inflammation. Bronchoconstriction per se may be associated with cough. While histologically those receptors that mediate the cough reflex are indistinguishable from those that mediate bronchoconstriction, recent evidence suggests that the cough receptors are functionally different from other irritant receptors and that cough may occur as a reflex that is independent of bronchoconstriction. Rapid and large lung volume changes can cause cough, as can physiologic effects such as laughter. Stretch receptors innervate slowly adapting fibers and do not cause cough. Bronchoconstriction is believed to be caused by activation of C-fiber and other receptors. The C-fiber receptors are highly sensitive to chemicals such as bradykinin, capsaicin, and hydrogen ions and form a complex unit of cough sensors in the airways. Alteration of local osmolality, such as that caused by an inhalant solution, can result in bronchoconstriction. Cough can also result from excessive respiratory water loss, whereas bronchoconstriction is believed to result from respiratory heat loss. Each can potentiate the other, although neither is dependent on the other for its action. Studies during sleep show that greater stimulation of the larynx is needed to produce cough in the rapid eye movement (REM) stage than in lighter stages of sleep, and in patients with chronic cough, less coughing occurs during REM than during non-REM sleep or waking periods.

Chronic Cough Due to UACS

Cough may be persistent with recurring bouts of bronchorrhea and rhinitis and postviral illnesses. Because of their superficial location, the sensory receptors in the upper airways make them easily susceptible to irritation. These rapidly adapting receptors release mediators and various components of the inflammatory cascade which can cause increased vascular permeability, airway hyperreactivity, and cough. Patients may also complain of a postnasal dripping sensation at the back of the throat. Examination of the pharynx may reveal a granular or cobblestone-like mucosa. Tenderness of the sinus areas may also be present.

GERD With or Without Microaspiration

Potential mechanisms of gastroesophageal cough include direct effect of reflux contents with stimulation of distal esophageal mucosal receptors, laryngeal and tracheobronchial afferents rather than actual pulmonary aspiration. The esophageal bronchial reflex travels through cholinergic efferent fibers in the tracheobronchial tree. In contrast, esophageal disorders such as diverticuli, achalasia, or hiatal hernia with reflux can result in cough secondary to microaspiration of esophageal contents into the airway. Further, it is speculated that coughing from any cause may further induce gastroesophageal reflux and hence create a vicious cycle.

ACE Inhibitor-Induced Cough

Activation of the arachidonic acid pathway, which increases prostaglandin or thromboxane synthesis, may play a role in the pathogenesis of cough seen in about 20% of patients using ACE inhibitors Genetic factors have also been implicated and women are affected more frequently than men. The lung contains a large amount of ACE, which is centrally involved in the metabolism of the inflammatory peptide bradykinin. Therefore, ACE inhibition would be expected to increase kinins and substance P levels in the lung. Bradykinin is known to sensitize somatosensory fibers, causing hyperalgesia and initiation of the cough reflex. Studies have shown that patients treated with thromboxane-receptor antagonists show reduction in cough within 2–3 days. Cough is generally not associated with the use of angiotensin II–receptor blockers as these agents do not exhibit the increased kinin effects of ACE inhibitors.

Heart Failure

Pump failure of the left heart causes a net backlog of fluid with decreased clearance and increased pulmonary capillary pressure. The increased pulmonary congestion causes interstitial and peribronchial edema, airway narrowing, and decreased total lung capacity. Pulmonary edema reduces the distensibility of the lung. Airway resistance is also increased. It is possible that reflex bronchoconstriction and stimulation of irritant receptors may also play a role. At the level of peripheral airways, peribronchial cuffing increases small airway resistance and results in intermittent deflation. All these mechanisms may contribute to initiating cough.

Chronic Infections & Bronchiectasis

Bronchiectasis is a disease involving bronchioles with mediator release leading to a cycle of infection and inflammation. Bronchiolar mucosal biopsy reveals infiltration by neutrophils and T lymphocytes; expectorated sputum has increased concentrations of cytokines such as interleukins and tumor necrosis factor-α and biomolecular enzymes such as elastase. Cylindrical or tubular bronchiectasis is characterized by dilated airways and is a residual effect of pneumonia or chronic infection. Varicose bronchiectasis is characterized by focal areas of constriction along with progressive dilatation of the airways resulting from structural defects. Cystic or saccular bronchiectasis is characterized by progressive dilatation of the airways resulting in large cysts and saccular structure with no air flow in the blind sacs of these bronchiectatic segments.

Immune-Mediated Diseases & Related Causes

Pulmonary involvement with connective tissue disorders such as rheumatoid arthritis and primary and secondary Sjögren's syndrome can cause chronic cough if associated with pulmonary fibrosis or upper airway involvement. Specifically, chronic cough due to Sjögren's syndrome due to mucosal dryness can be misdiagnosed as asthma or bronchitis and inspissation of secretions may lead to mucus plugging.

DIAGNOSTIC & CLINICAL CONSIDERATIONS

Since cough may occur in any pulmonary disease, it is usually considered a nonspecific symptom that may be accompanied by other related complaints such as chest pain and/or constitutional symptoms such as insomnia or urinary incontinence. Methods to assess intensity of chronic cough are not clearly defined or practical in clinical practice. At times, patients seek medical attention because of fear of an underlying serious disease. The onset, frequency, timing, and character of cough are good starting points in the evaluation of a patient with chronic cough. Clinical data as outlined in Table 2–2 are helpful in establishing a diagnostic plan. Trigger factors such as cold air, dust, fumes, allergen/environmental exposure, and cigarette smoke should be investigated if asthma is suspected. Rhinitis and nasal symptoms suggest an upper airway, nasal, or sinus cause. A careful history of medication use including ACE inhibitors and β-blockers should be sought. Chronic cough with daily sputum production that is present for more than 2 months in a patient with a smoking history is defined as chronic bronchitis. Bronchiectasis and cystic fibrosis usually cause large amounts of sputum with or

Table 2–2. Clinical clues and diagnostic steps in evaluation of chronic cough

Cause	Clinical data	Diagnostic tests
Aspiration pneumonia	Elderly, esophageal or neurologic disorders, history of sedation, or altered consciousness	pH probe, swallow studies
Asthma	Wheezing, postexercise shortness of breath aggravated by allergens and nonspecific irritants	Spirometric studies, methacholine challenge
Bronchogenic cancer	Change in cough, hemoptysis	Chest imaging, fiber optic bronchoscopy
Chronic bronchitis	Smoking history, chronic cough with sputum production	Pulmonary function tests
UACS and chronic sinusitis	History of postnasal drip mucopurulent sputum production, tender sinuses, and abnormal nasopharynx mucosa on ENT exam	Sinus x-rays, computed tomography
Foreign body aspiration GERD	Sudden onset, choking, localized wheeze History of heartburn, reflux symptoms, nocturnal cough, throat discomfort	Inspiratory and expiratory chest x-ray ENT examination pH probe, endoscopy
Postviral or RADS	Chronic, persistent symptoms aggravated by specific or nonspecific irritants	Transient or persistent spirometric abnormalities
Psychogenic	Daytime only with variable exacerbating factors	Diagnosis by exclusion
Pulmonary fibrosis	Nonproductive cough, dyspnea on exertion, "velcro" crackles, clubbing	Chest imaging, HRCT, pulmonary function tests with restrictive defect

Note: GERD, gastroesophageal reflux disease; HRCT, high resolution computed tomography; RADS, reactive airways dysfunction syndrome; UACS, upper airway cough syndrome.

without bronchial hyperreactivity. The association of hemoptysis, expectoration of copious amounts of purulent sputum, wheezing, orthopnea, and history of foreign body inhalation or repeated episodes of pneumonia may suggest a diagnosis of bronchiectasis. Positional bronchorrhea is also characteristic of bronchiectasis. Stress factors related to anxiety or psychosomatic disorders projecting as cough need to be kept in mind as part of the differential diagnosis. Symptoms of heartburn and nocturnal exacerbation of cough suggest GERD. History of chemical and/or noxious gas exposure/burns should be considered as these can cause chronic cough that may persist for months to years by causing airway inflammation and reactive airway dysfunction syndrome. Chronic pulmonary infections such as tuberculosis (TB), lung abscess, or necrotizing pneumonias cause chronic cough and sputum production. In such cases chest x-rays are usually abnormal. Bacterial tracheobronchitis or pneumonia may be a sequela or a cause of an acute exacerbation of chronic bronchitis and can result in cough of variable duration. Acute epiglottitis should be suspected if dyspnea, stridor, hoarseness, dysphagia, and increased salivation accompany cough. Tracheobronchial neoplasms may be manifested by cough with a normal or abnormal chest x-ray. This presentation can also be seen with a nonneoplastic bronchial tumor, foreign body obstruction, or stricture. Extrinsic bronchial or tracheal pressure secondary to a lymphoma or an aneurysm may cause a protracted cough. Obvious radiographic and clinical signs may indicate other identifiable causes such as connective tissue and immune mediated disorders that can cause pulmonary fibrosis.

Although the character, quantity, and timing of the cough are features noted in the evaluation of the patient, prospective studies show that GERD, UACS, and asthma are the most common causes of chronic cough regardless of the quantity of sputum production. They account for about 80% of the cases. The clinical profile that predicts these three main causes of chronic cough (ie, UACS, GERD, and asthma) in 99% of cases is (1) cough that is of at least 3 weeks duration and is persistently troublesome, (2) a nonsmoking patient, (3) a patient who is not receiving ACE inhibitors, and (4) a normal or nonspecific chest x-ray.

Listening to or eliciting the character of cough sounds has been historically helpful but is very observer dependent and not truly validated (Table 2–3). Types of cough sounds may be hoarse, barking, crisp, or staccato but rarely independently aid in reaching a diagnosis. The physical signs of chronic obstructive lung disease; the presence of digital clubbing, rhonchi, crackles, or localized wheezing; areas of tenderness in the sinuses; or signs of heart failure may be helpful in diagnosis. Detailed examination of the ears, nose, throat, tympanic membrane, and sinuses may reveal the source of irritation or a cobblestone oropharyngeal mucosa. Examination of the neck may show a mass or thyromegaly impinging upon the airways. Negative findings on chest examination do not preclude primary lung disease, and supplemental laboratory and radiologic examination may be required. Sputum studies for bacteriologic culture and cytologic analysis may be helpful if expectorated phlegm is purulent or the patient is at risk for lung cancer. Peripheral eosinophilia suggests allergy or asthma. An increased sedimentation rate suggests connective tissue disease or immune-mediated disorder or vasculitis. In the presence of facial pain, tenderness, and purulent or hemorrhagic drainage, sinus x-rays and computed tomography (CT) scans can confirm sinusitis. The presence of polycythemia, hypoxemia, or an abnormal chest x-ray may give further clues to underlying problems such as COPD. Conditions associated with cough and a normal or nonspecific chest x-ray are listed in Table 2–4. When the history, physical examination, or tests, including a chest x-ray, are not diagnostic, methacholine challenge and esophageal studies may be needed to further aid in diagnosis. A positive methacholine test result is consistent with hyperreactive airways, and though it is positive in a number of disorders other than asthma, a negative methacholine challenge test rules out asthma. Esophageal acid reflux can be assessed by a pH probe, endoscopy, or barium swallow. Generally, a negative pH test excludes reflux as a cause of chronic cough. Bronchoscopy has a low utility unless an endobronchial airway lesion such as bronchogenic cancer, tumor, or foreign body aspiration is suspected. Pulmonary function tests aid in

Table 2–3. Localization of cough and associated clinical characteristics

Cause	Clinical characteristics
Upper airway causes	
Tracheobronchitis	Associated with sore throat, upper airways symptoms
Foreign body aspiration	May be associated with signs of asphyxia/respiratory distress, or localized wheeze or stridor
Airway tumors	Nonproductive, occasional hemoptysis
Asthma	Chronic productive or dry cough with or without wheezing
Pulmonary infections	
Bacterial pneumonia	May be preceded by symptoms of upper respiratory infection, purulent cough
Atypical nonbacterial pneumonia	Paroxysmal cough with mucoid or blood-tinged sputum
Exacerbation of chronic bronchitis	Productive cough, associated shortness of breath
Bronchiectasis	Copious, foul-smelling, and multilayered purulent sputum; postural symptoms
Lung abscess	Copious, foul-smelling, blood-streaked, or purulent sputum
Tuberculosis or fungal infection	Persistent cough with mucoid sputum, may have associated hemoptysis
Pulmonary parenchymal inflammatory diseases	
Pulmonary fibrosis	Nonproductive, "dry" cough with or without dyspnea
Bronchogenic carcinoma	Nonproductive to productive cough with hemoptysis, may be associated with chest pain
Alveolar cell carcinoma	Variable, may be nonproductive or productive of watery mucoid copious sputum
Mediastinal lesions	
Mediastinal tumors	Cough may be positional with variable dyspnea
Aortic aneurysm	Brassy sound of cough
Nonpulmonary cardiovascular causes	
Left ventricular failure	Increased cough when supine, associated breathlessness especially with exertion
Pulmonary infarction	Cough, hemoptysis, chest pain, and dyspnea (any one or combination)

Table 2–4. Conditions with cough and a normal or nonspecific chest x-ray

Acute upper respiratory illness
UACS/postnasal drip/rhinitis/sinusitis
Tracheobronchitis/pertussis
Asthma or eosinophilic bronchitis
Early or mild bronchiectasis
Early or mild interstitial pulmonary fibrosis
GERD/esophageal disease/microaspiration
Tracheobronchial neoplasm or upper airway lesions
Psychogenic causes

Note: GERD, gastroesophageal reflux disease; UACS, upper airway cough syndrome.

reaching a diagnosis of asthma or restrictive lung disease. However, pulmonary function tests should be performed after the patient has recovered from an acute illness to exclude transient bronchial hyperreactivity. A CT scan of the chest may detect mediastinal masses, airway lesions interstitial lung disease, and bronchiectasis not usually evident on a chest x-ray.

MANAGEMENT PRINCIPLES

The principles of cough management are twofold. Symptomatic treatment of the troublesome or debilitating cough is the patient's primary concern. Specific measures directed at removing environmental triggers or reducing irritants such as smoking exposure are helpful. Nonspecific measures using centrally active antitussives or cough suppressant medications that reduce the sensitivity of irritant cough receptors form the mainstay of this medical approach. Use of antihistamines/nonsedating newer H1 blockers and inhaled nasal preparations are useful in cough due to UACS. Potential newer antitussive agents including peripheral opioid receptor and ion channel modulators are being studied, but are not yet in use in clinical practice. H2 blockers and proton pump inhibitors should be given a therapeutic trial when cough is suspected to be due to GERD. Inhaled steroids are useful in asthmatic/eosinophilic bronchitis. Understanding the possible origin of the cough-initiating mechanism is helpful. Coughing is ineffective when central obstructing lesions, reduced recoil, or severe peripheral resistance reduces flow rates. This situation is seen with endobronchial lesions, bronchial stricture, foreign body impaction, and patients with small tracheostomy tubes. Failure to cough adequately may lead to atelectasis, mucus obstruction, pneumonia, and bronchiectasis. In some conditions in which there is an associated increase in sputum production such as in bronchiectasis, protussive measures for increasing bronchial toilet may help in the long run. Chronic cough is not only physically and psychologically debilitating, but it can also lead to complications such as posttussive emesis, syncope, rib fractures, pneumomediastinum, pneumothorax, bullous emphysema, and abdominal hernias. An algorithm suggesting a diagnostic and management plan is shown in Table 2–5. If a careful methodological approach is adopted, a specific cause and successful treatment plan can be identified in more

Table 2-5. Algorithm for evaluation of new-onset cough

Step #1. History and physical examination—focus on the afferent limb of the cough reflex. Check for clues leading to diagnosis of asthma, GERD, bronchitis, bronchiectasis, or left ventricular failure

Step #2. If symptoms have been present for more than 3 weeks and the pathogenesis is not obvious, obtain a chest x-ray/CT scan
  If imaging is normal or the process changes noted are old, proceed to step 3
  If imaging is abnormal or patient is immunocompromised, proceed to step 8

Step #3. Remove aggravating factors or irritants and consider a therapeutic trial

Step #4. If UACS is suspected, institute empirical treatment. If there is no response, obtain sinus x-rays or a CT scan and/or allergy tests

Step #5. If asthma is suspected, perform pulmonary function tests. If the results are normal, perform a methacholine challenge

Step #6. If GERD is suspected, consider therapeutic trial and interventions. If no response, perform a 24-hour pH probe and do a swallow study

Step #7. If an upper airway or a large airway lesion is suspected, obtain ear, nose, and throat evaluation and consider bronchoscopic studies

Step #8. Treat the underlying cause and or consider other diagnostic tests

---

Note: CT, computed tomography; GERD, gastroesophageal reflux disease; UACS, upper airway cough syndrome.

than 80% of cases. This may be a slow empiric process, and multiple causes that account for about 25% of cases warrant a multifaceted treatment plan.

CLINICAL SCENARIOS

Case 1

A 35-year-old nursing student is seen by her physician for chronic nonproductive cough exacerbated by exercise, weather changes, and when she is playing with her children. She had little response to antitussives and other symptomatic treatment.

Physical Examination: Physical examination is normal, and her chest x-ray does not reveal any active disease. The pulmonary function tests show normal forced expiratory volume in the first second (FEV_1), normal forced vital capacity (FVC), and normal ratio. Her physician orders a methacholine challenge, which shows the following results:

	Baseline (L)	After 10 mg/mL methacholine inhalation (L)
FVC	4.80 (82%)	4.30
FEV_1	4.07 (87%)	3.00
FEV_1/FVC (%)	86	69

Discussion: This patient's diagnosis is hyperreactive airways dysfunction and cough-variant occult bronchial asthma. Cough can be one of the presenting symptoms of hyperreactive airways disease and bronchial asthma. This condition can remain undiagnosed until a provocation test is performed to induce bronchospasm, since baseline spirometric measurements may be normal. By convention, a 20% fall in FEV_1 is considered a positive result. A negative test result is useful to exclude the diagnosis of asthma in patients with chronic cough or exercise limitation and an otherwise normal spirometric analysis.

CLINICAL PEARL

Asthma may present as chronic cough without wheezing and a normal spirometry test should be followed by a methacholine challenge test to confirm this diagnosis.

Case 2

A 69-year-old man, nonsmoker with a history of coronary artery disease, hypertension, previous myocardial infarction, and an episode of acute respiratory distress syndrome during a previous hospitalization comes for a regular clinic follow-up. His medications include an ACE inhibitor for hypertension and nitroglycerine for chest pain as required. He says he is generally doing well except for increasing shortness of breath, infrequent episodes of paroxysmal nocturnal dyspnea, and increased cough at night since the last visit over 2 months ago.

Physical Examination: The physical examination reveals a S_3 gallop and bilateral basilar crackles. The chest x-ray shows an enlarged cardiac silhouette with increased vascularity. The electrocardiogram is unchanged from a previous study. Regular medications are continued with the addition of diuretic therapy. The patient responds well, and his symptoms of cough disappear.

Discussion: Among the common causes of chronic cough in a nonsmoker, ACE inhibitor–induced cough is a well-recognized entity. ACE inhibitors are commonly used in treating patients with hypertension, congestive heart failure, and diabetic nephropathy. However, these agents can cause a dry, hacking, nonproductive cough that may be paroxysmal and nocturnal. This cough can occur within a week of initiating therapy or can be delayed up to 4–6 months. In this clinical scenario, however, cough was due to acute left ventricular failure and vascular congestion. The symptoms of paroxysmal nocturnal dyspnea and the progressive shortness of breath in a patient with underlying heart disease are suggestive of pulmonary venous hypertension. Pump failure of the heart and altered hemostasis result in interstitial edema, lymphatic clogging, and perialveolar filling. Increased pulmonary capillary pressure and pulmonary edema cause cough along with shortness of breath and pedal edema.

CLINICAL PEARL

ACE inhibitors can cause chronic cough in patients with congestive heart failure who are on these agents. However, it is imperative to assess their cardiac function and treat heart failure aggressively, as paroxysmal cough may also reflect left ventricular dysfunction.

KEY CONCEPTS

① *Cough not only plays a major role in maintaining the defense of the airways and in clearing mucus and other foreign particles, but it can also spread disease and signify an underlying serious pathologic condition. Chronic cough is defined as cough persistent for three or more weeks and is a common problem seen in both pulmonary and general medical practice.*

② *In more than 90% of immunocompetent patients complaining of chronic cough who are not on ACE inhibitors and who have a nonlocalizing chest imaging, the cause is due to upper airway cough syndrome, gastroesophageal reflux disease with or without aspiration, or asthma.*

③ *Although it is a slow empiric process, a careful methodologic approach with review of associated symptoms and findings can lead to or rule out a specific cause, and a successful treatment plan can be implemented in more than 80% of cases.*

STUDY QUESTIONS

2–1.   A 64-year-old woman has a history of chronic bronchitis and chronic obstructive pulmonary disease (COPD) with repeated hospitalizations for acute exacerbations. Her most recent hospitalization was about 2 months ago, which resulted in her requiring mechanical ventilatory support and prolonged endotracheal intubation. She now comes in with increasing shortness of breath and a chronic, unrelenting, dry, hacking cough. On examination, she is hoarse, with intermittent stridor. She has inspiratory and expiratory rhonchi on lung examination with diminished breath sounds bilaterally. There is mild tachycardia but no gallop. Neck veins are not distended, and there is no peripheral edema. Her chest x-ray is normal. Her flow volume loop is shown below:

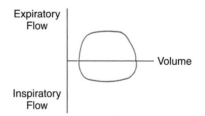

This patient's increased cough is most likely due to

a. exacerbation of her COPD/chronic bronchitis

b. underlying cor pulmonale secondary to COPD and pulmonary hypertension

c. tracheal stricture secondary to previous prolonged intubation

d. pulmonary edema

2–2. *A 56-year-old woman is referred for evaluation of chronic cough. She has recently migrated from Eastern Europe and has a positive purified protein derivative (PPD) test result of 11 mm. Other than cough she complains of generalized arthralgias and dryness of the eyes. She denies any fever or night sweats. Review of systems reveals symptoms of "chronic allergies" and "sinus congestion." Her chest x-ray and CT scan are normal and her sputum for bacterial culture, acid-fast bacillus, and fungal elements is negative.*

The possible causes of this patient's cough may be all of the following EXCEPT:

a. postnasal drip

b. occult asthma

c. smear-negative active TB

d. Sjögren's syndrome

SUGGESTED READING

Chung KF, Widdicombe JG. Cough. In: Murray JF, Nadel JA, Mason RJ, Boushey HA, eds. *Murray and Nadel's Textbook of Respiratory Medicine.* 4th ed. Philadelphia: Elsevier Saunders; 2005:831–847.

Hemoptysis

3

Juzar Ali

OBJECTIVES

▶ *Outline the various causes of hemoptysis and discuss the pathogenesis and pathophysiology in relation to the source of bleeding.*

▶ *Develop an algorithm for the diagnosis and management of hemoptysis and illustrate with clinical examples.*

GENERAL CONSIDERATIONS

Hemoptysis means coughing of blood and must not be confused with hematemesis or vomiting of blood. The incidence of hemoptysis varies widely and depends on the clinical setting. The duration of hemoptysis and the characteristics of expectorated blood may provide clues to its cause. The quantity of expectorated blood may range from blood-streaked sputum to a life-threatening amount. Although the designation is arbitrary, hemoptysis of 300 mL in 24 hours has been termed massive and could be life threatening because of the risk of aspiration, airway compromise, or associated hemodynamic collapse. Although fewer than 5% of all cases of hemoptysis are massive, mortality rates can be as high as 60%–75% in this group. Airway compromise may be life threatening even if hemoptysis is not massive in quantity. The unpredictability of recurrent hemoptysis, its poor correlation to parenchymal bleeding, and the absence of specific accurate predictors of outcome hinder its management. The rate of bleeding, associated ventilatory and hemodynamic derangements, and underlying comorbid conditions are major factors associated with poor outcomes in patients with hemoptysis.

ETIOLOGY

Worldwide, tuberculosis (TB) and bronchiectasis remain the most common causes of hemoptysis; other major causes are outlined in Figures 3–1 and 3–2. Although this list has essentially remained the same over the past 40 years, the rank order of the detectable causes in this list has changed due to the introduction of newer diagnostic techniques. The pathogenesis of bleeding and its pathophysiologic derangement depends on the underlying process (Table 3–1) and is described in

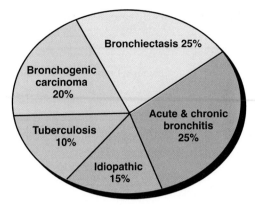

Figure 3-1. Some common causes of mild to moderate hemoptysis seen in an out-patient clinic setting.

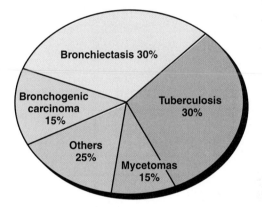

Figure 3-2. Some common causes of moderate to severe hemoptysis requiring inpatient hospital observation.

the following section. About 90% of the bleeding originates from bronchial circulation and its collaterals such as the axillary and intercostal vessels. The pulmonary circulation accounts for about 10% of all sources of hemoptysis. Various pathologic entities can be characterized by the predominant bleeding site and the structural defects associated with them (Table 3–2). The pathophysiology and pathogenesis of some of these clinical entities are discussed in the following sections.

PATHOGENESIS

Bronchiectasis

Bronchiectasis results from the destruction of the cartilaginous support of the bronchial wall by inflammation, infection, or alveolar fibrosis and traction.

Table 3–1. Classification of primary diseases in the differential diagnosis of hemoptysis

Pulmonary
  Airways disease: bronchitis, bronchiectasis, broncholith, adenoma, endobronchial hamartoma
  Infections: pneumonia, lung abscess, tuberculosis, fungal disease
  Vascular: pulmonary embolism, arteriovenous malformations
Cardiovascular
  Congestive heart failure, mitral valvular disease
Others
  Vasculitides
  Iatrogenic/traumatic
  Bleeding disorders/use of anticoagulants
  Substance abuse/drugs

Table 3–2. Etiology of hemoptysis: site and predominant circulation involved

Endobronchial site
  Chronic bronchitis
  Foreign body/broncholith
  Endobronchial mass/lesion
Bronchial circulation
  Bronchiectasis
  Chronic bronchitis
  Tuberculosis
  Mycetoma
  Pulmonary venous hypertension
  Bronchogenic carcinoma
Pulmonary circulation
  Cavitary tuberculosis
  Arteriovenous malformations
  Lung abscess
  Broncholiths
  Peripheral lung masses/carcinoma
  Radiation
  Iatrogenic
Diffuse capillary
  Diffuse alveolar damage
  Diffuse alveolar hemorrhage
  Idiopathic alveolar hemorrhage
  Autoimmune disorders/vasculitides
  Capillaritis

Acellular fibrotic strands replace small airways causing traction. This is accompanied by muscular hypertrophy, bronchomalacia, and architectural distortion. Most patients with massive hemoptysis have severe underlying necrotic, destructive, and fibrotic lung changes. Chronic purulent endobronchial infection also leads to suppurative tissue necrosis and generation of granulation tissue in the peribronchial region with bronchiectasis. The accompanying bronchial vessels undergo hypertrophy, with expansion of the submucosal vascular plexus and formation of bronchopulmonary anastomoses. The peripheral vessels are inflamed and this results in intense neovascularization and rupture of vessels which may initiate the onset of hemoptysis. A rich secondary vascular supply with anastomotic channels and increased pulmonary hypertension contributes to recurrent hemoptysis in these cases.

Tuberculosis

Intrapulmonary bleeding in TB may be multifactorial with attendant bronchiectasis depending on its acuity and site. Bleeding in TB may be due to necrosis of a small pulmonary artery or may result from rupture of vessels that run through or are tangential to the cavities resulting from chronic infection. At autopsy these patients have localized rupture of a dilated portion of the pulmonary artery traversing thick-walled cavities. These vessels are thought to be innocent bystanders caught up in the rim of inflammation and organization. Transient increases in pulmonary artery pressure may cause vascular rupture in a cavity. Tuberculous involvement of the vessel wall with local inflammation causes aneurysmal dilatation. The outer vessel is affected first, and the process of tissue destruction and replacement with granulation tissue progresses toward the lumen, leaving a weakened wall which bulges into an aneurysm called a Rasmussen aneurysm. As classically described, rupture of this aneurysm is a well-known albeit uncommon cause of massive hemoptysis.

Bronchogenic Carcinoma

About 7% of patients with bronchogenic cancer present with hemoptysis, and 20% have hemoptysis during the course of their illness. Squamous cell carcinoma is associated with an increased incidence of massive hemoptysis compared to other tumor types. However, there is no statistical correlation between cell types and frequency of hemoptysis. Massive bleeding is usually rare and mostly due to tumor erosion of large pulmonary vessels. Tumor necrosis and vascular rupture more commonly occur and cause small amounts of recurrent bleeding. Direct invasion of the pulmonary vasculature by tumor cells is rare. Metastatic disease in the lung from malignancies such as breast, kidney, colon, and esophageal cancer may extend directly into the tracheobronchial tree, resulting in hemoptysis. Endobronchial adenomas can bleed due to their vascular polypoid stalk and extend into the submucosa with their rich bronchial artery supply and cause hemoptysis because of their rich fibrovascular stroma and marked hypervascularity.

Chronic Bronchitis

Hemoptysis in chronic bronchitis arises from the superficial vessels in the bronchial mucosa. The bronchial arteries are increased in size and tortuosity in this condition. Increases in pulmonary artery pressure secondary to chronic obstructive pulmonary disease (COPD) and development of precapillary bronchopulmonary anastomoses may further aggravate the condition, leading to recurrent hemoptysis.

Pulmonary Mycetoma

Mycetomas occur in patients with preexisting cavitary or bullous lung disease resulting from old granulomatous disease such as TB or sarcoidosis. A mycetoma is a saprophytic fungal infection with necrotic cellular debris, mucus strands, and fibrin. *Aspergillus* species or mucormycosis may cause such a "fungus ball." Hemoptysis is a common symptom in mycetomas, but the pathogenesis is not clear. Although it has been speculated that hemolytic endotoxin, proteolytic enzymes, and microinvasion of fungus into the cavity wall may contribute to bleeding in pulmonary mycetoma, autopsy studies suggest that the bleeding may actually be due to friction of the fungus ball against the cavity wall. Pathologically, ulceration of cavitary lining, severe inflammation, increased number and congestion of capillaries, and fibrosis and thrombosis of bronchial and pulmonary arteries are seen. Abrasion of such capillaries with friction against the wall is the most likely cause of hemoptysis in these cases. Any change in position or change in the intrathoracic pressure can increase this movement and friction, thereby increasing the chance of bleeding.

Invasive Fungal Disease

Hemoptysis can also occur in invasive pulmonary fungal infection. In immune-compromised patients, bleeding and necrosis typically occur after the peripheral neutrophil blood count recovers, resulting in greater tissue inflammation and destruction. Pulmonary microangioinvasion by mycelial elements, which destroys parenchymal and vascular structures, causes infarction and hemorrhage. Fungal invasion of the pulmonary vasculature also results in thrombosis and distal ischemic necrosis and hemorrhage. *Aspergillus* and zygomycosis are the two major fungal groups causing this condition. In immunocompetent patients, endemic fungi may invade the lung, produce acute and chronic infection mimicking TB, and may cause hemoptysis. Fibrosing mediastinitis due to fungal infection, especially histoplasmosis, may cause hemoptysis by local destruction, fibrosis, vessel rupture, or related secondary pulmonary hypertension.

Broncholithiasis

Hemoptysis due to a broncholith is generally mild and considered benign because of its self-limiting nature. A broncholith is a calcified mediastinal lymph node(s) most commonly due to an infectious etiology. Histoplasmosis is the most frequent underlying cause of broncholithiasis in the United States. Other causes include TB, other fungal infections, actinomycosis, nocardiosis, and silicosis. Over time these calcified lymph nodes lead to external compression or erosion of the adjacent airways and vascular structures, causing obstruction and hemoptysis. A few cases of massive hemoptysis due to broncholithiasis have been described as a late complication resulting from erosion of broncholiths into the lung parenchyma, causing rupture of a pulmonary or bronchial artery, or from an aortotracheal fistula. Although there is no surrounding inflammation or bronchial artery collaterals, the broncholith is in close proximity to pulmonary veins. Healed, calcified peribronchial nodes may impinge on the bronchial lumen and erode vessels, resulting in pressure necrosis with fistula formation and hemoptysis.

Lung Abscess & Necrotizing Pneumonia

Lung abscess can cause hemoptysis when a necrotic cavity spreads directly into a surrounding vascularized lung. A large abscess may erode major pulmonary vessels resulting in massive hemoptysis. Formation of pseudoaneurysms or secondary filling of the abscess cavity will lead to recurrent hemoptysis. Pneumonia, especially with gram-negative bacteria and necrotizing infection, can lead to tissue breakdown and resultant alveolar damage and hemoptysis.

Cardiovascular Causes

Primary or secondary pulmonary hypertension from any congenital heart disease, such as Eisenmenger's complex, can result in hemoptysis. The long-standing state of high flow or pressure in the pulmonary artery circulation may lead to rupture of atheromatous plaques. In mitral stenosis, the primary site of bleeding is the bronchial veins; this bleeding is caused by increased capillary blood flow and pulmonary venous hypertension. Elevated left atrial pressure is transmitted back through the pulmonary veins to the capillaries, causing retrograde flow through the bronchopulmonary anastomoses, dilating the bronchial venous plexus. Blood is directed back to the right heart via azygos and intercostal veins. These prominent varices then may rupture in the presence of infection or increased intravascular volume or pressure.

Pulmonary Embolism

Hemoptysis in pulmonary embolism is generally of a mild to moderate nature. Embolism of pulmonary arteries follows detachment of a thrombus in the veins of the pelvis and lower extremities. Clinically, pulmonary embolism may be silent or massive, resulting in pulmonary infarction or cor pulmonale, severe shock, or sudden death. Hemodynamic alterations occur when emboli obstruct a significant portion of the pulmonary arterial bed. A resultant increase in pulmonary vascular resistance impedes right ventricular outflow and reduces left ventricular preload. The infarcted portion of the lung is solid, with air spaces filled with blood, and undergoes necrosis, organization, and ultimately fibrosis.

Vascular Anomalies

Vascular anomalies can be seen in cirrhosis, mitral disease, pulmonary schistosomiasis, and metastatic carcinomatosis. Sixty percent of primary arteriovenous malformations (AVMs) are associated with the hereditary hemorrhagic telangiectasia syndrome. Blood from multiple pulmonary arterial branches fills the cavernous spaces. The veins draining these spaces distend and become varicose. Degenerative changes result in the rupture of the venous walls and consequent hemoptysis. Ten percent of patients with AVM present with hemoptysis. Massive bleeds are rare.

Vasculitis & Alveolar Hemorrhagic Syndromes

Alveolar hemorrhage is a feature of many autoimmune diseases, vasculitides, drug- induced alveolar damage, and idiopathic systemic diseases. The vasculitides are defined as inflammation of the walls of the vessels with resultant reactive damage, leading to tissue ischemia and necrosis. In general, affected vessels vary in size, type, and location in association with the specific vasculitides. Vasculitis may occur as a primary process or may be secondary to another underlying disease. The bleeding results from diffuse vascular or endothelial injury. Other associated features may include thrombocytopenia. Hematologic malignancies with secondary thrombocytopenia and/or infection may result in occasional hemoptysis. Diffuse alveolar and vascular damage due to drugs, substance abuse, radiation injury, and infections and sepsis may also be responsible for pulmonary hemorrhage. Bleeding in these cases may be from the microvasculature and pulmonary capillaritis with no large-vessel involvement. Genetic connective tissue defects, autoimmune vasculitis, Goodpasture's syndrome, Wegener's granulomatosis, and idiopathic pulmonary hemosiderosis can account for some of the underlying processes.

Iatrogenic Causes

Iatrogenic causes of hemoptysis include traumatic lung injury due to transbronchial or transthoracic biopsy procedures or secondary to placement of a pulmonary artery catheter (PAC). Bleeding can also occur during a bronchoscopy. The majority of such events resolve spontaneously, but profuse bleeding can occur at times. Rupture of the pulmonary artery due to PAC placement may have a mortality rate of 50%. This complication most often occurs in individuals with pulmonary hypertension and is due to too distal a placement of the catheter with vascular rupture during balloon inflation. Infarctions related to PAC placement may bleed into the lung and are not necessarily associated with overt hemoptysis.

Cryptogenic Hemoptysis

Idiopathic or cryptogenic hemoptysis is a diagnosis of exclusion (Table 3–3) in which the cause remains undetermined despite the use of bronchoscopic evaluation and other diagnostic and radiologic techniques. Since there is an absence of either massive or fatal bleeding in these patients and they have a relatively good outcome, adequate pathologic studies are not available to delineate the pathogenesis.

Table 3–3. Disorders to exclude before diagnosing cryptogenic/idiopathic hemoptysis

Arteriovenous malformation	Emboli (pulmonary)
Aspiration	Eosinophilic granuloma
Bronchial adenoma	Hemosiderosis
Bronchiectasis	Lung sequestration
Catamenial (endometriosis)	Lymphangiomyomatosis
Cardiac (mitral stenosis)	

However, several explanations have been proposed. Acute and chronic bronchial inflammation is most frequently implicated as a cause of bleeding and dilated mucosal capillaries is the common bronchoscopic finding. These changes are unrelated to the patient's smoking history, clinical diagnosis of COPD, associated infection, or abnormal spirometric measurements. Occult bronchiectasis, especially "dry bronchiectasis" that is undetected on a routine chest x-ray and with a normal bronchoscopic exam may be another explanation. Rarely the finding of a subepithelial superficial bronchial artery may explain "cryptogenic" hemoptysis.

PATHOPHYSIOLOGY

The pathophysiology of hemoptysis varies with the extent, underlying cause, related comorbidities, and cardiopulmonary reserve. Mild hemoptysis produces little if any physiologic derangement but often results in significant psychological distress. Moderate chronic hemoptysis may lead to anemia. Acute severe hemoptysis may result in airway compromise and distal atelectasis, cough, shortness of breath, and wheezing. Alveolar flooding with blood produces severe shortness of breath and hypoxemia with lung compliance being markedly affected. Capillary bleeding associated with hemoptysis causes a syndrome similar to acute respiratory distress syndrome (ARDS) with hypoxemia, increased alveolar-arterial gradient, and resultant respiratory failure. Significant loss of blood may lead to reduction in circulatory volume and reduce cardiac output. Hemoptysis due to pulmonary emboli or infarction may be accompanied by acute right heart failure and shock. However, cardiovascular collapse is usually rare with most deaths due to asphyxiation.

DIAGNOSTIC & CLINICAL CONSIDERATIONS

History

The history of previous episodes may be an important diagnostic clue. Recurrent significant hemoptysis generally suggests an underlying pathologic condition. About 80% of patients presenting with massive hemoptysis have had one to four previous episodes of hemorrhage. The amount of blood loss, however, may give little indication of the severity and seriousness of the underlying process. The history establishes the duration, extent of bleeding, prior episodes, and presence of comorbid conditions and guides diagnostic considerations. A small amount of hemoptysis may occur during the course of a respiratory tract infection and may be of no clinical or prognostic significance, but this must be distinguished from serious bleeding. Patients with an underlying pulmonary infection will have purulent sputum mixed with blood, whereas those with TB, bronchogenic carcinoma, or pulmonary infarction will cough up frank blood without pus. Hemoptysis with putrid, foul-smelling sputum is seen with an anaerobic necrotizing infection or lung abscess. Some gram-negative pneumonia, such as that due to *Serratia,* may produce reddish sputum that is not truly hemoptysis. Pink, frothy sputum is characteristic of congestive heart failure or pulmonary edema. The pattern of hemoptysis may be a helpful sign in determining the cause. As a general observation, the most common cause of mild hemoptysis is chronic bronchitis, whereas massive hemoptysis is generally due to bronchiectasis, TB, or mycetoma. Patients with chronic bronchitis and bronchiectasis may have brief episodes of hemoptysis that recur over months or years. Recurrent hemoptysis with variable frequency may occur with an endobronchial lesion such as a bronchial adenoma not seen on a routine chest x-ray, whereas that occurring with regular monthly frequency in a female patient should raise suspicion of a menstrual-related event. This may be due to endometrial seeding in the lungs called catamenial (defined as occurring within 48 hours of menstruation) pulmonary disease. Other symptoms such as weight loss and anorexia preceding the actual bout of hemoptysis may point toward the diagnosis of carcinoma, and a history of night sweats, fever, and general ill health may point toward TB. Risk factors pertaining to travel, such as exposure to parasitic infestations, prolonged air travel, or history of trauma, should be determined and may provide help in reaching a diagnosis. Presence of multiorgan involvement, such as hematuria or skin lesions, may point toward connective tissue disorders or pulmonary renal syndromes such as Goodpasture's syndrome or Wegener's granulomatosis. It has been observed that ambulatory patients with mild hemoptysis remain the most enigmatic, whereas patients with massive hemoptysis most probably have an established diagnosis upon presentation. Generally speaking, massive hemoptysis is associated with inflammatory processes and rarely with malignancies, unless proximal airways, endobronchial lesions, or large blood vessels are involved, in which case the prognosis is unfavorable. Patients with undiagnosed mild hemoptysis who remain "idiopathic" at a 5-year follow-up have a favorable prognosis in the absence of persistent or recurrent bleeding.

Physical Examination

The physical examination should be done initially to quantify the volume of hemoptysis in an observed, controlled environment because estimation by the patient or a family member may be variable and erroneous. Patients are rarely able to accurately localize the exact site of the bronchopulmonary bleeding, and quantification of hemoptysis is difficult. The amount of bleeding may not be helpful diagnostically, but it determines to a large extent further management strategies dependent upon the integrity of the airways, level of consciousness, and hemodynamic stability of the patient. The presence of postural hypotension and tachycardia or tachypnea may suggest a compromised cardiovascular status. A febrile patient with chills suggests an underlying infection. Evaluating the upper airways is helpful in a comprehensive work-up, and noting the absence of skin lesions, such as ecchymoses and petechiae, and other signs of systemic illness may help in ruling out certain obvious causes or bleeding disorders before focusing on cardiopulmonary causes. Specific physical clues include digital clubbing, an oral or nasopharyngeal lesion, other bleeding sites, skin abnormalities, and specific cardiac or pulmonary auscultatory findings. Chest wall tenderness may suggest rib fractures or a traumatic cause, and a pleural rub suggests pleuritis or pulmonary infarction. Generalized wheezing or rhonchi may suggest obstructive airways disease such as chronic bronchitis, whereas a localized wheeze is a clue to an aspirated foreign body or a focal mass. Lung physical findings have to be interpreted with caution when hemoptysis occurs. Adventitious sounds on lung examination may represent a sequela to a bleed rather than its cause. Cardiac signs such as increased venous distention, murmurs, or a gallop may suggest heart failure, and a localized bruit over the lung field is a clue to an AVM.

Laboratory Tests

Laboratory studies helpful in evaluating patients with hemoptysis include a complete blood count. The presence of anemia signifies persistent blood loss or chronic bleeding diathesis. Hematuria with the presence of red blood cell casts in the urine suggests underlying renal pulmonary syndromes. A triad of hemoptysis, anemia, and alveolar infiltrates on chest x-ray is seen in idiopathic pulmonary hemosiderosis. The quantity of hemoptysis is not a reliable index of the degree of intrapulmonary hemorrhage. Other helpful diagnostic tests include sputum cytologic studies, sputum cultures, bleeding studies, blood chemistry analysis, serum serologic studies, and arterial blood gas studies. Hypoxemia and a high-probability ventilation-perfusion lung scan are consistent with and may be diagnostic of pulmonary embolism or infarction.

Imaging Tests

The chest x-ray remains the focal point of diagnosis. The chest x-ray may show an infiltrate or a mass that guides the next diagnostic step. However, changes seen on chest x-ray may represent aspirated blood from another site and possibly are a result of bleeding rather than its cause. However, it is important to remember that a nonlocalizing or normal x-ray does not preclude further testing or follow-up, especially if the patient has risk factors for an occult malignancy. The extent of the lung density or retained blood does not correlate with the amount of blood expectorated. Certain specific radiographic characteristics of diseases and disorders causing hemoptysis are helpful (Table 3–4). Specific diagnostic steps should be based on the probable source and site of bleeding and the underlying pathologic condition. Diffuse hemorrhage at the alveolar capillary level should be evaluated by serologic tests and may require an open or thoracoscopic lung biopsy for a specific diagnosis, whereas a localized disease usually warrants an endoscopic procedure. The CT scan is relatively more sensitive in detecting airway abnormalities not apparent on chest x-rays. It may confirm the findings of the chest x-ray or localize the bleeding source in those patients with a normal chest x-ray, especially in bronchiectasis. Other abnormalities seen on CT scan that may not be apparent on a chest x-ray include mycetoma and pulmonary nodules. High-resolution CT (HRCT) scanning is helpful in identifying bronchiectasis and central airway tumors or masses. Specialized multidetector CT angiography may be helpful in looking for vascular abnormalities such as AVMs and pulmonary arterial bleeds. The use of magnetic resonance imaging (MRI) techniques for the evaluation of hemoptysis is generally not helpful. The $\dot{V}/\dot{Q}$ scan and a spiral CT scan of the

Table 3–4. Causes, characteristics, and evaluation of hemoptysis

Cause	Source and pathophysiology	Chest x-ray	Specific diagnostic tests
Tuberculosis	Acute: necrosis of small arterioles Chronic: rupture of aneurysmal vessels, ectatic pulmonary vessels	Nodular/cavitary	Sputum cultures
Bronchiectasis	Bronchial vessel hypertrophy and expansion of submucosal plexus	May be normal, "tramline" shadows or cystic lesions	HRCT
Lung abscess	Parenchymal necrosis and formation of pseudoaneurysm	Cavitary lesion with air-fluid level	History of risk factors
Broncholith	Rupture of vessel and mucosa erosion with fistula formation	Hilar calcification	CT scan
Bronchogenic carcinoma	Tumor erosion of vessel, cavitary necrosis, vessel rupture	Mass lesion, or negative if in large airway	FOB, CT scan
Chronic bronchitis	Increased bronchial vascularity and tortuosity, development of precapillary anastomoses	Increased vascularity, signs of cor pulmonale	PFTs, FOB
Mycetomas	Friction of fungus ball within cavity with ulceration, inflammation,	Preexisting cavitary or bullous disease with double shadow or and capillary abrasion "ball" within cavity	CT scan if chest x-ray unclear
Invasive fungal infection	Microangioinvasion by fungus with thrombosis, necrosis, and hemorrhage	Diffuse interstitial or alveolar densities	CT scan, biopsy
Cardiovascular causes	Rupture of atheromatous plaques and arteriolar rupture with increased bronchopulmonary anastomoses	Signs of pulmonary hypertension	Echocardiogram, cardiac catheterization
Vascular (AVMs)	Distention and varicosity with degeneration and rupture of draining cavernous spaces	Solitary or multiple nodules	CT scan, pulmonary angiography

(continued)

Table 3–4. Causes, characteristics, and evaluation of hemoptysis *(continued)*

Cause	Source and pathophysiology	Chest x-ray	Specific diagnostic tests
Vasculitides and alveolar hemorrhagic syndromes			
Systemic lupus erythematosus	Alveolar hemorrhage, small-vessel vasculitis with capillaritis, granular IgG deposition along granular wall	Diffuse acinal filling	Glomerular nephritis, positive ANA
Goodpasture's syndrome	Alveolar hemorrhage with chronic inflammation, no vasculitis	Diffuse densities	Positive serum ABMA positive linear IgG in glomeruli
Wegener's granulomatosis	Necrotizing vasculitis with granulomatous inflammation	Nodular/cavitary parenchymal lesion	Positive cANCA, necrotizing glomerular nephritis, upper airway involvement
Nonspecific vasculitis	Small-vessel arteritis and capillaritis	Nonspecific	pANCA variable, necrotizing crescentic glomerular nephritis
Idiopathic pulmonary hemorrhage	Alveolar hemorrhage with interstitial fibrosis and hemosiderin-laden macrophages	Diffuse alveolar	Negative IgG deposits, diagnosis of exclusion

Note: ABMA, antibasement membrane antibody; ANA, antinuclear antibody; AVMs, arteriovenous malformations; cANCA, cytoplasmic antineutrophilic cytoplasmic antibody; CT, computed tomography; FOB, fiber optic bronchoscopy; HRCT, high-resolution computed tomography; IgG, immunoglobulin G; pANCA, perinuclear antineutrophilic cytoplasmic antibody; PFTs, pulmonary function tests.

chest may be diagnostic in pulmonary embolism or infarction but is not useful in localizing the source of bleeding when multiple abnormalities are present.

Other Specific Tests

Pulmonary function tests are helpful in distinguishing restrictive from obstructive lung disease and may help in identifying the pathophysiology of the underlying cause but do not directly aid in diagnosis. Bronchoscopy is indicated to assess the airways and to obtain histologic confirmation of specific diagnoses. The choice of rigid versus fiber optic bronchoscopy (FOB) or the use of both depends on the degree of bleeding, the location of the lesion, and the importance of maintaining a patent airway. The suction channel and suction capacity of most flexible fiber optic bronchoscopes are limited and make management of massive hemoptysis difficult. The decision to use the rigid bronchoscope, which permits efficient aspiration of blood and better tamponade of the bleeding site if needed, should be based on the underlying pathologic condition and the source and magnitude of the bleeding. The fiber optic scope passed through the lumen of the rigid bronchoscope yields better definition of the lesion with more peripheral airway visualization. The role of bronchoscopy or the type of bronchoscope used in lateralizing and localizing the site of bleeding in the lung or airways is not as controversial as the timing of the procedure itself. Active bleeding and sites of bleeding are visualized more commonly with early bronchoscopy done within 48 hours of the onset of bleeding. Although early visualization may help in determining the need for urgent intervention, it rarely alters the clinical outcome of the patient.

Hemoptysis with a normal or nonlocalizing chest x-ray poses an additional diagnostic challenge. Up to 30% of patients with hemoptysis have a normal chest x-ray. As shown in Figure 3–3, a systematic approach is helpful in the differential diagnosis. The presence of risk factors for malignancy such as a smoking history, exposure to environmental toxins, age greater than 40 years, and recurrent hemoptysis for a period greater than a week may dictate the need for bronchoscopy. In the absence of these risk factors of malignancy, the bronchoscopy findings are usually nondiagnostic or nonspecific, a specific bleeding site is rarely identified, and malignancy is rare. Moreover, in most patients with none of the risk factors outlined above who undergo a nondiagnostic bronchoscopy, a mean follow-up of 5 years revealed a benign course. In the majority of patients a normal

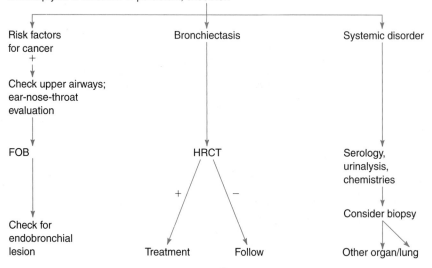

Figure 3–3. Algorithm for evaluation of hemoptysis in relation to normal or nonlocalizing chest x-ray. HRCT, high-resolution computed tomography.

bronchoscopy result effectively excludes a specific endobronchial cause of hemoptysis, and the prognosis for these patients is generally good. In such cases, pretest probability of cancer based on risk factors and the quantity and persistence of hemoptysis thus determines the need for a bronchoscopic evaluation. Patients without the above-mentioned risk factors can be safely followed if no other indications for the procedure are present. However, a chest x-ray with obscured central fields should not necessarily be considered normal in patients with hemoptysis. These patients may have central or larger airway lesions not clearly visible on chest x-ray, and the need for bronchoscopy should be assessed.

MANAGEMENT PRINCIPLES

The management of hemoptysis depends on the underlying cause and the volume of hemoptysis. On one hand, infrequent minimal hemoptysis does not require any specific control measures per se, but investigation of its underlying cause is warranted because even a small amount of hemoptysis may signal a potentially life-threatening episode. On the other hand, massive hemoptysis, regardless of its cause or underlying pathologic condition, necessitates aggressive management because it could be life threatening and its clinical course is unpredictable. The common cause of death in these cases is by asphyxiation, whereas blood loss and intractable hypoxemia may also contribute to increased mortality and morbidity. It may be helpful to focus on the anatomic site of hemoptysis and direct control measures toward the source of bleeding (Figure 3–4).

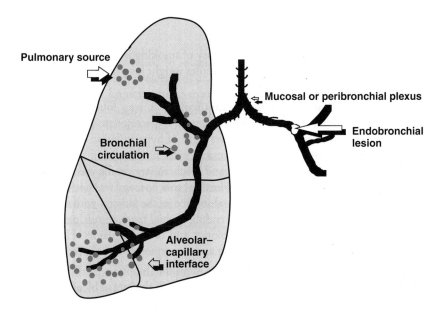

Figure 3–4. Focusing on the anatomic site of hemoptysis helps target management.

Physical Examination: Her pulse is 125 beats/min, her blood pressure is 90/60 mm Hg, and her temperature is 37.2°C (99°F). Her arterial blood gas studies show pH 7.47, P_{CO_2} 36, P_{O_2} 55, and O_2 saturation 89%. Her chest x-ray shows bilateral linear densities with a large round opacity in the right lung field within a cavity or bulla (Figure 3–6). A CT scan confirms a rounded opacity within a cavity consistent with a "fungus ball." Bronchoscopy confirms the bleeding site to be from the right upper lobe. Results of bronchial washings for culture, fungi, and mycobacteria are negative. The patient is treated conservatively with fluid management, broad-spectrum antibiotics, cough suppressants, and mild sedation. Initially she responds well, but 24 hours later has a recurrence of massive hemoptysis that required frequent suctioning even though her cough reflexes were good. However, she remains hemodynamically stable. Bronchial artery embolization (BAE) of her right lung is performed, resulting in the cessation of hemoptysis within 2 hours of the procedure. After a few days of observation and continued conservative treatment, she is discharged for outpatient follow-up.

Discussion: This clinical scenario illustrates the occurrence of massive hemoptysis due to a fungus ball/mycetoma in an underlying bullous/cavitary lesion. The primary cause of such a bullous or cavitary lesion is old granulomatous disease such as chronic inactive TB or sarcoidosis. The chest x-ray coupled with a CT scan is diagnostic of such a lesion. Bronchoscopic evaluation may be needed to confirm, lateralize, and localize the bleeding source in this case, especially in view

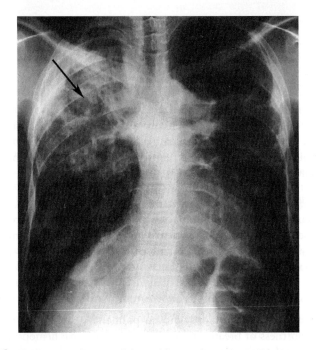

Figure 3–6. Chest x-ray showing bilateral linear densities in the upper zone with a rounded opacity within a cavity in the right upper zone (arrow).

of bilateral disease. In this case, BAE was performed successfully to control the bleeding. However, up to 20% of patients will have recurrent hemoptysis after BAE and may require multiple attempts due to anatomic variations and presence of collateral circulation responsible for the continued bleed.

CLINICAL PEARL

Regardless of the primary cause, massive life-threatening hemoptysis initially requires maintenance of airways, stabilization of hemodynamic parameters, and conservative supportive measures. Subsequently, specific therapeutic interventions such as BAE are indicated to control the bleeding.

KEY CONCEPTS

① *Pathophysiologic sequelae to hemoptysis vary with the extent and underlying pathogenesis and range from minimal derangement to life-threatening airway and respiratory compromise.*

② *While the management of hemoptysis depends upon the severity, location, and site of bleeding, attempts should be made to correct the underlying cause.*

STUDY QUESTIONS

3–1. A 59-year-old man with a history of 20–pack-years of smoking is referred for evaluation of mild intermittent hemoptysis of 6 months' duration. He was treated for TB in Vietnam. He denies any fever, chills, night sweats, or weight loss, and says that other than periodic hemoptysis mixed with moderate sputum, there has been no change in the character, intensity, and severity of cough. He is in no acute distress, appears generally healthy, and has no stigmata of chronic illness; his physical examination is unremarkable and his chest x-ray is normal. He is treated with antibiotics, and his hemoptysis resolves.

   Hemoptysis in this patient is most likely due to

   a. rupture of aneursymal bronchiectatic vessels related to TB

   b. neovascularization and traction bronchiectasis

   c. increased submucosal and mucosal bronchial edema and tortuosity of vessels secondary to chronic bronchitis.

   d. cavitary necrosis and tumor bed erosion related to bronchogenic carcinoma

3–2. A 29-year-old woman with a history of frequent "pneumonia" in the past is seen with complaints of moderate to massive hemoptysis. She has been treated with frequent antibiotic courses in the past. She is now coughing up large amounts of purulent sputum and is febrile. On examination she is in moderate distress with tachypnea. She has digital clubbing and crackles are heard in the left lower zone of her lung posteriorly. Her chest x-ray shows multiple small cystic shadows with air-fluid levels in the left lower zone Her laboratory data are normal except for mild anemia and moderate hypoxemia. Sputum shows numerous white blood cells with mixed flora, predominantly gram-negative organisms and a few fungal hyphae.

All the following statements regarding this patient are correct EXCEPT

a. the most likely diagnosis is bronchiectasis;

b. hemoptysis in this case is due to vascular hypertrophy and submucosal bronchopulmonary vascular anastomoses;

c. hypoxemia and anemia are unusual in this case;

d. invasive pulmonary aspergillosis with microinvasion of vessels and surrounding tissue destruction is causing this degree of hemoptysis.

SUGGESTED READING

Fitzgerald FT, Murray JF. Chapter 18. In: Murray JF, Nadel JA, Mason RJ, Boushey HA, eds. *Murray and Nadel's Textbook of Respiratory Medicine.* 4th ed. Philadelphia: Elsevier Saunders; 2005.

Noncardiac Chest Pain

4

Michael Stumpf & Kevin Reed

OBJECTIVES

▶ List the various organ systems that are responsible for causing chest pain, describe the diseases of the respiratory, musculoskeletal, and gastrointestinal systems that cause chest pain, and elucidate how to differentiate them.

▶ Explain the pathophysiology and pathogenesis of common causes of chest pain other than coronary artery disease and describe the evaluation of patients with these diseases.

▶ Evaluate and critique neuropsychiatric causes of chest pain.

GENERAL CONSIDERATIONS

Chest pain is a very common symptom that can result from a number of causes and may denote serious or life-threatening diseases such as acute coronary syndrome (ACS), pulmonary embolism, and tension pneumothorax. Conversely, it may result from a disorder that may not be life threatening but may be disabling because of the patient's anxiety about the discomfort. Because of the potential seriousness of the complaint of chest pain, it should prompt immediate evaluation. Identification of the correct cause requires a thorough understanding both of the patient's symptoms and of the differential diagnosis of disorders that can cause chest pain.

Coronary artery disease (CAD) remains the leading cause of death in the United States. For this reason, the immediate priority in evaluating a patient with chest pain is to assess for CAD as the cause of the pain (Figure 4–1). The process begins with a history and physical examination, but the physician must appreciate the limitations of history and physical examination in distinguishing the cause of chest pain. Evaluation for ACS, or chest pain caused by myocardial ischemia, often includes a number of laboratory tests such as cardiac enzyme levels, exercise testing, echocardiography, computed tomography (CT) angiography, and thallium scintigraphy. One third of patients initially evaluated for ACS in the emergency department are discharged or released after 36 hours of observation without the diagnosis of acute ischemia. When the cause remains unclear after these tests, the patient is often assessed with coronary arteriography. A number of risk factors

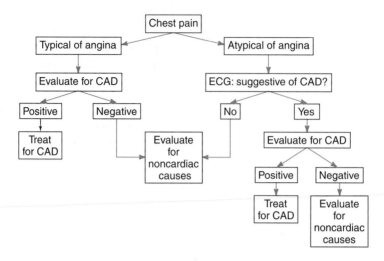

Figure 4–1. The evaluation of chest pain begins with a history and is initially directed at eliminating coronary artery disease (CAD) as the cause of chest pain. If the results of the evaluation are negative for CAD, the evaluation should proceed to search for other causes. "Noncardiac causes" include all causes of chest pain other than CAD and may include some causes referable to the heart (see text). See Figure 4–2 for the evaluation of noncardiac causes of chest pain. ECG, electrocardiogram.

predict the chances of an abnormal angiogram. However, of patients who undergo coronary arteriography, 20%–30% have normal or near-normal coronary arteries, and the cause of their chest pain remains unclear. About 80% of this group continues to have chest pain for 10 years or more and 50% remain disabled because of chest pain.

Determining the cause of chest pain not due to CAD is often difficult (Figure 4–2). Various studies have demonstrated that common causes include gastrointestinal (GI), musculoskeletal, pulmonary, and psychological disorders, as well as cardiac causes other than CAD. This chapter reviews these disorders and discusses approaches to the diagnosis.

PATHOPHYSIOLOGY OF CHEST PAIN

The pathophysiology of chest pain is variable. The lung, for example, can have pain arising from stimulation of the mucosa of the trachea and main bronchi, whereas the lung parenchyma along with the visceral pleura is insensitive to painful stimuli as it is not innervated by nociceptive receptors. The tracheobronchial tree and lungs are innervated by autonomic afferent and efferent pathways. These include afferent pathways for the cough, stretch and irritant receptors in the central airways, but seldom include afferent pathways for pain. Pain originating from the tracheobronchial tree is presumably mediated by type C fibers or through the vagal pathway. Pain receptors in the parietal and diaphragmatic pleural surfaces are derived from the intercostal nerves; irritation of these areas results in

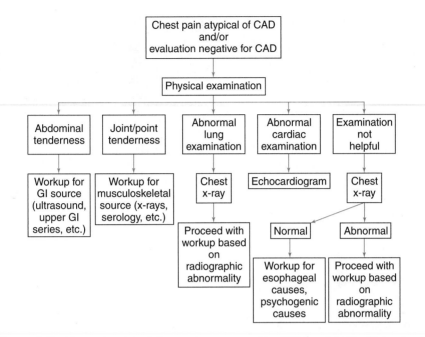

Figure 4–2. The evaluation of chest pain not caused by CAD is guided by history and physical examination. Additional tests may be ordered to aid with the diagnosis. See the text for a description of abnormal cardiac and pulmonary examination findings in patients with chest pain. GI, gastrointestinal.

pain in the adjacent chest wall. The central portion of the diaphragm is supplied by the phrenic nerve, and pain in this area is often perceived in the ipsilateral shoulder. It is the inflammation in the adjacent parietal pleura that causes chest pain. Distension of pulmonary vascular structures with stimulation of mechanical receptors from pressure overload states such as those seen in pulmonary hypertension and valvular stenosis may initiate pain in these conditions.

Disorders of the chest wall secondary to trauma, inflammation, or fibrositis of the muscle bone articulations occurs and can produce superficial or deep somatic pain. The pain perception is initiated by nociceptors that can detect thermal, mechanical, or chemical changes above a certain threshold. The pain fibers travel via the spinal cord to the brain, specifically the somatosensory cortex and the limbic system. Radiculitis along the cutaneous distribution of the involved intercostal nerves can cause pain with associated hyperalgesia or anesthesia of the surrounding skin. Vascular compression and obstructive lesions affecting the sympathetic chain and stellate ganglion can lead to pain when the thoracic outlet area is affected either by tumor or other infiltrative disorders. The neurobiology of pain associated with cardiac and pericardiac structures is not clear and the chemical transmitters and sensory pathways that travel through the cardiac nerves, sympathetic ganglia, and the dorsal thoracic roots are not well understood. Pain attributed to mitral valve prolapse syndrome cannot be explained on the basis of mitral regurgitation, and autonomic and neuroendocrine dysfunction may be a possible cause. The pericardium contains few afferent pain fibers except in the diaphragmatic portion through the phrenic nerves. This results in pain referred to the area of the trapezius muscle and associated pleural pain is not uncommon. Vascular rupture with hematoma formation causes pain in aortic dissection.

Mechanical and thermoreceptors activated by stretch, chemical irritants, and stimulated through the vagal and sympathetic chain result in pain originating in the esophagus. Sensation from both the esophagus and the heart is transmitted to the central nervous system through the sympathetic and parasympathetic systems. The sympathetic or spinal afferents are primarily responsible for the sensation of esophageal pain. Centrally, the nociceptive primary afferents terminate on neurons in specific layers of the dorsal horn of the spinal cord. Convergence of multiple visceral afferents from both the heart and esophagus onto the same dorsal horn probably explains the difficulty in distinguishing between esophageal and cardiac pain.

PULMONARY CAUSES OF CHEST PAIN

Pleurisy & Pleural Effusion

Inflammation of the pleura (pleurisy or pleuritis) may be caused by a number of disorders (see Table 4–1). Pleurisy is typically characterized by fever, cough, dyspnea, and pleuritic chest pain (pain that varies with the respiratory cycle). Physical examination may reveal a pleural friction rub on the involved side, and a pleural effusion, which is usually an exudate, may be evident on chest x-ray. Pleurisy is more a syndrome than a true disease and is often associated with infections, neoplasms, or various connective tissue diseases, the most common of which is systemic lupus erythematosus. In some cases, pleurisy is the initial manifestation of lupus. When this occurs, the diagnosis of lupus is not usually immediately apparent. Lupus pleuritis is usually associated with fever, cough, dyspnea, and a pleural friction rub, and it tends to be recurrent. It is seen in both idiopathic and drug-induced lupus. The diagnosis of lupus pleuritis is made by pleural fluid analysis and serologic testing.

The differential diagnosis of pleural effusions is broad, and as discussed in greater detail in Chapter 11, the cause of pleural effusions must always be investigated, most often with thoracentesis. Patients with pleural effusions often present with dyspnea and with chest pain that may be sharp or dull in character. On physical

Table 4–1. Pulmonary causes of chest pain

Pleurisy and pleural effusion
Malignant mesothelioma
Pneumothorax
Pneumomediastinum
Diffuse parenchymal lung disease
Pulmonary embolism
Pulmonary hypertension

examination, breath sounds are diminished and the chest is dull to percussion over the effusion. Above the effusion, the lung is atelectatic, and bronchial breath sounds are heard. Chest x-ray confirms the presence of an effusion. The most common causes for pleural effusions causing pain are infectious and neoplastic but the differential is extensive. Residual pleural scarring and persistently abnormal chest x-ray findings are common after resolution of the pleural effusion.

Malignant Mesothelioma

Malignant mesothelioma has a classic presentation with pleural effusion with chest pain that may be referred to the ipsilateral shoulder or upper abdomen and that is typically constant rather than pleuritic in nature. The majority of patients with mesothelioma have a remote history of asbestos exposure; the latent period between asbestos exposure and the development of mesothelioma is 20–40 years. Smoking does not increase the risk of malignant mesothelioma as it does for most pulmonary neoplasms.

Physical examination may only reveal findings consistent with a pleural effusion. A pleural effusion, which may be massive, and pleural thickening are almost always evident on chest x-ray. The diagnosis is made with pleural biopsy. Malignant mesothelioma is difficult to distinguish histologically from adenocarcinoma, and for this reason many experts suggest that an open pleural biopsy is required for diagnosis. A percutaneous needle biopsy yields very small fragments of tissue and is often inadequate to allow differentiation of mesothelioma from adenocarcinoma. Pathologic distinction may be confirmed by electron microscopy and immunocytochemistry.

Pneumothorax

Chest pain is seen in up to 90% of patients with pneumothorax. The pain of pneumothorax is often anterior or radiating to the ipsilateral shoulder and is almost invariably associated with dyspnea. The diagnosis of spontaneous pneumothorax may be suspected based on the history of a sudden onset of unilateral chest pain, often pleuritic in nature, associated with sudden (and often worsening) dyspnea. Pneumothoraces are often described as primary or secondary. Primary pneumothoraces are classically seen in tall, thin young males without previous history of lung disease. The presumed etiology is the rupture of apical blebs and there is a high rate of recurrence. Secondary pneumothoraces occur in patients with known structural lung diseases (COPD, LAM, etc) or trauma including iatrogenic trauma such as complications from central venous access insertion. In patients on mechanical ventilators, worsening hypoxemia and increasing airway pressures suggest the possibility of pneumothorax.

Physical examination often reveals diminished or absent breath sounds and hyperresonance to percussion on the affected side of the chest. If the pneumothorax is large enough or is under tension, the trachea may be deviated away from the side of the pneumothorax. With a tension pneumothorax, the patient may become hypotensive because of decreased venous return to the heart resulting from increased intrathoracic pressure and will require emergency treatment.

The diagnosis of pneumothorax is confirmed with chest x-ray (see Chapter 11). However, a tension pneumothorax is usually easy to diagnose by history and physical examination alone, and delaying treatment until a chest x-ray can be obtained may result in a fatal outcome.

Pneumomediastinum

Pneumomediastinum is air within the mediastinum. The most common cause of pneumomediastinum is alveolar rupture with dissection of air along the bronchovascular bundle toward the hilum and into the mediastinum. Common causes include severe asthma attacks and with repeated Valsalva maneuvers during childbirth. Pneumomediastinum can also be the presenting sign of an esophageal rupture. The presenting symptom of pneumomediastinum is often substernal chest pain with radiation to the neck. The hallmark physical sign is Hamman's sign, which is a grating sound heard over the precordium due to bubbles of air in the mediastinum. Hamman's sign is usually synchronized with the heartbeat and is best heard with the patient in the left lateral decubitus position. Subcutaneous emphysema in the neck, face, and upper chest may also be present. Radiographic imaging is the confirmatory tests.

Diffuse Parenchymal Lung Disease

Diffuse parenchymal lung disease (DPLD) is an unusual cause of chest pain because of the lack of nociceptive receptors in the lung parenchyma. Pain caused by DPLD is usually due to inflammation of the pleura; thus, the pain is typical of pleurisy or of the major airways. The history is extremely important in developing the differential of DPLD with emphasis on exposures to drugs, occupations and hobbies, and symptoms of connective tissue diseases. The physical examination may be helpful with findings such as crackles and clubbing. The diagnosis is often made by radiographic imaging (CXR and high-resolution CT scanning) but the ultimate diagnosis is made by biopsy and histology. Chest pain caused by inflammation of the trachea and main stem bronchi is felt in the midline of the anterior chest or in the neck, and may be perceived as a dull, aching pain or as a burning pain. There are no specific physical findings associated with pain caused by this mechanism, but the history may suggest the diagnosis of inhalation of an irritant substance or acute tracheobronchitis.

Pulmonary Embolism

Chest pain is reported to occur in 60%–80% of patients with pulmonary embolism although dyspnea is the more common symptom. The cause of the pain is felt to be secondary to stretch on the proximal arteries, right ventricular strain or from pleurisy secondary to pulmonary infarction. The diagnosis of pulmonary embolism is difficult to make on clinical grounds alone, and clinical suspicion is correct no more than one third of the time. Nonetheless, pulmonary embolism is suspected in any patient who has the sudden onset of dyspnea, chest pain, hypoxemia, and a feeling of impending doom. Predisposing conditions include the components of Virchow's triad which include venous stasis, intimal injury, and hypercoagulable states.

Physical examination is rarely helpful in the diagnosis of pulmonary embolism, although in some patients with massive pulmonary emboli, a right ventricular third heart sound (S_3) may be heard, and jugular venous distention may be present. Most pulmonary emboli arise from deep veins in the lower extremities, and physical examination may reveal edema, erythema, and tenderness in a lower extremity, although these findings are unreliable.

Subtle signs of pulmonary embolism on the chest x-ray, including a pulmonary infiltrate, pleural effusion, and elevation of the hemidiaphragm, are sometimes present. However, confirmation of the diagnosis requires further testing including ventilation-perfusion scans, CT angiography, and pulmonary angiograms.

Pulmonary Hypertension

Pulmonary hypertension is sometimes associated with chest pain. The chest pain of pulmonary hypertension usually does not cause chest pain until it is advanced enough to cause right ventricular ischemia. The ischemia is caused by right ventricular pressure overload from increasing pulmonary vascular resistance. The classic description of pulmonary hypertension was primary versus secondary but the most accepted description is that of the World Health Organization (WHO) which divides it into five groups. Physical examination of a patient with severe pulmonary hypertension typically reveals a right ventricular lift and a loud pulmonic component of the second heart sound (P_2). In the presence of right ventricular failure, jugular venous distention and peripheral edema are usually present. Enlarged pulmonary arteries are apparent on plain chest x-rays or chest CT scans in advanced pulmonary hypertension. There may be evidence of right ventricular enlargement on an electrocardiogram (ECG). Echocardiography or right heart catheterization and direct measurement of pulmonary artery pressure are required to make a definitive diagnosis of pulmonary hypertension.

GI CAUSES OF CHEST PAIN

General

After CAD has been ruled out, the differential diagnosis of chest pain should include GI disorders. GI causes of chest pain can be divided into esophageal and nonesophageal categories (Table 4–2). While gastroesophageal reflux disease (GERD) and esophageal motility disorders are the most common etiologies, a new entity known as functional chest pain of presumed esophageal origin has emerged. The evaluation of GI causes of chest pain can be difficult due to the close proximity of the esophagus and heart as well as the similar neural nociceptor pathways both organs share. Both organs are innervated by the vagus nerve and thoracic spinal nerves which transmit pain and pressure sensations to the hypothalamus. As a result, clinical presentation does not distinguish cardiac pain from GI pain but certain symptoms and signs may suggest a GI etiology. Provided the patient does not present with alarm symptoms, pharmacologic therapy is the preferred method of diagnosis and treatment. Invasive diagnostic testing is reserved for refractory symptoms. The diagnosis and management of GI causes of chest pain are outlined in Figure 4–3.

Gastroesophageal Reflux

GERD is the most common cause of noncardiac chest pain. Transient relaxation of the lower esophageal sphincter (LES) allows gastric acid to enter the esophagus resulting in inflammation and sometimes ulceration of the esophageal mucosa. Common exacerbating factors include medications such

Table 4–2. Gastrointestinal causes of chest pain

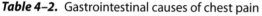

Esophageal	Nonesophageal
GERD	**Acute pancreatitis**
Motility disorders	Peptic ulcer disease
Nutcracker esophagus	Biliary tract disease
Diffuse esophageal spasm	Splenic flexure syndrome
Hypertensive lower esophageal sphincter	
Achalasia	
Nonspecific motor disorder	
Functional chest pain of presumed esophageal origin	

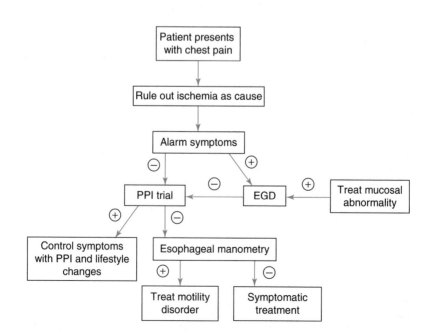

Figure 4–3. Diagnostic algorithm for esophageal chest pain. PPI, proton pump inhibitor; EGD, upper G1 endoscopy.

as NSAIDs; foods, such as chocolate, caffeine, and alcohol; pregnancy; and hiatal hernia.

GERD may present as chest pain, cough, asthma, and hoarseness. Chest pain is considered an atypical presentation but has been reported in up to 37% of patients. The character of the chest pain may be sharp, stabbing, burning, or dull and boring. Often symptoms are worse at night or in a supine position. The initial diagnostic and therapeutic intervention, in the absence of alarm symptoms (Table 4–3), is to place the patient on a trial of proton pump inhibitor therapy. If symptoms improve, the physician can be confident in diagnosing GERD. If there is no improvement, further diagnostic tests such as radiographic upper GI series, endoscopy, ambulatory pH monitoring, and evaluation for motility disorders are required.

Esophageal Dysmotility

While esophageal dysmotility is the leading cause of noncardiac chest pain in patients without GERD, it is relatively uncommon. Studies have demonstrated that esophageal manometry is normal in 70% of patients with non-GERD-related noncardiac chest pain. Both nutcracker esophagus and hypertensive LES have been recognized as the most common causes of non-GERD noncardiac chest pain. Evaluation with manometry should be performed after GERD has been ruled out.

The chest pain may mimic angina in location and character. Like angina the pain may radiate to the neck, arm, and shoulder. Initially, esophageal spasm was thought to be the cause of chest pain in dysmotility disorders. Recently, however, esophageal hypersensitivity and abnormal pain perception has emerged as the mechanism. Therefore, pain modulation has become the mainstay of therapy while smooth muscle relaxation may provide transient relief of symptoms (Table 4–4).

Table 4–3. Alarm symptoms

Early satiety
Weight loss
Initial symptoms of GERD in patients over 45
Anemia

Table 4–4. Therapy for functional chest pain of esophageal origin

Pain modulation
Antidepressants (Imipramine, Trazadone, SSRIs)
Theophylline
Anxiolytics (Alprazolam, Citalopram)
5-HT$_3$ antagonists (Odansetron)
Muscle relaxants
Calcium channel blocker
Nitroglycerin
IV antispasmodic (cimetroprium bromide)
Sildenafil

Note: SSRIs, selective serotonin reuptake inhibitors.

NUTCRACKER ESOPHAGUS

Nutcracker esophagus is not a disease but a term used to describe a manometric finding of high amplitude peristaltic contractions in the distal 10 cm of the esophagus. Not all patients with nutcracker esophagus have chest pain but recent studies have shown that it is more common in patients with higher average distal peristaltic contractions. Studies have also shown an overlap with this finding and hypertensive lower esophageal sphincter.

HYPERTENSIVE LOWER ESOPHAGEAL SPHINCTER

Hypertensive LES is defined as a resting, midrespiratory lower esophageal pressure greater than 45 mm Hg. Some patients with a hypertensive LES also have incomplete relaxation. Similar to diffuse esophageal sphincter DES, hypercontracting motility abnormalities appear to be frequently associated with either high resting LES pressures or incomplete relaxation. Little is known about the potential pathophysiologic mechanisms in these hypercontractile disorders.

Functional Chest Pain of Presumed Esophageal Origin

Noncardiac chest pain with no apparent explanation can be classified as functional chest pain of presumed esophageal origin. This diagnosis of exclusion can only be made after GERD and esophageal dysmotility have been ruled out. Multiple studies with balloon distention and acid stimulation have demonstrated that patients with this disorder have lower perception thresholds for pain and altered central processing of intraesophageal stimuli. This is also the proposed pathophysiology of GERD and dysmotility-related chest pain. Psychologic comorbidities such as depression and anxiety are common in patients with functional chest pain. Therefore, in addition to symptomatic relief, patients may also benefit from cognitive behavioral therapy, antidepressants, or anxiolytics if indicated.

Other GI Disorders

Acute pancreatitis, peptic ulcer disease, and biliary tract disease typically cause abdominal pain but often cause chest pain. The pain may result from distention of the involved hollow organs or from inflammation of the involved organs and nearby structures. These conditions are often diagnosed based on history, physical exam, laboratory tests, and radiographic evaluation. Therapy is disease specific and symptoms are often relieved when their underlying medical conditions are treated.

MUSCULOSKELETAL CAUSES OF CHEST PAIN

 Musculoskeletal chest pain accounts for approximately 10%–15% of emergency room visits per year. They are often diagnosed by history and reproduction of pain by palpation on physical exam (Table 4–5).

COSTOCHONDRITIS

Costochondritis is a condition characterized by diffuse pain and tenderness at the costochondral or costosternal junctions. The upper costal cartilages are most

Table 4–5. Musculoskeletal causes of chest pain

Fibromyalgia
Costochondritis
Tietze's syndrome
Lower rib pain syndrome
Sternalis syndrome
Xiphoidalgia
Pancoast tumor
Trauma
Herpes zoster

frequently involved. There is no associated erythema, swelling, or heat at the sites of tenderness.

Although this is a common diagnosis of chest pain, the causes are poorly understood. Diagnosis is based on history and the ability to reproduce the pain upon palpation. The course is typically self-limiting with occasional exacerbations. Persistent symptoms should prompt an evaluation for fibromyalgia.

LOWER RIB PAIN SYNDROME

This condition is also known as rib-tip syndrome, slipping rib, twelfth rib, and clicking rib and is characterized by lower chest or upper abdominal pain. The pain is typically reproduced upon palpation of a tender spot on the costal margin. A definitive cause has not been found but some reports implicated hypermobility of the anterior end of the costal cartilage.

The diagnosis can be made by either direct palpation or the reproduction of pain when curling fingers under the rib and gently pulling it forward. Majority of patients with this condition are women with a mean age of 40. The treatment is supportive with pain persisting for more than 4 years in a majority of cases. Patients with this condition often undergo frequent, extensive work-ups for chest pain despite having a diagnosis of lower rib syndrome.

STERNALIS SYNDROME

The sternalis syndrome is localized tenderness directly over the body of the sternum or sternalis muscle. Palpation typically causes bilateral radiation of pain. Diagnosis is based on reproduction of pain upon palpation and may be aided by radiographic changes and increased uptake on bone scanning. The syndrome is generally self-limited and is not associated with persistent symptoms.

TIETZE'S SYNDROME

Tietze's syndrome is a closely related variant of costochondritis. It is a benign but painful condition characterized by predominately unilateral and tender nonsuppurative swelling and erythema of the cartilaginous articulations of the anterior chest wall. The pain is described as sharp, intermittent, and stabbing. The cause is unknown but some patients have described antecedent upper respiratory infections and excessive coughing prior to symptoms. Biopsy reveals chronic inflammatory fibrosis.

XIPHOIDALGIA

Xiphoidalgia is characterized by pain and tenderness over the xiphoid process of the sternum. It is closely related to costochondritis and may be acute or chronic. Symptoms can be exaggerated by eating a heavy meal or bending movements. Reproduction of pain over the xiphoid is specific and diagnostic. Analgesics or analgesic-steroid injections are often curative.

FIBROMYALGIA

Fibromyalgia is an inflammatory disorder characterized by diffuse musculoskeletal pain associated with characteristic multiple bilateral symmetrical tender points. The common locations of tender points in the chest wall are the midpoint of the upper fold of the trapezius and the origin of the pectoralis from the second rib lateral to the costochondral junction. Patients with fibromyalgia often have associated symptoms of morning stiffness, sleep disturbance, irritable bowel syndrome, headache, and depression. Fibromyalgia has been increasingly recognized as a cause of chest pain mimicking angina pectoris. The diagnosis is made by demonstrating 11 out of 18 predefined paired tender points on physical exam.

PANCOAST TUMOR

Pancoast tumor is a superior sulcus primary lung tumor that often invades the brachial plexus or nearby bony structures. It most commonly occurs in the right lung and causes pain that is often localized to the shoulder and medial border of the scapula at its onset. With progression of the tumor, the pain may extend along the distribution of the ulnar nerve with atrophy of the muscles of the arm and hand on the involved side. The tumor may involve the sympathetic chain and stellate ganglion producing Horner's syndrome (miosis, anhidrosis, and ptosis). The diagnosis of Pancoast tumor is often suspected after clinical examination and chest x-ray and is confirmed with CT scan or magnetic resonance imaging.

HERPES ZOSTER

Herpes zoster is a syndrome caused by reactivation of the varicella-zoster virus. The syndrome consists of pain and eruption of a vesiculopustular rash, classically limited to one dermatome. The pain may be severe and is often described as burning sensation over the affected area. Thoracic dermatomes are frequently involved, and chest pain is a common complaint. The diagnosis of herpes zoster is made by physical exam which is positive for a vesicular rash involving a dermatome. The involvement of multiple dermatomes should raise the suspicion of immunosuppression. There is no treatment but antiviral medications can be used to suppress reoccurrences.

TRAUMA

Trauma as a cause of chest pain is easily diagnosed by history and physical exam. The pain is localized to the site of the injury and the onset is typically acute. Pain may result from soft tissue contusion, skeletal injuries, or damage to underlying structures. There is generally tenderness over injured muscles and ribs and palpation elicits point tenderness. Unrecognized trauma, such as that caused by coughing or sneezing, may sometimes result in musculoskeletal injury.

CARDIAC CAUSES OF CHEST PAIN OTHER THAN CAD

There are a number of cardiac causes of chest pain that are not due to left ventricular ischemia and CAD, but which should be considered in the differential diagnosis of chest pain (Table 4–6). Although the purpose of this chapter is to discuss noncardiac chest pain, it is imperative to mention a few cardiac causes that routine testing for the evaluation of CAD may fail to diagnose.

Pericardial Disease

Pericarditis, which is the inflammation of the pericardium, causes chest pain that is usually substernal, pleuritic, and intermittent. The pain is classically worse when lying down and relieved by sitting up and leaning forward. Causes of pericarditis include infections, neoplastic infiltration of the pericardium, rheumatologic disorders, uremia, and drugs. Most infectious cases of pericarditis are due to viruses or bacteria, but rarely are they caused by fungi or parasites. Often no causative agent can be identified. The pathognomonic sign of pericarditis is a friction rub heard on cardiac auscultation. The classic description is a rough three component sound consisting of a presystolic, systolic, and diastolic component. The ECG often shows diffuse ST segment elevation (multiple coronary artery distributions) and PR segment depression.

Postcardiac Injury Syndrome

Postcardiac injury syndrome is characterized by the onset of fever, leukocytosis, elevated erythrocyte sedimentation rate, pleuropericarditis, and parenchymal infiltrates following a latency period after myocardial or pericardial injury. Postcardiac injury syndrome is thought to be an immunologic reaction to injury of the mesodermal pericardial cells and blood in the pericardial space. It typically occurs within 4–6 weeks following the injury and causes chest pain that is sometimes indistinguishable from angina. Postcardiac injury syndrome has been described following myocardial infarction (Dressler syndrome), chest trauma, cardiac surgery, pacemaker implantation, and angioplasty. The incidence of postcardiac injury syndrome is much higher following surgical procedures than after acute myocardial infarction. Although symptoms usually develop within a few

Table 4–6. Cardiac causes of chest pain other than coronary artery disease

---

Pericardial disease
Postcardiac injury syndrome
Myocarditis and cardiomyopathy
Mitral valve prolapse
Aortic dissection

---

weeks after the causative event, they have occurred up to 1 year later. The treatment is usually a trial of corticosteroids.

Myocarditis & Cardiomyopathy

The pain of myocarditis often resembles angina or, in up to 40% of patients, may be similar to pericardial pain because of associated pericarditis. Alternatively, patients may have no pain but may present with the development of congestive heart failure. The initial symptoms may resemble a viral syndrome and often patients are ill for more than a week before symptoms referable to the heart dominate the clinical picture. In most cases, an infectious cause is presumed but is often never confirmed. Infectious causes of myocarditis include a wide variety of viruses as well as *Rickettsia*, other bacteria, and protozoa. Radiation, uremia, and toxins such as lead or chemotherapeutic agents may also cause myocarditis. The diagnosis is often made with clinical history and physical, serology, echocardiography, and occasionally with myocardial biopsy.

Mitral Valve Prolapse

The majority of patients with mitral valve prolapse are asymptomatic, but there are some chest pain syndromes including panic attacks that may occur with this condition. The pain often differs from angina in character and duration. They also commonly complain of palpitations due to tachyarrhythmias. The classic physical exam finding is a midsystolic click with or without a murmur on auscultation. An echocardiogram is often used to confirm the diagnosis. Although many causes of the pain have been proposed, none has been confirmed.

Aortic Dissection

Chest pain is the hallmark of aortic dissection. It is present in over 90% of patients, and its onset is abrupt, reaching maximal intensity shortly after commencing, compared to myocardial pain which crescendos over several minutes. Anterior ripping or tearing chest pain with radiation to the intrascapular regions is the most common complaint. The location of the pain may be helpful in determining the site of the dissection, although it is not diagnostic. Anterior pain is more common in ascending aortic dissections, and posterior pain is more common in descending aortic dissections. There may be difficulty in distinguishing the pain of aortic dissection from that of myocardial infarction. However, the diagnosis of aortic dissection is favored when the pain is maximal in the intrascapular regions. Additional findings suggesting aortic dissection include pulse deficits, a new murmur of aortic insufficiency, an absence of electrocardiographic signs of acute myocardial infarction, and the presence of a widened mediastinum on chest x-ray. Diagnostic procedures include a chest CT scan with contrast and transesophageal echocardiography. Aortography is no longer required for diagnosis but may be necessary to determine appropriate therapy.

The primary event in nontraumatic aortic dissection is tear of the aortic intima. The cystic medial necrosis of the aorta leading to aortic dissection is a pattern of injury and repair consequent to acute or chronic hemodynamic forces. About 20% of the population with acute aortic dissection has cystic medial necrosis. Hypertension is the most common associated finding in 95% of this population, and it may play a role in the formation of an intramural hematoma. This usually occurs after an intimal tear with hemorrhage in the medial layer. The dissection may move antegrade or retrograde and form a false lumen with partial or complete thrombosis. Associated conditions include coarctation of the aorta, Marfan syndrome, or congenital bicuspid valves. Trauma from deceleration injuries can cause acute aortic dissection.

NEUROPSYCHIATRIC CAUSES OF CHEST PAIN

Chest pain is a common presenting symptom of psychiatric disorders accounting for up to 30% of patients presenting to the emergency room with chest pain. The pain is difficult to differentiate from ischemic causes of chest pain because ischemic chest pain is often accompanied by anxiety. Neuropsychiatric chest pain is often recurrent and disabling to the patient. However, when the diagnosis is made, the pain is usually treatable.

Generalized Anxiety Disorder

General anxiety disorder (GAD) is a psychiatric disorder characterized by excessive, often irrational, anxiety and worry. Patients find it difficult to control the symptoms which could cause a significant impairment of daily functioning. Typically somatic complaints such as chest pain prompt medical evaluation. The chest pain may also be accompanied by tingling of the lips, dry mouth, and carpopedal spasms. A carefully obtained history will usually uncover a stressful event that precipitated the attack. Diagnosis is made after ruling out medical conditions and fulfilling certain criteria established by the *DSM-IV* manual. Treatment includes behavioral therapy, selective serotonin reuptake inhibitors SSRIs, and anxiolytics.

Panic Disorder

In contrast to patients with GAD, patients with acute panic disorder have a more dramatic presentation. These patients present with the onset of chest pain after the inception of a panic attack. They describe difficulty breathing and a sensation of panic, fear, and palpitations. Typically the chest pain is nonexertional. The features of a classic panic attack are so characteristic that the chest pain is easily attributed to the attack. Most attacks last only a few minutes. In young patients there is no need for an extensive work-up, but in older patients the work-up should be guided by the clinical situation and the patient's risk factors for CAD.

MANAGEMENT PRINCIPLES

With the pathogenesis and pathophysiology of chest pain being so variable, it is imperative to assess the underlying process to guide its management. Symptomatic treatment of chest pain due to musculoskeletal disorders with anti-inflammatory agents and pain medications is sufficient since the underlying process is usually self-limiting.

Pain associated with neurasthenic disorders and neuropsychiatric causes best responds to a combination of psychopharmacologic agents and psychosocial support. Organic causes, however, such as the various cardiopulmonary or gastroenterologic disorders outlined above mandate a thorough and complete work-up and specific treatment.

CLINICAL SCENARIOS

Case 1

A 36-year-old woman with no previous medical history presents with complaints of sharp anterior chest pain. The pain began approximately 3 weeks ago, but she did not seek medical attention. She describes the pain as substernal, sharp, and lasting for 1–3 minutes. The pain is not related to exertion. Upon further questioning, she also admits to worsening exertional dyspnea over the past 6 months to a year. She takes no medications and denies tobacco, alcohol, or illicit drug use.

Physical Examination: Her physical examination is remarkable only for cardiac findings that include a left lower parasternal systolic lift, a physiologically split second heart sound, and a loud P_2. There is also a II/VI systolic murmur at the left lower sternal border that is accentuated with respiration. Her lungs are clear and her peripheral pulses are normal. The chest x-ray reveals prominent pulmonary arteries. Her ECG shows negative deflection of the QRS complex in lead I, indicating right axis deviation.

Discussion: Based on her age, sex, and lack of risk factors, CAD is very unlikely in this patient. However, based on the physical examination, chest x-ray, and ECG, the most likely diagnosis is pulmonary hypertension. An echocardiogram in this case would show a dilated right ventricle with elevated pulmonary artery pressures. If other causes of secondary pulmonary hypertension such as congenital heart disease or recurrent pulmonary emboli are ruled out, this case is consistent with a diagnosis of primary pulmonary hypertension.

CLINICAL PEARLS

- Pulmonary hypertension may present with chest pain.
- The physical findings of a parasternal/precordial lift, a loud second heart sound with $P_2 > A_2$, a murmur of tricuspid insufficiency, and a right ventricular lift can help with the diagnosis.
- Secondary causes of pulmonary hypertension, including congenital heart defects, pulmonary emboli, connective tissue diseases, pulmonary parenchymal diseases, and HIV infection should be ruled out.
- Chronic obstructive pulmonary disease is a common cause of pulmonary hypertension, but is rarely severe.

Case 2

A 50-year-old physically active man (nonsmoker) with a past history of hypertension presents to the emergency department with complaints of pressure-like substernal chest pain with radiation to the left shoulder. The pain has occurred several times at rest and has been intermittent, lasting 2–3 minutes. It has not occurred with exertion. There are no associated symptoms. The pain is relieved with sublingual nitroglycerin in the emergency department. His only medication is an antihypertensive agent.

Physical Examination: His physical exam is normal and his ECG shows T-wave inversion in the precordial leads.

Discussion: This man is at risk for myocardial infarction based on his age and his history of hypertension. The character of his pain is typical of angina, but unlike angina it has occurred at rest. His initial work-up is negative for ACS. He subsequently undergoes a thallium stress test that shows no evidence of myocardial ischemia and his coronary arteriography is normal. He is subsequently referred to a gastroenterologist for evaluation of his chest pain. His work-up includes endoscopic examination with normal results, but esophageal manometric measurements reveal abnormally high distal esophageal pressures and prolonged duration of contraction. He is diagnosed with nutcracker esophagus. Treatment with long-acting nitrates resolves his symptoms.

CLINICAL PEARLS

- Distinguishing esophageal from cardiac chest pain is often impossible by history.
- Nutcracker esophagus is the most common motility disorder causing chest pain.
- Classic findings of nutcracker esophagus are distal esophageal pressures greater than 180 mm Hg and duration of contraction greater than 6 seconds.

KEY CONCEPTS

Pain arising from a cardiopulmonary source is difficult to evaluate due to overlapping of its origin and location with other causes such as esophageal disorders.

Musculoskeletal chest pain is usually not significant and can be diagnosed by careful history and physical examination.

Management of chest pain depends on the underlying cause that must be determined by a careful diagnostic work-up. This is especially applicable to chest pain due to cardiac and pulmonary causes.

STUDY QUESTIONS

4–1. A 60-year-old man with a history of hypertension presents to the emergency department with a complaint of severe anterior chest pain that started 2 hours ago. The pain radiates toward his back and is associated with shortness of breath and diaphoresis. His history is significant for smoking two packs of cigarettes per day for 20 years and occasional alcohol use. On physical examination, his blood pressure is 255/130, his heart rate is 145 beats/min, and his respiratory rate is 26 breaths/min. His cardiac rhythm is regular and he has an S4. There is a II/VI diastolic decrescendo murmur heard at the second right intercostal space. The remainder of the findings upon physical examination is normal.

The first test that should be ordered is

a. chest x-ray

b. ECG

c. serum lipase measurement

d. echocardiogram

e. stool test for occult blood

4–2. A 23-year-old man presents to the emergency department complaining of sudden onset of left-sided pleuritic chest pain and dyspnea while he was lifting a heavy object. On physical examination he appears to be in distress, diaphoretic, and tachypneic. His blood pressure is 88/50, and his heart rate is 140 beats/min. He has markedly diminished breath sounds with hyperresonance to percussion over his left hemithorax.

The first thing to do in this case would be to

a. obtain an immediate chest x-ray;

b. give a small dose of a β-adrenergic blocking drug to slow the heart rate;

c. place a nasogastric tube to evaluate for blood in the stomach;

d. have the patient breathe into a paper bag;

e. insert a small chest tube on the left side.

4–3. A 35-year-old man with a history of well-controlled hypertension presents to the emergency room with a complaint of substernal chest pain that began 2 hours ago after eating dinner. The pain does not radiate and is not associated with shortness of breath, nausea, or vomiting. Similar pain has occurred after meals and at night but is usually relieved with antacids. His history is significant for smoking one pack of cigarettes a day for 10 years, occasional alcohol use, and no illicit drug use. His father had a myocardial infarction at age 50 and his mother is healthy. His blood pressure is 160/90, heart rate is 90 beats/min, and respiratory rate is 20 breaths/min. Other than mild distress, his physical exam is normal. Cardiac rhythm is regular and cardiac enzymes are negative. If you suspect gastroesophageal disease as the cause for his chest pain, what is the most appropriate next step in diagnosis.

a. exercise stress test

b. 24-hour pH monitoring

c. EGD

    d. PPI trial

    e. esophageal manometry

4–4. A 40-year-old woman presents to your clinic after completing two months of proton pump therapy for GERD. This is her second trial of therapy and she reports no relief of symptoms despite compliance with medications and diet. You decide to perform esophageal manometry and determine she has high amplitude peristaltic contractions in the distal 10 cm of the esophagus. You instruct her to continue the PPI and you add which additional medication to her:

    a. intravenous Cimetroprium bromide

    b. calcium channel blocker

    c. nitroglycerin

    d. Sildenafil

    e. SSRI

4–5. A 40-year-old woman presents to the emergency room with a complaint of chest pain and dry cough for one day. The pain is characterized as stabbing with radiation to the back and is not associated with nausea or vomiting. This is her first episode of chest pain and she is concerned that it is a heart attack considering the extensive history of coronary artery disease (CAD) in her family. She has smoked 2 packs of cigarettes a day for 20 years, drinks 2 glasses of wine each night with her dinner, and denies illicit drug use. Her blood pressure is 140/90 mm Hg, heart rate is 70 beats/min, and respiratory rate is 22 breaths/min. On physical exam you notice the patient sitting forward on the edge of the bed and you hear a grating sound upon auscultation of the heart. What do you expect to see on her EKG?

    a. normal sinus rhythm

    b. diffuse ST elevations and PR depressions

    c. ST elevations in leads II, III, and aVL with T-wave inversions

    d. alternating of QRS axis between beats

    e. left ventricular hypertrophy

4–6. A 40-year-old woman presents to the emergency room with the complaint of substernal chest pain lasting 2 days. She is well known to the emergency room physicians and has been evaluated for chest pain multiple times without finding a cause. Her EKG and cardiac enzymes are negative and after reviewing her records you notice that her GI work-up, including EGD and empiric proton pump inhibitor therapy, has been negative in the past. Vital signs are stable. The pain is located directly over her left seventh rib and when you curl your fingers under her rib and pull, she retracts in pain. Which of the following is the correct diagnosis?

    a. Xiphoidalgia

    b. Tietze syndrome

    c. Costochondritis

    d. Lower rib pain syndrome

    e. Herpes zoster

4–7. A 65-year-old man presents to the emergency room with a 2-day history of left-sided chest pain. He says the pain began as throbbing in nature and has recently started burning. When asked to locate the pain, he traces a band from his axilla to his anterior chest. Upon examination you notice an erythematous area with

overlying vesicular lesions. You inform him of his diagnosis. What is the most accurate statement regarding his diagnosis?

a. Cure less common in immunocompromised patients

b. Caused by a bacteria

c. Reduce duration of symptoms with medications

d. He has to be hospitalized to receive proper treatment

SUGGESTED READING

Murray JF, Gebhart GF. Chest pain. In: Murray JF, Nadel JA, Mason RJ, Boushey HA, eds. *Murray and Nadel's Textbook of Respiratory Medicine.* 3rd ed. Philadelphia: WB Saunders; 2000:567–584.

Lung Sounds

Ross S. Summer & Jason M. Konter

OBJECTIVES

- ▶ *Understand the pathogenesis and pathophysiology of normal and abnormal breath sounds.*
- ▶ *Recognize the implications of abnormal sounds in individuals with specific lung disease.*
- ▶ *Formulate a differential diagnoses for the causes of various abnormal lung sounds.*

ORIGIN OF NORMAL BREATH SOUNDS

Breath sounds result, in large part, from turbulent airflow. Turbulent airflow occurs when the orderly arrangement of particles in laminar flow becomes disrupted. During respiration, this can occur when airflow reaches a critical velocity such as during forced expiration or when airflow is physically disrupted as occurs at airway branch points.

During auscultation, breath sounds are heard best over the trachea and central airways. These sounds, appropriately named tracheal or bronchial breath sounds, consist of high- and low-frequency sounds. In the periphery of the lung, higher pitched components are more attenuated than lower pitched ones, resulting in the muffled quality of normal alveolar breath sounds. Listening to alveolar breath sounds (also called vesicular sounds), the expiratory phase sounds shorter (a 3:1 inspiratory:expiratory ratio) because expiration is a passive process resulting in lower flow rates and less turbulence. The inspiratory:expiratory ratio (1:3) heard over the central airways better approximates the actual time spent in each phase of the respiratory cycle (Figure 5–1).

PATHOPHYSIOLOGY OF ABNORMAL LUNG SOUNDS

Abnormal breath sounds include sounds of differing intensity, duration, or quality when compared to those of the normal respiratory cycle. Qualitative differences in breath sounds are collectively called adventitious breath sounds. The three most common types of adventitious breath sounds are wheezes, rhonchi, and crackles. Other less frequent sounds heard on auscultation are squeaks and a pleural rub.

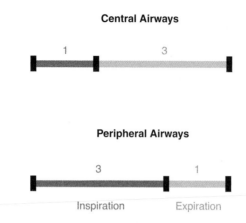

Figure 5–1. Inspiratory-expiratory ratio during auscultation.

Intensity of Breath Sounds

Care must be taken when assessing the significance of variations in the intensity of lung sounds. Bilateral and unilateral decreases in breath sounds can be of great clinical significance, but some asymmetry of sound intensity is common in normal lungs secondary to minor differences in regional airflow.

Significant differences in the intensity of breath sounds provide valuable insights into the pathologic state of the lung. In general, sound travels better through liquid than it does through air; thus, pathologic states resulting in increased airway fluid (ie, consolidation by blood, water, or pus) facilitate the transmission of breath sounds (Table 5–1). This means that there is more transmission of sound through a pneumonic than through a normal lung, allowing one to identify areas of consolidation by using physical examination techniques such as egophony (nasal or bleating sound), bronchophony, and whispering pectoriloquy. Egophony, which means "goat sound," refers to the high-pitched bleating sound "ay" heard over consolidated regions of lung as the patient repeats the sound "ee." Compared to normal lung, in consolidated regions, a higher pitched sound will be better heard and allows for recognition of a spoken phrase such as "ninety-nine." This is termed bronchophony. Whispering pectoriloquy involves having the patient whisper a word or phrase that contains several high-pitched components. A useful phrase such as "one, two, three" spoken as a whisper by the patient is heard more loudly by the examiner. Whispering pectoriloquy is also characteristic of a large cavity and may be heard above the level of a pleural effusion.

Since sound travels less efficiently through air, it makes sense that decreases in the intensity of breath sounds will be detected in diseases characterized by hyperinflation of the lung (eg, asthma, emphysema, or chronic bronchitis). Importantly, decreases in breath sounds can also result from various other mechanisms (Table 5–1), including failure of air to enter the lungs (airway obstruction) and processes that increase the distance between the lung and chest wall (effusion).

Table 5–1. Changes in the intensity of breath sounds

Increased	Decreased
Increases in airway fluid	**Increased lung volume**
Pneumonia	Hyperinflation
Pulmonary hemorrhage	Asthma
ARDS	Emphysema/bullous disease
Congestive heart failure	Chronic Bronchitis
Increased air entry/turbulence	**Decreased air entry**
Hyperventilation	Hypoventilation
Mouth breathing	Airway obstruction
	Phrenic nerve injury
	Muscle weakness
	Lung collapse
	Increased distance of lung from chest wall
	Obesity
	Pleural thickening
	Pneumothorax
	Empyema
	Hemothorax
	Transudative effusion

Note: ARDS, acute respiratory distress syndrome.

Duration of Breath Sounds

As mentioned in the section on normal breath sounds, the typical inspiratory:expiratory (I:E) ratio heard during auscultation of the peripheral lung is 3:1. Decreases in this ratio can occur in various diseases of the airway (asthma, chronic obstructive pulmonary disease [COPD], or tracheal stenosis) in which the passage of air is obstructed, prolonging expiratory time. This finding is especially pronounced in emphysema, where the loss of alveolar attachments produces much greater expiratory versus inspiratory obstruction (see the flow volume loops in Chapter 1). In a patient with an acute asthma attack or significant exacerbation of COPD, this auditory ratio is often reversed. Along with the I:E ratio, another simple bedside maneuver used to assess airway obstruction is to measure forced expiratory time (the time required for an individual to reach residual volume when expiring from total lung capacity) by auscultation over the trachea at the level of the suprasternal notch; any value greater than 6 seconds suggests airway obstruction. In a study examining the usefulness of this maneuver, prolonged forced expiratory time was found to correlate well with obstruction as measured by spirometry.

Wheezes

Wheezes are high-pitched musical sounds thought to result from the movement of air through a segment of airway oscillating between the point of closure and a partially open state. High-pitched musical sounds are produced when the caliber of the airway is significantly narrowed and as the airway walls oscillate. The pitch of the wheeze is dependent on the elasticity of the walls and the flow velocity. This is especially applicable in expiratory wheezes. The mechanism of inspiratory wheezing is not clear, though it seems to be related to turbulent airflow through a narrowed lumen.

Wheezes are caused by a variety of disease processes (Table 5–2), and the timing of a wheeze within the respiratory cycle may provide clues as to the diagnosis (Figure 5–2). For example, wheezes heard throughout the respiratory cycle are highly suggestive of either asthma or a fixed airway obstruction, whereas the detection of a loud pan-inspiratory wheeze (ie, stridor) of constant pitch is invariably associated with an extrathoracic (laryngeal or tracheal) airway obstruction. End-expiratory wheezes are entirely nonspecific and have been detected in bronchiolar

Table 5–2. Etiology of wheezes and stridor

Upper airway	Lower airway	Parenchymal
Intrathoracic airway obstruction	Asthma	Pulmonary edema
Tumor	Emphysema	
Airway stricture	Chronic bronchitis	
Extrathoracic airway obstruction	Acute tracheobronchitis	
Laryngeal edema	Bronchiectasis	
Vocal cord paralysis	Bronchiolitis	

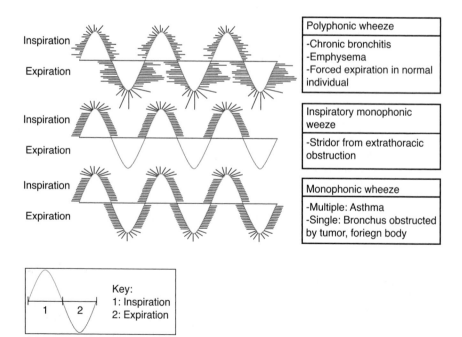

Figure 5–2. Wheeze within a respiratory cycle.

disease (asthma or bronchiectasis), structural disease (mucus plugging), and processes occurring within the alveolar space (pulmonary edema).

The complexity (monophonic or polyphonic) of audible wheezes may also suggest specific disease states. Monophonic wheezes consist of a single note whereas polyphonic wheezes are made up of several dissonant notes. An example of a single monophonic wheeze is the single tone created by a bronchus occluded by a tumor. The stenosis is fixed, so the pitch and timing remain constant. Similarly, a fixed obstruction of the upper airway (neck and upper trachea) results in the production of a monophonic wheeze. Wheezes generated by upper airway obstructions should be referred to as stridor and can be distinguished from fixed lower airway obstructions based on their predominance during inspiration. The presence of stridor should immediately prompt a careful evaluation of the upper airways.

Disease states that have complex wheezing patterns are those that produce polyphonic or multiple monophonic wheezes. Multiple monophonic wheezes occurring simultaneously is a classic finding in asthma. In such cases multiple airways are narrowed to the point of near closure. Each wheeze consists of a single pitch and varies in duration and timing. Polyphonic wheezing is the result of dynamic compression of the airways and is mainly found in either COPD or normal subjects during maximal forced expiration. Finally, care must be taken when using the presence or absence of wheezing as a diagnostic tool for assessing airway obstruction. It is important to note that the production of a wheeze requires adequate airflow rates. Severe airway obstruction significantly impairs airflow and thereby retards, or even eliminates, the ability to generate a wheeze.

Rhonchi

Rhonchi are easily distinguished from wheezes in that they are low-pitched honking or groaning sounds. Rhonchi are thought to result from the movement of air past bronchi partially obstructed by thick secretions. Rhonchi are found in any disease state associated with increased airway secretions (eg, pneumonia, chronic bronchitis, tracheobronchitis, asthma exacerbation, and cystic fibrosis). This pathophysiologic mechanism for the generation of rhonchi explains why these sounds frequently disappear, or change character, following a cough.

Crackles

Crackles result from the abrupt opening of previously closed airways. Consistent with this mechanism, crackles typically predominate in the lung bases, where the transpulmonary pressure is lowest and the parenchyma less distended.

The sound of crackles has been likened to the opening of a Velcro strap or the rubbing of hair together. Various disease states are associated with crackles on auscultatory exam (Table 5–3).

Like wheezes, the timing of crackles during the respiratory cycle may provide insight into the pathologic state of the lung (Figure 5–3). For example, isolated early inspiratory crackles have been associated with various obstructive lung diseases (asthma, chronic bronchitis, and emphysema) and can also be found in healthy individuals lying supine or beginning inspiration from below the

Table 5–3. Differential diagnosis of crackles

Early inspiratory	Mid- to late-inspiratory
Dependent atelectasis	Bronchiectasis
Bronchitis	Restrictive lung diseases
Asthma	Asbestosis
Emphysema	Idiopathic pulmonary fibrosis
	Sarcoidosis
	Scleroderma lung disease
	Pulmonary edema

Early inspiratory crackles
-Dependent atelectasis
-Bronchitis
-Asthma
-Emphysema

Mid-late inspiratory crackles
-Bronchiectasis
-Restrictive lung disease
   -Asbestosis
   -Idiopathic pulmonary
    fibrosis
   -Sarcoidosis
   -Scleroderma lung disease
-Pulmonary edema

Key:
1: Early Inspiration
2: Mid-Late Inspiration
3: Expiration

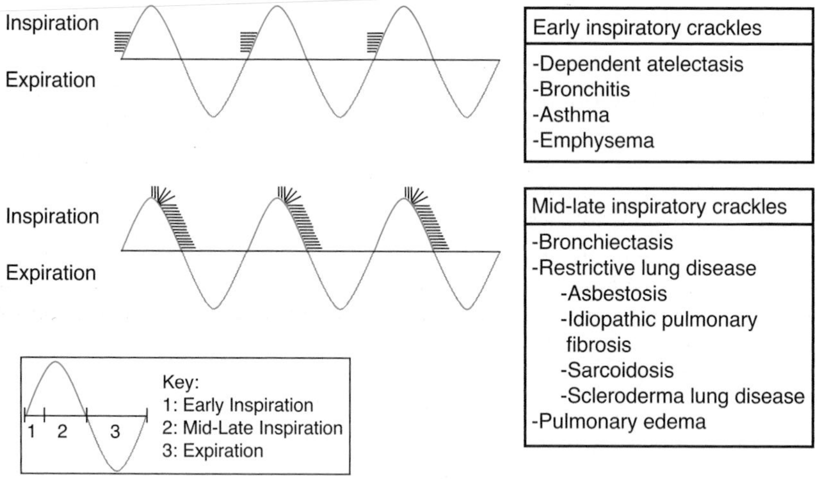

Figure 5-3. Inspiratory crackles.

functional residual capacity. Mid- to late-inspiratory crackles are typically found in restrictive lung diseases such as idiopathic pulmonary fibrosis and end-stage sarcoidosis.

Although crackles are not invariably associated with lung pathology, they are only rarely found in healthy individuals breathing from end-tidal volume, and should always be considered pathologic if they persist after a deep inspiration to total lung capacity.

Squeaks

Squeaks are brief wheeze-like sounds at the end of inspiration caused by the sudden opening of closed airways followed by rapid oscillation of the airway wall termed "airway flutter." They are high pitched in nature with a variable duration and are often accompanied by crackles. These sounds are heard in conditions causing increased retractile forces such as pulmonary fibrosis, bronchiectasis, or bronchiolitis.

Pleural Rub

Normally the small amount of pleural fluid separating the visceral and parietal pleura allows the lung to move smoothly without touching the chest wall. However, when pleural surfaces are inflamed and thickened, a friction rub may be produced that is characteristic of pleural inflammation and usually associated with pleuritic pain. This sound can be imitated by rubbing the palm of one hand lightly and slowly over the dorsum of the other hand. It has a scratchy and creaking character and may be confused with coarse crackles or an extra sound originating from the movement of the chest wall. Typically, a pleural rub is heard both at the end of inspiration and at the beginning of expiration, but can occur in any one phase and even with the presence of a large pleural effusion.

DIAGNOSTIC & CLINICAL CONSIDERATIONS

The presence of a rare or occasional sound of differing intensity, duration, or quality when compared to the patient's normal respiratory sounds is usually not significant. Attempts should be made to have the patient take several deep breaths and cough, and persistent isolated sounds not associated with any past or present historical clinical event should be reassessed at another examination. Clearly abnormal and persistent sounds should be evaluated in the context of the entire history and physical examination and further assessed by pulmonary function tests or roentgenographic studies. This is illustrated in the clinical examples below.

CLINICAL SCENARIOS

Case 1

A 65-year-old male smoker (150–pack-years) presents to the hospital with the subacute onset of shortness of breath. He states that his shortness of breath started approximately 6 months prior to this visit. He admits to occasional dry cough, but denies fever, chills, or night sweats. On review of systems, the patient states he has lost approximately 20 lb unintentionally and has been bothered by pain in this left scapular area.

Physical Examination: On physical exam he is in no apparent distress with normal vital signs and oxygen saturation of 92% on room air. Neck exam demonstrates tracheal deviation to the right. Jugular venous pressure is normal. The left hemithorax is dull to percussion throughout. Auscultation of the lungs reveals diminished breath sounds on the left with an overall prolonged expiratory phase. Other aspects of the physical examination are normal except for a trace of pedal edema.

Laboratory data reveal a normal white blood cell count and a slight microcytic anemia. Electrolytes are normal except for increased serum calcium.

Discussion: In this case the patient presents with the subacute onset of shortness of breath and the physical examination is helpful. The finding of a prolonged expiratory phase in the context of the patient's extensive smoking history is very suggestive of an underlying obstructive lung disease. Also, the unilateral decrease in breath sounds is indicative of a pleural effusion, pneumothorax, or atelectasis. Associated findings on percussion are also helpful. Since dullness to percussion is not a finding in pneumothorax, this patient either has a pleural effusion or atelectasis as the cause of his symptoms. To distinguish between these processes requires that one understand how an effusion and atelectasis affect the position of mediastinal structures. Large effusions tend to push mediastinal structures away, whereas atelectasis tends to pull mediastinal structures toward the pathologic side. Since in this case the patient's trachea is deviated to the right (away from the affected side), this suggests that the cause for the patient's shortness of breath is a large pleural effusion. This patient has a large pleural effusion caused by a carcinoma of the lung. Moreover, a metastatic lesion from this primary tumor was also responsible for the patient's left scapular pain.

CLINICAL PEARL

In this case, associated physical signs and findings on percussion help to delineate causes of decreased breath sounds on lung examination.

Case 2

A 55-year-old woman with a history of coronary artery disease, smoking, and diabetes mellitus presents with sudden onset of chest pain and shortness of breath. She states that pain started suddenly after she had finished dinner and at first thought it was heartburn. Over-the-counter antacids have provided no relief. She also admits to nausea, but denies vomiting, fever, or chills. Shortness of breath started about half an hour later, and steadily progressed. She states it was the shortness of breath which prompted her to come to the hospital.

Physical Examination: Physical examination revealed an obese middle-aged woman. She appeared uncomfortable and was in moderate respiratory distress and using her accessory muscles of respiration. Vital signs were pulse 120 beats/min, respiratory rate 32 breaths/min, blood pressure 118/80 mm Hg, temperature 37.2°C, and oxygen saturation 90% on room air. Neck exam revealed an elevated jugular venous pressure. Lung exam revealed bilateral crackles two thirds of the way up the chest with bilateral wheezing. A faint II/VI systolic ejection murmur was heard on the cardiac exam. The abdominal exam demonstrated mild tenderness without rebound or guarding. Trace lower extremity edema was also noted.

Laboratory data revealed a white blood count of 10,000/mm³ with no left shift. Initial cardiac enzymes were normal. Arterial blood gas measurements on room air showed pH 7.46, Pco_2 32 mm Hg, and Po_2 55 mm Hg. ECG showed sinus tachycardia with ST elevations in II, III, aVF, lead I, and aVL.

Discussion: In this case the history suggests that the patient is experiencing a myocardial infarction. Although the patient does not have classic chest pain, it is well established that women and diabetics can commonly present with atypical symptoms. In this case, the ECG confirms the diagnosis of inferolateral myocardial infarction. The management of patients during a myocardial infarction focuses on increasing the oxygen supply and decreasing the oxygen demand of the heart. Despite these goals, the information gathered during the lung exam can provide valuable insight that aids in the management of the patient. For example, in our patient we detect crackles and wheezes, findings consistent with pulmonary edema secondary to myocardial pump failure. These findings direct us immediately to use diuretics along with supplemental oxygen in the care of this hypoxic patient. Although the pathogenesis of wheezes in pulmonary edema is not clear, it likely results from an increase in peribronchial fluid, which causes airway compression. Finally, crackles in patients with myocardial infarction also have important prognostic value. The extent of crackles (base to apex) within the lung directly correlates with the severity of myocardial injury and portends a worse outcome for the patient.

CLINICAL PEARL

Physical signs on lung examination are helpful diagnostically and for follow-up of the patient's clinical condition. The extent of crackles may correlate with the severity of disease.

KEY CONCEPTS

Recognizing the pathophysiology of abnormal lung sounds assists the clinician to focus on the underlying pathogenesis of the disease process and direct its management.

Coupled with a comprehensive history, auscultation of breath sounds forms an important part of lung examination. It helps to initiate the evaluation of a respiratory problem and provides clues of a change in the clinical condition of a patient.

 STUDY QUESTIONS

5-1.   Which of the following diseases are characterized by wheezes heard during inspiration?
  a. congestive heart failure
  b. asthma
  c. tracheal stenosis
  d. right main stem obstruction by tumor
  e. chronic bronchitis

5-2.   A unilateral decrease in the intensity of breath sounds is characteristic of all of the following except
  a. paralyzed diaphragm
  b. empyema

  c. right main stem obstruction

  d. right middle lobe pneumonia

  e. pneumothorax

5–3. All of the following are causes of mid- to late-inspiratory crackles relative to total lung capacity except

  a. asbestosis

  b. idiopathic pulmonary fibrosis

  c. dependent atelectasis

  d. pulmonary edema

  e. bronchiectasis

SUGGESTED READINGS

Bickley LS, Szilagyi PG. *Bates Guide to Physical Examination and History Taking.* 9th ed. Philadelphia: Lippincott Williams & Wilkins; 2007.

Pasterkamp H, Kraman S, Wodicka G. Respiratory sounds, advances beyond the stethoscope. *Am J Respir Crit Care Med.* 1997;156:974–987.

SECTION 2
Disease/Disorder Based

Obstructive Lung Disease   6

David A. Welsh & Dwayne A. Thomas

OBJECTIVES

▶ *Define airway obstruction and understand its pathophysiologic relationship to various disease processes.*

▶ *Review the clinical features of the various diseases that present with airway obstruction.*

GENERAL CONSIDERATIONS

Airway obstruction can be defined as any abnormal reduction in airflow. Resistance to airflow can occur anywhere in the airway from the upper airway to the terminal bronchi and is characteristic of asthma and chronic bronchitis. Although diseases that cause airway obstruction have a common physiologic effect, their pathogenesis and pathophysiologic mechanisms may be quite different. Airflow limitation may also be the result of loss of elastic recoil due to tissue destruction, as seen in emphysema. Despite this distinction in pathogenesis and pathophysiology, the diseases are sometimes difficult to distinguish clinically. This chapter will focus on asthma, chronic obstructive pulmonary disease (COPD)/emphysema, and bronchiectasis with some reference to other causes of obstructive lung disease and emphysema.

ASTHMA

 Asthma is a chronic inflammatory disorder of the airways in which many inflammatory cells play a role, including mast cells, lymphocytes, neutrophils, and eosinophils. This airway inflammation leads to widespread but variable airflow obstruction that is reversible either spontaneously or with treatment. Asthma is also characterized by increased airway responsiveness to various physiologic and environmental stimuli, such as exercise, cold air, dust mites, and animal dander.

More than 5% of children under the age of 18 have experienced an asthma attack. Because of its prevalence, the health care burden of asthma is substantial, both in terms of costs and of morbidity. While overall mortality is low and has been relatively stable over the past several decades, specific populations, such as African Americans, have a much higher risk of poor outcomes. Any mortality attributable to asthma is alarming as this is largely preventable with appropriate therapy.

Etiology & Pathogenesis

Much has been learned through autopsy studies on patients who have died with severe asthma. Common features include not only occlusion of the airway by mucous plugging, but also the presence of inflammatory cells, including neutrophils, eosinophils, and lymphocytes. Smooth muscle hypertrophy and hyperplasia are present, along with denuded airway epithelium and subepithelial thickening.

More recently, the pervasiveness of inflammation has been confirmed in bronchial biopsies from patients with mild asthma. While neutrophils are not predominant in these cases, activated eosinophils, mast cells, and lymphocytes are found variably throughout the tracheobronchial tree. Basement membrane collagen deposition and epithelial injury can also be found.

The cycle of inflammation characteristic of asthma begins with sensitization upon inhalation of an allergen. Dendritic cells, which are antigen-presenting cells, migrate to regional lymph nodes where antigen is introduced to resident T and B lymphocytes. The B cells are induced to begin immunoglobulin E (IgE) production by interleukin-4 (IL-4) and interleukin-13 (IL-13) secreted by the T cells. The IgE can then be bound by IgE receptors on airway mast cells (Figure 6–1).

Upon reexposure, the IgE bound to mast cells complexes with the allergen and activates the cell. Activation is followed by the release of histamine, leukotrienes, and cytokines that mediate the physiologic effects of asthma and perpetuate the inflammation.

Among the cytokines produced, several, notably IL-4, IL-5, and granulocyte macrophage-colony stimulating factor, recruit eosinophils to the lung, prolong their survival, and stimulate production of mediators such as major basic protein (MBP) that can injure the bronchial mucosa, induce bronchospasm, and perpetuate the proinflammatory state.

The mechanisms predisposing certain individuals to develop asthma are unknown. Current evidence supports a paradigm referred to as the "hygiene hypothesis." This theory proposes that environmental exposures early in life dictate the development of immune responses that manifest clinically as allergy and asthma.

Helper CD4⁺ T cells can be subdivided into Th1-type cells, which produce IL-2 and interferon γ and participate in cell-mediated immunity, or Th2-type

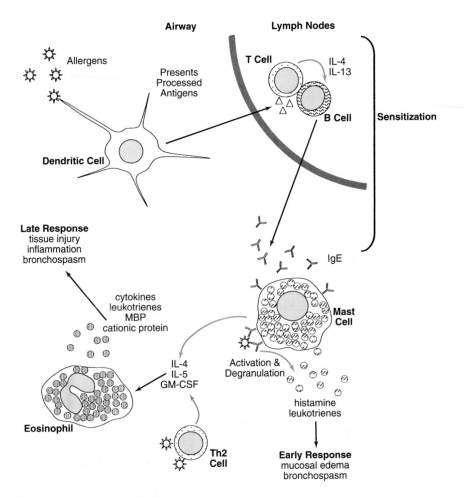

Figure 6–1. Asthma pathogenesis.

cells, which produce IL-4, IL-5, IL-10, and IL-13 and direct allergic inflammation. The hygiene hypothesis suggests that newborns are skewed toward a Th2 phenotype and need early environmental exposures to allow the development of Th1 immunity and to balance the response to future antigen exposure. Both nature and nurture may have a role in the development of asthma. Early life exposure to measles, hepatitis A, infections due to day care contacts, or contact with older siblings, and even in utero presentation of antigens may induce the Th2 → Th1 shift, but the magnitude of the shift is likely influenced by genetic factors.

The hereditary aspects of asthma are complex, with over a hundred genes implicated in various studies. Although atopy plays a major role, not all patients demonstrate that clinical phenotype. The presence of rhinitis with or without positive skin tests is associated with a substantial increase in asthma symptoms.

Pathophysiology

Acute allergic asthma has classically been divided into early and late phases. Within minutes of reexposure to a trigger, receptor activation on mast cells induces degranulation and release of histamine, leukotrienes, and other bronchoconstrictors. Smooth muscle contraction and mucosal edema cause the airway obstruction that is responsible for symptomatic asthma. This phase usually resolves within an hour.

A second peak in symptoms, beginning 4–6 hours after exposure and lasting up to 24 hours, characterizes the late response. The symptoms are often more severe. Eosinophil-mediated inflammatory damage is primarily responsible, but other cell types can be involved.

Acute bronchoconstriction and airway edema, along with mucus plug formation, are responsible for increased resistance to airflow. There is narrowing of almost all airways, but small bronchi 2–5 mm in diameter are most affected. Functional residual capacity (FRC) often increases because expiratory times are prolonged and increased inspiratory effort reduces pleural pressure. The increase in FRC places the muscles of respiration at a mechanical disadvantage. These factors increase the work of breathing during an acute attack.

Because of the inhomogeneity of the obstruction, ventilation-perfusion mismatch occurs, compromising gas exchange. In contrast to COPD, asthmatics vigorously compensate for this by hyperventilation. Therefore, although mild to moderate hypoxemia is common, most patients are hypocapnic during exacerbations. The development of hypercapnia signals impending respiratory arrest. With treatment, symptoms can resolve quickly, but abnormalities in pulmonary physiology often persist for weeks.

Despite the episodic nature of the disease with normal spirometry between attacks, asthmatics do not have normal airways between exacerbations. Inflammation can be found even while asymptomatic, and the airways are hyperresponsive to bronchoconstrictor challenge with histamine or methacholine.

It is becoming increasingly clear that unchecked inflammation in asthma has long-term consequences. The chronic inflammatory state leads to deposition of connective tissue and marked basement membrane thickening can occur. This then leads to irreversible airway obstruction and remodeling of airways. An accelerated decline in lung function has been observed in asthma patients, which may be aggravated by tobacco smoking, that can result in clinical and pathophysiologic features similar to COPD.

Diagnostic & Clinical Considerations

Extrinsic, or allergic, asthma usually starts in childhood, and patients have elevated serum IgE levels and positive skin-prick test results for common inhalant allergens. Intrinsic, or nonallergic, asthma typically is of later onset, and patients have negative skin test results for common allergens. Asthma symptoms are variable and tend to follow a circadian rhythm, with the greatest airway narrowing between the hours of 3 and 5 am in the majority of patients.

Triggers of asthma include a host of factors. These include antigens secreted by house dust mites, pollen (eg, grass, ragweed, and tree), molds, exercise, cold air, air pollution (eg, sulfur dioxide), perfumes, upper respiratory tract infections (particularly viral), and drugs (eg, β-blockers and aspirin). This list is not exhaustive and only gives examples of some of the known triggers. The initial evaluation should always include a detailed history regarding potential triggers.

Typical asthma symptoms include wheezing that is most noticeable on expiration; dyspnea, along with a sensation of chest tightness; and cough secondary to increased airway sensitivity. Cough may actually be the presenting symptom in some patients, particularly children.

The findings on physical examination vary depending on the severity of the episode, but are absent between episodes of asthma. Wheezing is usually heard near the end of expiration in mild asthma, but is present throughout the entire respiratory cycle when the episode is severe (see Chapter 5). The absence of respiratory sounds is indicative of impending respiratory failure and collapse. The respiratory rate is increased, and there is an interruption of speech, as well as the use of accessory muscles of respiration. Tachycardia (higher than 110 beats/min) and *pulsus paradoxus* (greater than 10 mm Hg difference in blood pressure during inspiration and expiration) are physical findings associated with a severe, acute asthma flare.

The spirometric changes in obstructive airways disease demonstrate a reduction in the forced expiratory volume in the first second (FEV_1) with a low ratio of the FEV_1 to the forced vital capacity (FEV_1:FVC) (Figure 6–2). However, obstructive physiology is not unique to asthma. Additional supportive evidence of asthma is the reversibility of airflow obstruction demonstrated by a 12% improvement with an absolute increase of 200 mL in the FEV_1 after inhalation of a bronchodilator. Complete reversal is expected but not always seen in patients with more severe disease.

Measurement of the peak expiratory flow (PEF) rate is another simple way to assess airflow variability. Its diurnal variation is approximately 15%, it can be measured

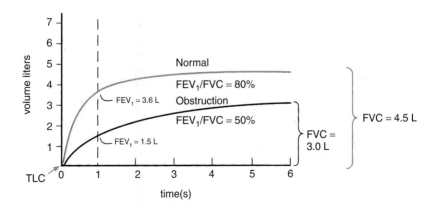

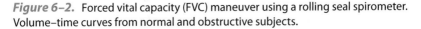

Figure 6–2. Forced vital capacity (FVC) maneuver using a rolling seal spirometer. Volume–time curves from normal and obstructive subjects.

simply and easily at home, and it may aid in assessing the response to therapy. If confusion remains, a methacholine challenge test can be conducted to determine the degree of airway hyperresponsiveness. The concentration of methacholine required to cause a 20% decline in the FEV_1 (PC_{20}) is recorded, and if it is less than 4 mg/mL, the result is considered positive (a PC_{20} of 4–16 mg/mL is considered borderline).

A diagnosis of asthma may be established by the history of recurrent symptoms, reversible airflow obstruction on spirometry, and the exclusion of other diagnoses.

Management Principles

With appropriate asthma management, the disease can usually be controlled. Asthma must first be viewed as a chronic inflammatory disease, and therefore controlling airway inflammation must be emphasized. The goal is to control the disease so that the patient can function normally. Therapy should be guided by the severity of disease and should include education so the patient may become an active participant in the management of his or her disease. Poorly controlled asthma should be viewed as a failure of therapy, and a change in the treatment plan is warranted. This approach is more important now that chronic inflammation is believed to lead to a progressive decline in airway function.

The recommended pharmacologic therapy for asthma control revolves around a stepwise approach; treatment should be instituted at an intensity expected to control symptoms and then reassessed frequently and modified up or down in a stepwise fashion. If asthma symptoms are intermittent and mild, a short-acting β-agonist on an as-needed basis is all that is typically necessary. Low-dose inhaled corticosteroids should be instituted if asthma symptoms are mild but persistent. Moderate, persistent asthma usually requires the addition of a long-acting inhaled β-agonist bronchodilator. Combination therapy has been found to be more effective than increasing the dose of inhaled steroid. Severe, persistent asthma may necessitate the use of higher inhaled corticosteroid doses, leukotriene inhibitors, theophylline, or even oral steroids. It must be emphasized that *scheduled* short-acting β-agonists or long-acting β-agonists *without* concomitant corticosteroids should be avoided as some studies have found an increase in mortality with their use.

Central to the treatment of asthma is trigger avoidance. Short-term triggers, such as exercise and cold air exposure, need not be avoided because they are not believed to alter airway inflammation. Therapy should be maximized so that symptoms are controlled with exercise and airway cooling. It is more important to avoid triggers that lead to chronic airway inflammation, such as dust mites and household pets, since exposure to these triggers can lead to permanent airway changes if inflammation is not adequately controlled. Exposure to known triggers should be controlled more effectively so they no longer cause symptoms.

Patients with known triggers confirmed by allergen testing may be candidates for immunotherapy. Allergen immunotherapy is recommended only for asthmatics who have had a specific allergen identified and have persistent symptoms despite appropriate therapy. Asthmatics with poorly controlled disease may benefit from monoclonal anti-IgE antibody omalizumab trial.

With severe symptoms or acute flares, rapid control can be achieved with systemic steroids. Antibiotics are ineffective except when used for comorbid conditions like bacterial pneumonia or purulent bronchitis. Common reasons for failing to control symptoms include poor compliance or inhaler technique and persistent environmental triggers.

CHRONIC OBSTRUCTIVE PULMONARY DISEASE

COPD is the fourth leading cause of mortality in the United States, and the number of affected individuals is projected to increase worldwide in the future. The Global Initiative for Chronic Obstructive Lung Disease (GOLD) defines COPD as "a disease state characterized by airflow limitation that is not fully reversible. The airflow limitation is usually progressive and associated with an abnormal inflammatory response of the lungs to noxious particles or gases."

Etiology & Pathogenesis

Although COPD was frequently subdivided into chronic bronchitis and emphysema in the past, it is now recognized that most patients have elements of both conditions. Chronic bronchitis, which is defined clinically as cough with sputum production for 3 months a year for 2 consecutive years, is associated with hypertrophy of mucus glands and increased number of goblet cells in the more central airways and peribronchiolar fibrosis in the more peripheral airways. Emphysema is the destruction of alveolar walls and airspace enlargement without significant fibrosis (see Table 6–1 for a description of the subtypes of emphysema).

The injury pathways leading to these changes are incompletely understood and likely multifactorial. Cigarette smoke or air pollutants initiate inflammatory cell infiltration of the respiratory epithelium which is composed of macrophages, neutrophils, and CD8[+] lymphocytes (Figure 6–3). Eosinophils are absent except during acute bronchitis exacerbations, and the intensity of the inflammatory response

Table 6–1. Emphysema pathological subtypes

Centriacinar
 This is the most common subtype and is associated with long-term cigarette smoking. There is a predilection for the upper lung zones with disease beginning in the respiratory bronchioles and extending peripherally. Focal disease is seen in coal workers' pneumoconiosis.
Panacinar
 The entire alveolar unit is uniformly affected in this subtype. The lower lobes are predominantly involved. This subtype is most commonly seen with α-1 antitrypsin deficiency and some inherited connective tissue disorders, but is also found in advanced smoking-related emphysema.
Distal acinar
 The distal structures, alveolar ducts, and sacs are involved here. Apical subpleural blebs are common and may cause spontaneous pneumothorax. The typical patient is a tall, slender, young male. Airflow can sometimes be well preserved in this form of emphysema. This type may be seen in HIV infection or with substance abuse.

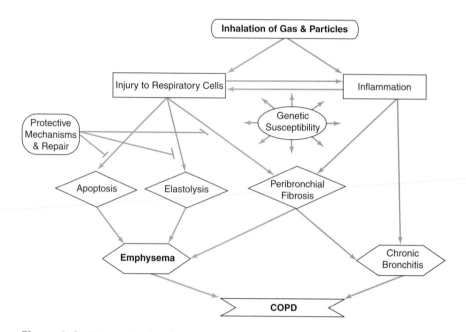

Figure 6–3. Schematic of pathogenesis of chronic obstructive pulmonary disease (COPD).

is much lower than in asthma. There is significant interindividual variability in the response to the inhalants. First-degree relatives of COPD patients are more likely to have airflow obstruction suggesting a genetic predisposition. Indeed, polymorphisms in the tumor necrosis factor and heme oxygenase-1 genes have been associated with an increased risk of COPD.

Generation of proteases, reactive oxygen species, and other toxic substances by the inflammatory cells may then degrade the connective tissue substratum of the lung. In the peripheral airways, the response to injury includes collagen deposition and scar formation. This is different than in the alveolar space. Here destruction of elastin fibers along with epithelial and endothelial cell apoptosis leads to loss of the alveolar walls without scar formation. Thus, abnormal repair mechanisms are a likely component of COPD pathogenesis.

An imbalance between proteases and counterbalancing antiproteases has long been thought to be central to the development of emphysema. This is supported by the ability to produce emphysema in animal models by the instillation of elastase and by the observation that individuals who are deficient in α_1-antitrypsin suffer from premature-onset emphysema. α_1-Antitrypsin is a serum protein produced by the liver that is responsible for the inhibition of neutrophil elastase. The inability to convincingly demonstrate an imbalance between proteases and antiproteases in the lungs of most other patients with COPD has raised questions about this hypothesis. However, quantum proteolysis may be occurring on a level that we are currently unable to measure in these patients.

Pulmonary vascular changes are evident in progressive COPD. The loss of the pulmonary capillary bed correlates with the loss of alveolar surface area in emphysema. Hypoxic pulmonary vasoconstriction resulting in intimal thickening, smooth muscle cell hypertrophy, and connective tissue formation further contributes to the development of pulmonary artery hypertension and right heart failure. This condition is known as *cor pulmonale.*

Pathophysiology

Mucus hypersecretion and ciliary dysfunction lead to a productive chronic cough that is often the first sign of disease. Pooling and inspissation of mucus can lead to airway obstruction, especially during acute exacerbations.

Along with airway secretions, several other mechanisms are thought to contribute to the development of airflow obstruction in COPD. Peribronchiolar fibrosis creates a fixed obstruction in the smaller airways. Mucosal edema due to inflammatory infiltration worsens the obstruction by encroachment on the lumen. All airways exhibit some degree of smooth muscle tone which, because of the already narrowed diameter, may be a factor in obstruction.

The alveolar wall destruction central to emphysema is also important in the development of airflow limitation. Alveolar septae adjacent to bronchioles serve to tether the airway open. As lung parenchyma is lost, the elastic recoil of the lung diminishes and the forces keeping the airway open are compromised. This is especially evident during expiration as lung volumes get smaller and airway tethering is reduced even in the nondiseased state.

Resistance to airflow alone cannot fully explain the exercise limitation that invariably accompanies advanced COPD. In fact, dyspnea and exercise capacity correlate poorly with FEV_1. A much stronger correlation exists with the extent of lung destruction as assessed by computed tomography (CT) or diffusion capacity.

The airway obstruction does, however, indirectly impact exercise capacity. Obstruction becomes more pronounced during exhalation as lung volume and elastic recoil diminish. When severe, patients may be unable to completely expel their tidal volume before the next breath. This "breath stacking" increases the FRC and reduces the inspiratory capacity. Rapid respiratory rates and increased tidal volumes during exercise exacerbate the problem. This is known as *dynamic hyperinflation.*

The pathophysiology of COPD extends beyond the lung. The lung disease is associated with circulation of a variety of potentially detrimental mediators. Combined with the frequent occurrence of hypoxia, deconditioning, and malnutrition, these substances result in a systemic disease process characterized by hypermetabolism, myopathy of skeletal muscle, and psychiatric disturbances, along with cardiovascular and renal disease.

Diagnostic & Clinical Considerations

The symptoms attributable to COPD only become evident after a prolonged period with progressive loss of pulmonary function or after being unmasked by an acute exacerbation. This is because of the enormous physiologic reserve of the respiratory system. In order to identify affected individuals earlier, the National Lung Health Education Program recommends spirometry for all current or former smokers ≥45 years old or anyone with chronic cough, dyspnea, or wheezing.

Tobacco smoking accounts for 80%–90% of the risk of developing COPD and is therefore considered its primary cause. However, for reasons that are unclear, only approximately 15% of cigarette smokers develop clinically significant COPD. α_1-Antitrypsin deficiency, an inherited disease, accounts for approximately 1% of the cases of COPD. Testing should be performed for those with premature-onset emphysema, in those with COPD without recognizable risk factors, and siblings of an affected individual.

Environmental pollution is now recognized to account for a significant percentage of COPD cases worldwide. In addition to considering urban air quality, an evaluation for potential occupational exposure to dusts and chemicals is also warranted.

Human immunodeficiency virus (HIV) infection accelerates the development of emphysema in patients who also smoke. Individuals who present with a premature onset of COPD should be considered for HIV testing.

The most common presenting symptoms are shortness of breath with or without wheezing, cough, and mucus production. Symptoms are initially episodic, and acute exacerbations are characterized by an increase in sputum production and purulence. The presence of wheezing is not critical to the diagnosis, and the sputum need not be purulent.

As the disease progresses, there is an increase in the frequency of exacerbations, which include an increased cough, hypoxemia, purulent sputum, and dyspnea. With severe disease, chronic hypoxemia and hypercapnia may also be present. These conditions may lead to erythrocytosis, morning headaches (from the hypercapnia), cor pulmonale, lower extremity edema, and weight loss secondary to increased work of breathing.

The abnormal findings upon physical examination of the chest are a direct result of airway obstruction and air trapping. Decreased breath sounds, prolonged expiration, wheezing, and distant heart sounds are all common findings in COPD patients. If the disease is particularly severe, the patient may use accessory muscles of respiration and pursed lip breathing to improve respiratory efficiency. Cyanosis may also be present.

The chest x-ray reveals evidence of hyperinflation with flattening of the diaphragms, elongation of the cardiac silhouette, and an increased retrosternal air space (Figure 6–4). If present, bullae appear as radiolucent areas of various sizes surrounded by thin, hairline shadows.

Pulmonary function tests are necessary for diagnosis and assessment of the severity of disease. The diagnosis of COPD requires a postbronchodilator FEV_1:FVC ratio <70%. The FEV_1 is a measure of the severity of airflow obstruction, and normal values are based on the patient's age, race, sex, height, and weight. The GOLD criteria for COPD staging are presented in Table 6–2.

FEV_1 normally decreases approximately 20–30 mL per year with age. This decrease is accelerated in smokers and appears to be related to the degree of

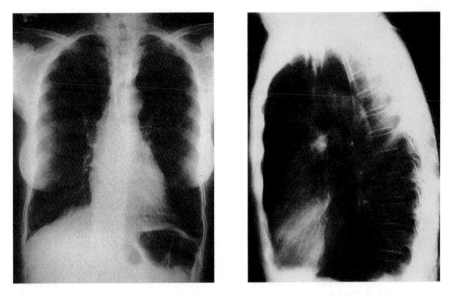

Figure 6–4. Chest x-ray revealing hyperinflation in the posteroanterior view with flattening of the diaphragms most evident on the lateral film. Note the elongation of the cardiac silhouette and the increased retrosternal air space on the lateral film.

Table 6–2. GOLD COPD staging criteria

Stage	Symptoms	Spirometry
Stage 0 (At risk)	Chronic cough, sputum	Normal $FEV_1/FVC \geq 70\%$ $FEV_1 \geq 80\%$
Stage 1 (Mild)	With or without cough, sputum, dyspnea	$FEV_1/FVC < 70\%$ $FEV_1 \geq 80\%$
Stage 2 (Moderate)	With or without cough, sputum, dyspnea	$FEV_1/FVC < 70\%$ $50\% \geq FEV_1 < 80\%$
Stage 3 (Severe)	With or without cough, sputum, dyspnea	$FEV_1/FVC < 70\%$ $30\% \geq FEV_1 < 50\%$
Stage 4 (Very severe)	With or without cough, sputum, dyspnea	$FEV_1/FVC < 70\%$ $FEV_1 < 30\%$ or $FEV_1 < 50\% + PaO_2 \leq 60$ or $PaCO_2 \geq 50$ mm Hg

cigarette consumption. With smoking cessation, only a small amount of lung function returns, typically less than 75 mL, but the rate of decline slows to a rate similar to that of nonsmokers (Figure 6–5).

Lung volumes can show an increase in the total lung capacity, FRC, and residual volume, indicating air trapping (Figure 6–6). The single-breath diffusion capacity, a measure of gas transfer across the alveolar membrane, is decreased

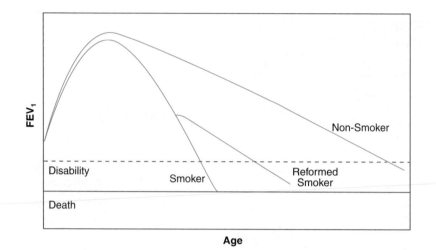

Figure 6–5. Impact of smoking on lung function over time. All people lose function with aging beyond ~25 years of age, but do not become symptomatic until very late in life. Susceptible smokers lose lung function at a variable but accelerated rate. Smoking cessation returns the individual nearly to the normal rate of decline, postponing disability and death. (Adapted from Fletcher C, Peto R: The natural history of chronic airflow obstruction. *Br Med J.* 1977;1:1645–1648.)

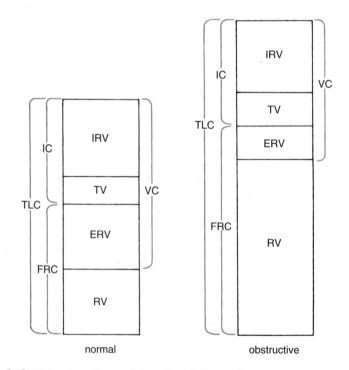

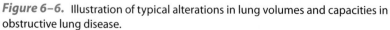

Figure 6–6. Illustration of typical alterations in lung volumes and capacities in obstructive lung disease.

in proportion to the severity of disease. It is reduced as a result of the loss of the alveolar capillary bed and a reduction in effective alveolar surface area for diffusion. Hypoxemia develops as the disease progresses, and hypercapnia increases in frequency with an FEV_1 of less than 1 L.

A variable number of patients with COPD will have a significant increase in the FEV_1 (12%, with a minimum change of 200 mL) in response to an inhaled β-agonist. As many as 60% of COPD patients will respond when tested on multiple occasions. The absence of a response on any single test should not prevent the use of an inhaled bronchodilator.

Management Principles

Smoking cessation is key to successful management if the patient is still smoking. Abstinence can decrease mucus production, reverse small airway changes, and reduce the annual rate of decline in the FEV_1. Even brief reminders by the physician will increase quit rates. Pharmacologic support including nicotine replacement and bupropion, an aminoketone antidepressant, has been shown to be an effective adjuvant.

Annual influenza vaccination is also indicated for all patients. This can reduce morbidity and mortality by ~50% in COPD patients. The pneumococcal vaccine should probably also be given every 5 years, although strong evidence in support of this is lacking.

The majority of therapy for COPD is symptom directed. Treatment is initiated with bronchodilators. Both β-agonists and anticholinergics are effective in reducing dyspnea, increasing exercise capacity, and improving quality of life. Inhaled short-acting agents such as albuterol and ipratropium bromide are usually begun first for mild and variable symptoms. Long-acting agents such as salmeterol and/ or tiotropium may be added for persistent symptoms. Systemic bronchodilator therapy should be avoided as effective inhaled therapy is available.

Pulmonary rehabilitation should be undertaken for patients who remain limited in their activities of daily living. Successful programs are multidimensional and include cardiovascular exercise, training muscles of respiration, nutritional support, instruction on optimal inhaler technique, and education about the disease and its management. Rehabilitation does not change the airflow limitation, but has been shown to increase exercise capacity and quality of life and reduce hospitalizations.

Inhaled corticosteroids may reduce exacerbations and improve quality of life, but only in those with moderately severe disease. Their use in COPD is much more controversial than their use in asthma. There is no role for the chronic administration of systemic steroids in COPD.

Several studies have demonstrated the beneficial effects of long-term oxygen therapy. Its appropriate use has been shown to reduce morbidity and prolong the survival of hypoxemic patients with severe COPD. Some of its most important effects have been the alleviation of cor pulmonale, improved cardiac function, and improved exercise performance. At least 16 hours of continuous oxygen supplementation daily is required to impact survival.

Surgical options including bullectomy, lung volume reduction surgery, and lung transplant may be useful in highly selected patients. α_1-Antitrypsin replacement therapy should be reserved for individuals with hereditary deficiency and a marked reduction in circulating levels.

The treatment of acute exacerbations differs from that for chronic disease, which is described above. Antibiotics improve outcomes if ≥1 of the following symptoms are present: increased dyspnea, increased sputum production, or increased sputum purulence. Systemic steroids hasten recovery and reduce relapse rates, but should not be used for longer than 2 weeks because of an increased incidence of adverse effects. Noninvasive positive pressure ventilation (ie, mechanical ventilation applied via a face mask) is indicated for patients with respiratory failure associated with exacerbations.

BRONCHIECTASIS

Bronchiectasis is defined as an abnormal permanent dilation of bronchi. The definition has recently been modified to include the clinical description of chronic daily production of mucopurulent sputum. First described by Laënnec in 1819, bronchiectasis is an uncommon condition whose prevalence has declined coincident with improvements in health care.

Etiology & Pathogenesis

Although a definitive etiology is commonly not identified, the destruction of the muscular and supporting tissue of the bronchial and bronchiolar walls that characterizes bronchiectasis is usually the end result of another underlying pathologic condition. Clinical entities associated with bronchiectasis are summarized in Table 6–3.

Childhood immunization against respiratory pathogens has dramatically reduced the incidence of bronchiectasis in developed nations; however, infection is still the major etiology of bronchiectasis in older individuals and in underserved areas. Necrotizing pneumonias, tuberculosis, pertussis, and HIV infection are common culprits.

Several congenital or inherited conditions also lead to bronchiectasis, including primary ciliary dyskinesia. In this condition, alterations in the structure of the cilia make them immotile, inhibiting the mucociliary clearance of bacteria and promoting the development of chronic sinusitis and bronchiectasis. A subset of this disease is Kartagener's syndrome, in which situs inversus is present in addition to bronchiectasis and sinusitis. Cystic fibrosis accounts for nearly half of all cases of bronchiectasis in children and young adults.

Other less common causes include interlobar sequestration, bronchial obstruction, central bronchiectasis associated with allergic bronchopulmonary aspergillosis, and Young's syndrome (chronic sinopulmonary infection and azoospermia).

Pathophysiology

Bronchiectasis is often categorized by the appearance of the airway (cylindrical or tubular, varicose, or saccular). However, this anatomic classification does not

Table 6–3. Conditions associated with bronchiectasis

Infection
  Necrotizing pneumonia (eg, *Staphylococcus aureus*)
  Tuberculosis
  Mycobacterium avium (eg, Lady Windermere syndrome)
  Childhood infections (eg, pertussis, measles)

Immune deficiency
  Hypogammaglobulinemia
  Chronic granulomatous disease
  Human immunodeficiency virus infection
  Posttransplantation

Inflammatory
  Inflammatory bowel disease (eg, Crohn's disease, ulcerative colitis)
  Rheumatoid arthritis
  Sjögren's syndrome
  Systemic lupus erythematosus
  Allergic bronchopulmonary aspergillosis

Injury
  Inhalation (eg, chlorine)
  Aspiration pneumonitis

Anatomic
  Endobronchial obstruction (eg, tumor, foreign body)
  Extrinsic compression (eg, lymphadenopathy)
  Tracheobronchomegaly
  Middle lobe syndrome

Congenital
  Cystic fibrosis
  Yellow nail syndrome
  α-1 Antitrypsin deficiency
  Pulmonary intralobar sequestration
  Marfan's syndrome
  Ciliary dyskinesia syndromes (eg, Kartagener's, primary ciliary dyskinesia)

---

appear to correlate with either the etiology or the clinical characteristics of the disorder.

It may be more useful to subdivide bronchiectasis into focal and diffuse disease. A common cause of focal disease appears to be bronchial obstruction. It interferes with bronchial mucus clearance, which can lead to infection, inflammation, and tissue destruction. The bronchial obstruction may be due to an intraluminal process such as a tumor or aspirated foreign body, extraluminal compression, or torsion. Diffuse bronchiectasis can represent the progression of recurrent infection in an area of focal disease or can be the result of multilobar pneumonia or a systemic disorder.

Although the pathogenesis varies according to the predisposing condition, infection is a key component of all of these conditions. Proteolytic enzymes secreted by polymorphonuclear leukocytes directly destroy tissue. Purulent secretions are also believed to contain enzymes (collagenases and elastases) that may also contribute to tissue destruction. Once tissue is destroyed, the process is irreversible. Recurrent infection and perpetuation of an inflammatory state by cytokine overexpression causes clinical exacerbations and progressive disease.

Airway destruction and inflammation most often leads to obstructive physiology; however, the parenchymal injury can also produce a restrictive lung defect.

Diagnostic & Clinical Considerations

Cough and sputum production (usually purulent) occurs in 90% of all patients with bronchiectasis. Recurrent infections are common and are associated with wheezing, cough, fever, weight loss, and hemoptysis. Sputum volumes are usually large, and in some cases may be more than 500 mL/d. However, such volumes are less common now that antibiotic therapy is regularly prescribed.

On physical examination, persistent crackles that begin early in inspiration are present over the affected segments. Diffuse rhonchi and wheezing can be auscultated. With extensive disease breath sounds are decreased with dullness to percussion. If the destruction is widespread and the patient is hypoxemic, digital clubbing and cor pulmonale may also be present.

Bronchiectasis should be suspected in anyone with a chronic cough productive of purulent sputum, but the diagnosis is based on the demonstration of anatomic alterations in the bronchial tree. In the early phases, the chest x-ray may be normal. Signs of bronchiectasis on a plain chest x-ray include tubular shadows called "tram tracks," which are the result of thickened bronchial walls, fibrosis, and localized alveolar destruction or collapse.

High-resolution computed tomography (HRCT) scans have replaced bronchographic studies as the gold standard for diagnosis since they provide adequate definition of the airways. Diagnostic findings include nontapering airways and airways ending with dilations. The pathognomonic finding on HRCT is the *signet ring sign* in which the bronchial diameter is ≥1.5× larger than the accompanying vessel in cross-section (Figure 6–7). Pulmonary function tests usually show airway obstruction and air trapping because of the premature closing of the bronchi. The FVC, FEV_1, and FEV_1:FVC are reduced, and the residual volume is increased. Patients commonly are responsive to bronchodilators and have an abnormal methacholine challenge test.

Management Principles

Although intervention for bronchiectasis is not as well studied as interventions for asthma or COPD, identifying and treating acute exacerbations, reducing chronic bacterial colonization and inflammation, controlling bronchial hemorrhage, and treating the underlying predisposing conditions are the mainstays of bronchiectasis care.

Patients are often chronically colonized with bacteria such as *Haemophilus influenzae, Pseudomonas aeruginosa, Streptococcus pneumoniae,* and *Branhamella catarrhalis.* Bronchial hygiene and scheduled intermittent oral or inhaled antibiotics have been shown to decrease microbial burdens in some patients. These

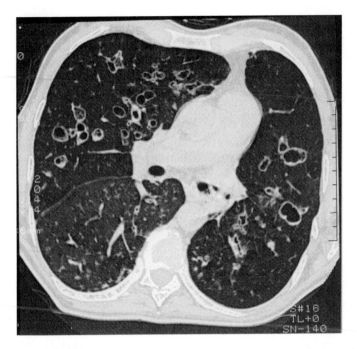

Figure 6–7. Computed tomographic scan showing bronchiectasis with signet ring sign.

measures, as well as inhaled corticosteroids, may reduce airway inflammation and destruction and may also limit the progression of disease.

Obviously management of the specific underlying condition will depend on the disease process. Examples include monthly immunoglobulin transfusions for those with IgG subclass deficiency and immunomodulatory agents for connective tissue disease. Cystic fibrosis has been found to respond to aerosolized dornase alfa and tobramycin as well as oral anti-inflammatory agents.

If bronchoconstriction is present, the use of an inhaled β-agonist is also appropriate. Smoking cessation and oxygen supplementation are also important. All patients should receive pneumococcal vaccine and an annual flu vaccine.

Evaluation of localized bronchiectasis by bronchoscopy or virtual CT images to rule out an endobronchial cause is warranted. Surgical resection is indicated in only a minority of patients, typically those who have severe localized disease or significant hemoptysis. Hemoptysis is now commonly managed by bronchial artery embolization. Lung transplantation is an option in some patients with end-stage disease.

CLINICAL SCENARIOS

Case 1

A 38-year-old woman under your care with a history of asthma since age 13 is evaluated because of persistent episodes of shortness of breath and wheezing.

These episodes require short-acting β-agonist rescue ~5 times per week and wake her from sleep ~3 times per month. She has recently purchased a cat for her 9-year-old daughter that she refuses to give up. She has been taking her inhaled corticosteroids as prescribed. On physical examination, her blood pressure is 110/70, her respiratory rate is 22 breaths/min, her pulse is 80 beats/min, and her temperature is 37°C (98.6°F). She is 94% saturated by pulse oximetry. She is alert and awake in no obvious respiratory distress. Her lung sounds are clear. The rest of her exam is unremarkable. Spirometric testing reveals an FEV_1 of 90% of predicted.

Discussion: This patient's symptoms would place her in the "mild, persistent" asthma classification, which would dictate initial treatment with low-dose inhaled corticosteroids and an as-needed short-acting β-agonist. However, she is experiencing symptoms *on treatment*. Therefore, advancing to combination therapy with a long-acting β-agonist is indicated. While they are useful, leukotriene inhibitors appear to be less effective than long-acting β-agonists. Combination therapy is superior to higher doses of steroids. Immunotherapy may be useful with continued exposure to a specific allergen, but should be reserved until pharmacologic therapies have been optimized.

CLINICAL PEARL

Based on symptoms, the management of asthma warrants a step-up in combination therapy rather than simply doubling the dose of inhaled corticosteroids. Immunotherapy can be considered when a specific antigen has been identified.

Case 2

A 49-year-old man with a known history of COPD presents to the emergency department with a depressed level of consciousness evolving gradually over the past week. His wife notes that his breathing has become faster and more labored. He quit smoking 10 years ago.

Physical Examination: Upon arrival at the hospital, the patient is noted to be lethargic and tachypneic, with a respiratory rate of approximately 35–40 breaths/min. Rhonchi and tubular breath sounds are heard over the entire left chest. Moderate peripheral edema is noted. Arterial blood gas readings are as follows: pH 7.23, P_{CO_2} 72 mm Hg, and P_{O_2} 38 mm Hg. The chest x-ray reveals hyperinflation without cardiomegaly, pulmonary edema, or infiltrates. The patient is intubated and placed on mechanical ventilation with a respiratory rate and tidal volume set to normalize the P_{CO_2} and P_{O_2}. Within minutes he becomes hypotensive.

Discussion: This patient has (sub)acute on chronic respiratory failure. He likely has an FEV_1 < 1 L and cor pulmonale. His hypercapnia and hypoxia are due to ventilation-perfusion mismatch. Ventilating him to achieve a normal P_{CO_2} and P_{O_2} would require a rapid respiratory rate and/or high tidal volumes. Superimposed on his expiratory airflow obstruction and preexisting gas trapping, this would result in dynamic hyperinflation. Intrathoracic pressure will increase, decreasing the venous return to the right heart and compromising preload, leading to a fall in cardiac output and hypotension.

Myocardial infarction, acute bronchospasm, and pulmonary embolus are within the differential diagnosis, but are less likely to coincide with the initiation of positive pressure ventilation. This patient's disease was due to α_1-antitrypsin deficiency. While the majority of COPD is smoking related, it is important to remember that there are other causes.

CLINICAL PEARL

While mechanical ventilation may be needed to treat respiratory failure, it is often associated with secondary effects such as decreased venous return and decreased cardiac output.

KEY CONCEPTS

   Although characterized clinically by episodic symptoms and bronchospasm, asthma is primarily an inflammatory disease of the airway.

   COPD is chronic obstruction to airflow that is only partially reversible. In addition to the resistance to airflow, obstructive lung disease may increase work of breathing through increases in FRC which limit inspiratory capacity.

The abnormal, permanent bronchial dilation that defines bronchiectasis is the end result of a variety of insults and injuries to the airway wall.

STUDY QUESTIONS

6–1. Eosinophils are present in the airways of patients with
   a. asthma
   b. COPD
   c. asthma and COPD
   d. bronchiectasis
   e. none of the above

6–2. In patients with COPD, which of the following correlate most poorly with exercise capacity and quality of life?
   a. FEV1
   b. inspiratory capacity
   c. diffusing capacity
   d. dyspnea
   e. activity of daily living questionnaires

SUGGESTED READINGS

Barker AF. Medical progress: Bronchiectasis. *N Engl J Med.* 2002;346:1383–1393.

Barnes PJ, Drazen JM, Rennard SI, Thomson NC, eds. *Asthma and COPD: Basic Mechanisms and Clinical Management.* 2nd ed. London: Academic Press; 2002.

Bone RC. Bronchiectasis. In: Bone RC, Dantzker DR, George RB, Matthay RA, Reynolds HY, eds. *Pulmonary and Critical Care Medicine: Obstructive Diseases.* St. Louis: Mosby-Year Book; 1997.

Owens GR. Chronic obstructive pulmonary disease. In: Bone RC, Dantzker DR, George RB, Matthay RA, Reynolds HY, eds. *Pulmonary and Critical Care Medicine: Obstructive Diseases.* St. Louis: Mosby-Year Book; 1997.

Parenchymal Lung Disease

Leonardo Seoane & Carol M. Mason

OBJECTIVES

- ▶ *Understand the physiologic derangements that lead to diffuse parenchymal lung diseases.*
- ▶ *Integrate the pathophysiology of diffuse parenchymal lung diseases to understand clinical disease presentations.*
- ▶ *Understand the therapy and prognosis of diffuse parenchymal lung disease.*

GENERAL CONSIDERATIONS

Definition

Diffuse parenchymal lung diseases (DPLDs) are a heterogeneous group of nonneoplastic disorders resulting from damage to the lung parenchyma by varying patterns of inflammation and fibrosis. These disorders are also known as interstitial lung diseases, but these injuries not only involve the interstitium (the space between the epithelial and endothelial basement membranes), but also the air spaces, peripheral airways, and blood vessels, and therefore DPLD is a more appropriate term. One of the problems of dealing with DPLDs is that the terminology for different histopathologic entities and clinical syndromes has become confusing and is littered with acronyms. For idiopathic fibrosis alone there are more than 20 synonyms. An international multidisciplinary committee has standardized the classification of idiopathic interstitial pneumonias. The terminology put forth by the committee will be used here (Figure 7–1).

Normal Structure & Function

The basic structural unit of the lung is the alveolar-capillary membrane, which is the site of respiratory gas exchange. In the terminal air spaces of the lung, the pulmonary capillaries are closely apposed to the alveolar walls, giving the pulmonary circulation a large surface area where gas exchange can take place. The overall alveolar surface area is approximately $100–140$ m^2, an area at least 50-fold greater than the surface area of the skin. The alveolar-capillary membrane is normally a delicate structure

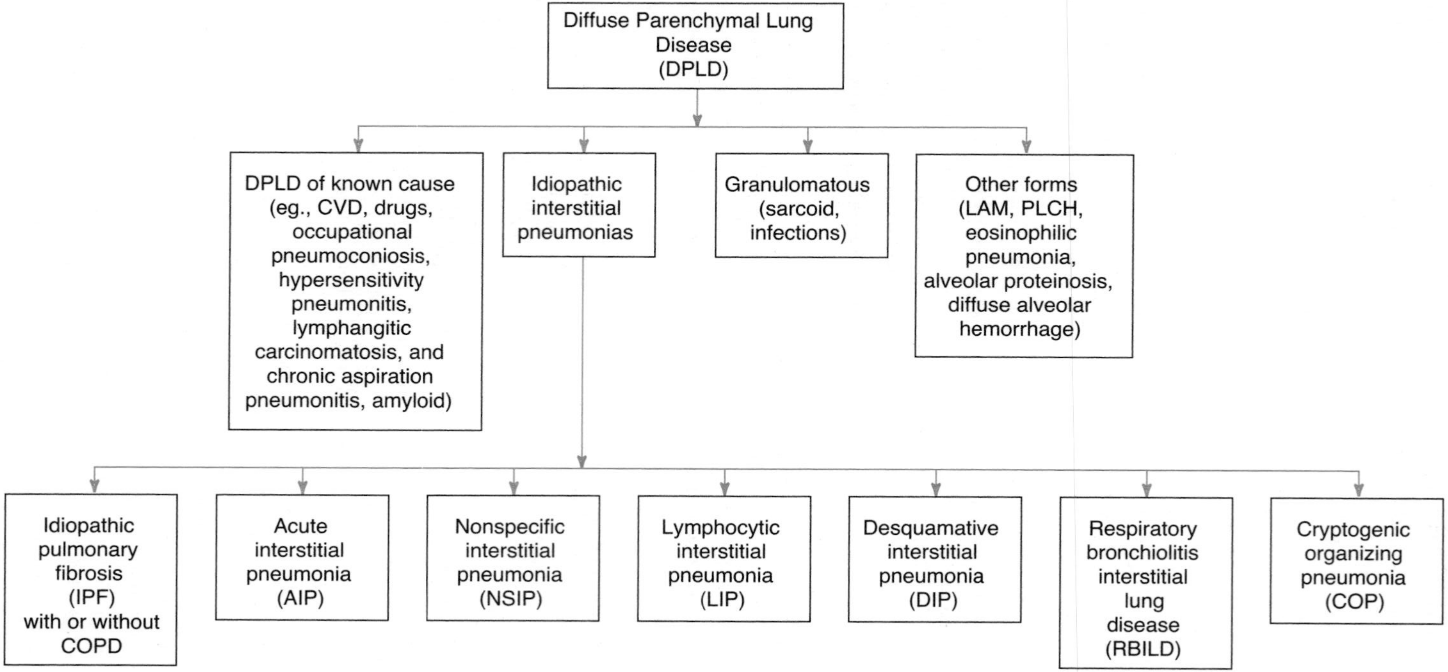

Figure 7–1. Classification of diffuse parenchymal lung diseases (DPLDs). CVD, cardiovascular disease; LAM, lymphangioleiomyomatosis; PLCH, pulmonary Langerhans cell histiocytosis; COPD, chronic obstructive pulmonary disease. (Modified with permission from the American Thoracic Society/European Respiratory Society International Multidisciplinary Consensus Classification of the Idiopathic Interstitial Pneumonias. *Am J Respir Crit Care Med.* 2002;165:277–304.)

composed of the alveolar epithelium (primarily type I alveolar squamous epithelial cells), the epithelial basement membrane, the interstitial stroma, the endothelial basement membrane, and the capillary endothelium. Type I alveolar epithelial cells constitute more than 90% of the alveolar surface area. Also present in the alveolar spaces are type II alveolar epithelial cells, which are the progenitor cells of type I cells during gestation and after several types of lung injuries. Type II pneumocytes reside at the corners of the alveolar septae, and due to their cuboidal shape they constitute only a small portion of the alveolar surface area (less than 10%), although they outnumber the type I cells by two-fold. They are the cells responsible for production and storage of surfactant, which forms a thin layer on the alveolar surface. Thus, for gas exchange to occur, oxygen must diffuse from the alveolar space through the surfactant layer, the epithelial cell, the epithelial basement membrane, the interstitial tissue, the endothelial basement membrane, the endothelial cell, the plasma, and the red blood cell membrane and cytoplasm to reach the molecule of hemoglobin that will bind it for transport. Carbon dioxide follows the pathway in the opposite direction to reach the alveolar space, from which it is exhaled. In the normal lung, the alveolar-capillary unit (ie, a representative alveolar septum) is of the order of 8–12 µm in thickness which, given the rapid rates of diffusion of oxygen and carbon dioxide, does not pose a significant barrier to gas exchange (Figure 7–2). Also present in the alveolar spaces are the resident scavenger cells of the lung, the alveolar macrophages. These cells are mobile phagocytes that roam the alveolar surfaces and represent the initial line of defense against invading pathogens or toxins. If unable to clear the offenders, they are also quite active metabolically and are capable of initiating inflammatory responses to the offending agent.

ETIOLOGY & PATHOGENESIS

Several patterns of lung injury can occur. If the injury is related to a distinct exposure or clinical scenario, such as a severe toxic inhalational exposure or an episode of bacterial septic shock or severe pancreatitis, widespread alveolar damage may result from the inflammatory reaction, with cellular activation and release of inflammatory mediators. The histologic pattern is known as diffuse alveolar damage (DAD). The clinical correlate of this lung injury is the acute respiratory distress syndrome (ARDS), which is characterized by severe respiratory distress. There is extensive endothelial and epithelial destruction, with flooding of the alveolar spaces with inflammatory exudates. This pattern occurs acutely regardless of the cause of the damage. There is disruption of the epithelial layer of type I alveolar pneumocytes, resulting in exposed basement membrane, as well as defects in surfactant function and synthesis (Figure 7–3). With loss of surfactant function, increases in surface tension may result in localized areas of alveolar collapse or atelectasis; these areas may contribute to ventilation-perfusion mismatching and shunt or shunt-like states. Accompanying the destruction of the alveolar-capillary barrier, there is exudation of inflammatory proteinaceous material into the air spaces, with fibrin deposition and the formation of hyaline membranes. Inflammatory cells, including polymorphonuclear leukocytes and mononuclear cells, are recruited (in response to chemotactic agents released during the

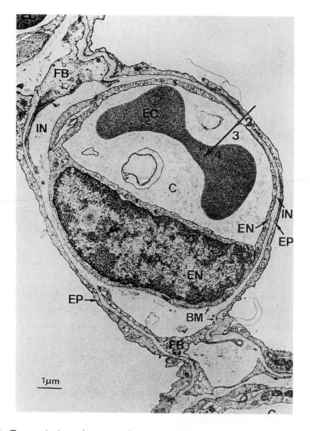

Figure 7–2. Transmission electron photomicrograph of the normal alveolar-capillary structure. Structures shown in this cross-section are the capillary (C) with an endothelial cell (EN, including nucleus), an alveolar epithelial cell (EP), the thin interstitial space (IN), the basement membrane (BM), and fibroblast processes (FB). As oxygen diffuses from the alveolus into the bloodstream, it traverses the alveolar-capillary barrier (2), the plasma (3), and the erythrocyte (4). (Reproduced with permission from Weibel E and *Respiration Physiology*, Vol. 11; Weibel ER. *Morphometric Estimation of Diffusion Capacity*, pp 54–75, 1970/71 with kind permission of Elsevier Science NL, Sara Burgerhartstraat 25, 1055 KV Amsterdam, the Netherlands.)

inflammatory process) into the alveoli within hours of the inciting injury. This process differs from acute bacterial pneumonia, which is characterized by influx of primarily polymorphonuclear leukocytes with a fibrinous exudate and possibly a component of hemorrhage. Necrosis may occur in severe cases. However, acute bacterial infections generally present with sufficiently distinct clinical signs and symptoms that they are not often confused with interstitial pneumonitis.

When acute lung injury results from a well-defined insult that occurs at a specific time, the histologic pattern of the alveolar injury is more homogeneous than would occur if the insult were ongoing or even of a chronic, recurring nature. In the first

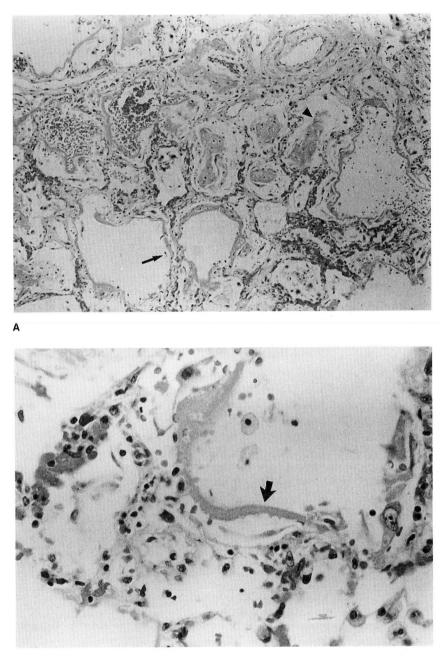

A

B

Figure 7–3. Histopathology of diffuse alveolar damage (DAD). **A.** Low-power view reveals thickening of alveolar septae from edema and inflammatory infiltration (arrow), and alveolar space hemorrhage and fibrin membrane formation (arrowhead). **B.** Higher power view of hyaline membrane (arrow).

instance, a lung biopsy would reveal most of the injury to be in the same stage (initial acute exudative phase or a reparative phase), with relatively less heterogeneity than when the injury is of an ongoing nature. Ongoing injury may occur with the repeated administration of drugs or radiation, which are toxic and provoke the injury. In such a situation, the histopathologic picture is that of acute injury superimposed on various phases of the reparative process. Idiopathic pulmonary fibrosis (IPF) (in which the inciting agent cannot be identified) is characterized by ongoing injury in the setting of the repair process that results in fibrosis and scarring rather than restoration of normal architecture. Recent studies suggest that the fibrotic responses in the lung relate to dysregulated immune or inflammatory responses. Alveoli are lost in this process of ongoing inflammation and scar formation (Figure 7–4). Therefore, the histologic hallmark of IPF is usual interstitial pneumonia (UIP). UIP is characterized by temporal heterogeneity. The histology is a heterogeneous appearance with alternating areas of normal lung, interstitial inflammation, fibrosis, and honeycomb change. Scattered foci of proliferating fibroblasts (fibroblastic foci) are also present. These represent areas of active fibrosis.

DAD and pulmonary fibrosis constitute one response of the lung to injury, but other patterns can occur. Many inciting agents have been described as resulting in a pattern of lung injury known as organizing pneumonia with or without organization within the bronchioles (polypoid bronchiolitis obliterans). This pattern was formerly known as bronchiolitis obliterans with organizing pneumonia. An idiopathic variety has been described as cryptogenic organizing pneumonia (COP). In this injury, the primary site of damage is the bronchiolar epithelium, and the

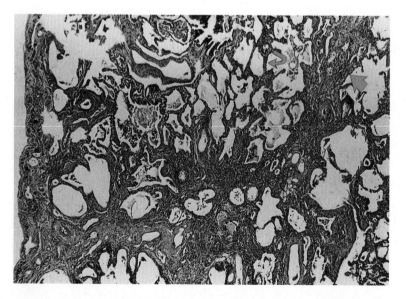

Figure 7–4. Histopathology of idiopathic pulmonary fibrosis (IPF). Features are destruction of alveolar structures and thickened alveolar septae (curved arrow), with inflammatory cell infiltration and fibrosis (large arrow).

injury results in the formation of connective tissue plugs within the terminal bronchioles, which can also extend distally to fill the alveolar ducts (Figure 7–5). Rather patchy in nature, an inflammatory exudate consisting of mononuclear cells in the peribronchiolar areas accompanies the fibrosis that occurs in bronchioles and alveolar ducts. Macrophages in the alveoli adjacent to involved areas may accumulate and take on a foamy appearance, simulating the appearance of lipoid pneumonia. An important feature of organizing pneumonia is that the lesions are all uniform in nature, suggesting that they are temporally homogenous. In order for the diagnosis of organizing pneumonia to be confirmed, it must be the predominant pattern on biopsy with the appropriate clinical presentation. Histologic changes of organizing pneumonia may be seen in the setting of other types of injury, including DAD and IPF. However, for the diagnosis of this distinct entity to be made, it must be the predominant histopathologic pattern.

Another pattern of lung injury is bronchiolitis obliterans, also known as constrictive bronchiolitis. This pattern of injury only involves the bronchioles and is not a true DPLD. Most commonly recognized following organ transplantation (lung, heart-lung, and bone marrow transplantations), constrictive bronchiolitis can also occur as an idiopathic disorder, accompanying collagen vascular diseases, after infections, or as a result of drug or toxin exposure. Bronchiolitis obliterans has been associated with exposure to the artificial butter flavoring Diacetyl among workers in a microwave popcorn plant. Histopathologically, this injury is characterized by peribronchiolar mononuclear cell inflammatory infiltration and concentric fibrosis of the terminal bronchioles (Figure 7–6). If this process is progressive, it leads to narrowing and gradual obstruction at the bronchiolar

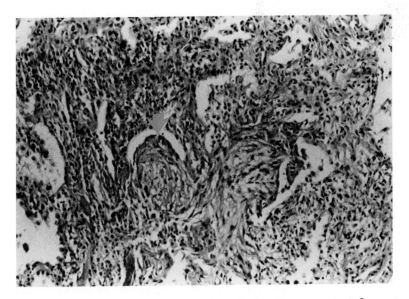

Figure 7–5. Histopathology of proliferative bronchiolitis. Note extensive inflammatory infiltrate and connective tissue plugs filling the lumens of terminal bronchioles (arrow).

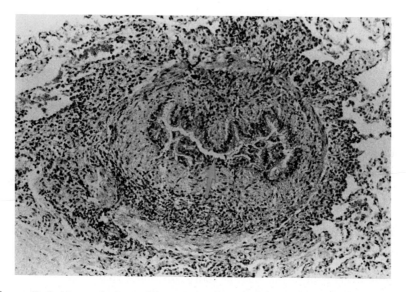

Figure 7–6. Histopathology of constrictive bronchiolitis. High-power view of terminal bronchiole concentrically narrowed with near obliteration of airway lumen (arrow). (Modified and reproduced with permission from Colby TV: Bronchiolar pathology. In: Epler GR, ed. *Diseases of the Bronchioles.* New York, Raven Press, 1994, pp 77–100.)

level. Histopathologic changes are usually limited to the bronchioles, and there is little involvement of the distal parenchyma. Chronically, there may be accompanying bronchiolar dilatation with mucus stasis. Because of the tendency for this disorder to occur in conjunction with organ transplantation, hypotheses of the cause have been developed. Bronchiolar epithelial injury may underlie the process, either due to alloimmune-dependent and/or non-alloimmune mechanisms that result in injury and inflammation of the epithelial cell and subepithelial structures resulting in fibrosis of the small airways. However, the pathophysiology remains uncertain. If the injury is progressive and uninterrupted, excessive fibroproliferation due to ineffective epithelial regeneration and severe small airway obstruction may result, which is often refractory to current therapies.

Another response of the lung to insult is the formation of granulomatous inflammation. While usually seen in the setting of certain infections (eg, tuberculosis or fungal infections), pneumonitis due to hypersensitivity to antigens may also result in the formation of granulomas. In addition, an idiopathic variety known as sarcoidosis may occur. Presumably a reaction to an antigen, recognized or not, this disease is accompanied by widespread granuloma formation (involving lymph nodes, spleen, liver, skin, and/or the eyes). The lung is frequently involved. Granulomatous inflammation characteristically is patchy in distribution and includes components of granulomas and mononuclear cell alveolitis as well as areas of fibrosis. A granuloma is a structure composed of epithelioid cells derived from monocytes and macrophages and is presumably formed by the cell-mediated reaction to an antigen. It has a small nodular center composed of mononuclear cells and fibroblasts with or without necrosis (necrosis is typically not a feature of sarcoidosis, but may accompany infectious causes) (Figure 7–7). Special stains may reveal the presence of organisms within the granuloma in the infectious granulomatous diseases, and tissue culture may result in growth of the organism. In

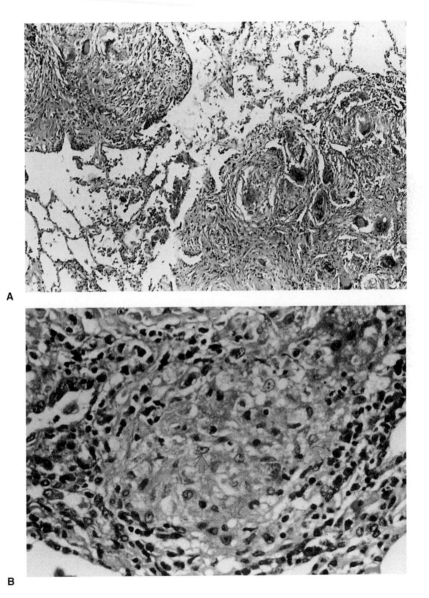

Figure 7–7. Histopathology of granulomatous inflammation due to sarcoidosis. **A.** Low-power view of granuloma formation within the lung parenchyma. Note multinucleated giant cells (arrows). **B.** High-power view of a single granuloma composed of epithelioid cells (arrow) with surrounding mononuclear inflammation (curved arrow).

addition, surrounding epithelioid cells, lymphocytes, and multinucleated giant cells formed by fusion of the epithelioid cells located in the interstitium, but they can be primarily located within the vasculature, as can be seen in several types of vasculitis. Depending on the cause of the disorder, granulomas may resolve or fibrosis may occur via the accumulation of collagen from fibroblasts as the disease activity wanes.

Within the first several days to 1 week after the injury occurs, repair processes are initiated. To repair the damaged alveolar epithelium, type II pneumocytes proliferate and cover the exposed basement membranes where type I pneumocytes have been damaged and lost, and they also form an epithelial layer over fibrin and hyaline membranes. The inflammatory exudate in the alveolar spaces and septae is also infiltrated by fibroblasts. Following fibrinolysis of proteins in the alveolar space, proteoglycans and a new collagenous extracellular matrix are deposited. Initially, there is deposition of fibronectin, an integral component of the intercellular matrix, followed by deposition of type III collagen, type I collagen, and elastin. Accompanying these changes is resorption of exuded proteins, blood, and edema. After lining the alveolar surfaces, the type II pneumocytes differentiate into type I cells as resolution of the injury takes place. Ideally, the end result of the repair process is the restoration of normal alveolar structure and function. However, several outcomes of the repair process may occur: there can be restoration of normal alveolar architecture or overexuberant fibrosis with scarring and loss of the damaged alveolar air spaces. The extent of the original injury and the phenotype of the host may determine whether repair and restoration of normal alveolar architecture occur (more limited injury) or whether fibrosis and destroyed alveolar spaces result (more extensive injury). The outcome may be residual restrictive physiologic changes if injury is mild or respiratory failure and death if the injury is more severe.

PATHOPHYSIOLOGY

Exposure to injurious agents may cause derangements in the structure of the alveolar-capillary unit, which may adversely affect the lung's primary function of gas exchange. Individual units may be destroyed, vastly reducing the overall number in the lung. Such destruction also occurs in emphysema and is probably due to chronic excessive protease activity in the terminal air spaces. Alternatively, the lung can be exposed to an injurious agent that incites an inflammatory reaction in the alveolar space and septal wall (alveolitis). Once this reaction is in progress, one of two outcomes may result: elimination of the offending agent with resolution of the injury and inflammation, or persistence of the injury with resultant development of fibrosis. Which pathway is followed, as well as the extent of the injury, determines the ultimate outcome of the inflammatory reaction and has long-term prognostic implications as well.

After the inciting agent is initially encountered, the ensuing reaction or host response to the insult varies, based on the composition and quantity of the foreign substance. Many agents have been described as inducing alveolitis, including infectious microbes, toxic substances (ozone, inorganic dusts, and other pollutants), radiation, many chemotherapeutic agents, and even oxygen in high inspired concentrations. Alveolitis can also result from systemic disturbances, such as autoimmune diseases, with accompanying vasculitis due to immune (antigen–antibody) complex deposition or cell-mediated immune responses. The pulmonary vasculature including the capillaries may be affected, and alveolitis may occur. Because of the normally delicate nature of the alveolar-capillary unit, damage may occur on either the epithelial or the endothelial surface, depending on whether the insulting agent is inhalational or hematogenous in origin. The lung, however, has a limited number of ways in which it can react to injuries, and many of the inflammatory responses follow common pathways regardless of the nature of the stimulus.

When damage occurs to either the type I alveolar epithelial cell or the capillary endothelial cell, edema and cell membrane disruption are usually the initial responses. This is followed by inflammation either from the inciting agent itself or from cellular damage. Repair processes begin and granulation tissue may form. Fibrosis then develops or resolution occurs. Any disruption of the normally delicate structure of the alveolar-capillary unit will result in thickening of the unit and some degree of impairment of gas exchange due to impaired diffusion. In the initial stages, this might be quite mild and evident only on exertion as a widening of the alveolar-arterial oxygen gradient ($P_{A}O_{2} - P_{a}O_{2}$). In more severe instances, gas exchange abnormalities may occur at rest and respiratory failure may result, such as occurs in ARDS. Usually pulmonary hypertension occurs at the end stage of progressive disease. Characteristically, the interstitial parenchymal abnormalities are characterized by alveolar septal thickening, loss of lung compliance, and absence of airflow obstruction. Depending on the severity of alveolar involvement, alveolar air spaces may be lost as repair processes result in incorporation of damaged alveoli into the interstitium of the lung. Accordingly, lung volumes are reduced, resulting in restrictive patterns of abnormalities on pulmonary function testing. All of the pathophysiologic derangements that occur due to DPLDs are nonspecific with regard to the cause of the process. In other words, the injury patterns of the lung are limited and represent the outcome of common pathways resulting from a variety of insults. Pulmonary function tests aid in confirming the diagnosis of DPLDs, assessing the severity and/or progression of the process, and following response to therapy.

Lung volume testing usually reveals reductions in total lung capacity, vital capacity, and functional residual capacity, but residual volume usually remains relatively preserved (Figure 7–8). Expiratory flow rates are normal or slightly supranormal due to the effect of the fibrotic parenchymal disease "tethering" open the airways and supplying increased elastic recoil to generate airflow. Airflow obstruction, while not a feature of the most common interstitial parenchymal processes, may be present in patients with a history of extensive tobacco use (who make up more than 50% of patients in most series of IPF). When present, an obstructive ventilatory defect may lead to a combined obstructive- restrictive process, which may mask or minimize the restrictive defect secondary to the interstitial process. COP and sarcoidosis usually cause restrictive abnormalities due to "drop-out" of involved alveolar units, which do not contribute to measured lung volumes or capacities.

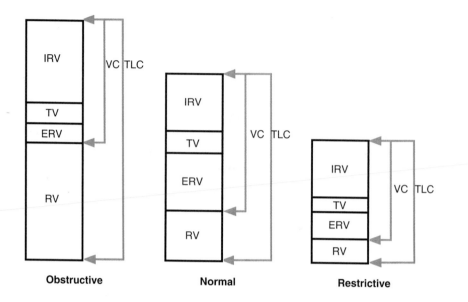

Figure 7–8. Illustration of normal lung volumes and volumes representative of obstructive disease and restrictive disease. ERV, expiratory reserve volume; IRV, inspiratory reserve volume; RV, residual volume; TLC, total lung capacity; TV, tidal volume; VC, vital capacity.

DPLDs also affect the static compliance of the lung, which is defined as a change in lung volume resulting from a given change in transpulmonary pressure. Interstitial injury and fibrosis result in a reduction of compliance due to remodeling of alveolar architecture and increased elasticity or elastic recoil of the lung. Elastic recoil is the inverse of compliance; it is the property of the lung that opposes inflation. Thus, fibrotic processes increase elastic recoil and reduce the compliance of the lung. A typical compliance (pressure/volume) curve is shown in (Figure 7–9), where compliance is defined as the slope between two points on the curve. Reductions in compliance result in a shift of the curve downward and to the right. Thus, for any given change in transpulmonary pressure, there is a smaller change in volume than in a normal lung, accompanied by a reduction in total lung capacity. This is a result of the increased elastic recoil of the lung that occurs with alveolar septal destruction and/or fibrosis. Any condition that makes the lung stiffer or opposes inflation will result in increased elastic recoil, loss of compliance, and more inspiratory work of breathing for the patient. Because lung compliance and chest wall compliance are in series, changes in the chest wall itself (eg, severe kyphoscoliosis or morbid obesity) can also result in alterations in total compliance. Measurement of lung volumes may help differentiate loss of chest wall compliance from loss of lung parenchymal compliance. DPLD usually results in a significant decrease in the residual volume with relative preservation of the expiratory reserve volume. The opposite is usually seen in patients with a decrease in chest wall compliance.

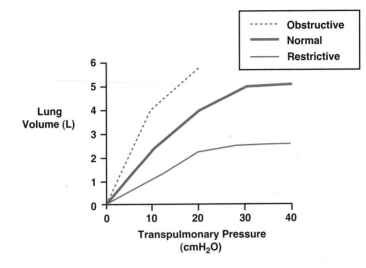

Figure 7-9. Representative normal static lung compliance curve and curves for restrictive and obstructive lung diseases. Restrictive diseases shift the curve downward and to the right, and obstructive diseases shift the curve upward and to the left.

Arterial blood gas analysis may demonstrate abnormalities, particularly in patients with progressive, severe interstitial inflammation or fibrosis. Initially, resting blood gas measurements may be normal, with hypoxemia developing during exercise. Resting hypoxemia may also occur, usually with normal or low arterial carbon dioxide pressure (P_{CO_2}). Widening of the $P_{AO_2} - P_{aO_2}$ is commonly present. Hypercapnia is an unusual finding but may occur if respiratory failure supervenes. Oxygenation abnormalities are probably due to a combination of ventilation and perfusion mismatching (due to the parenchymal abnormalities) and to diffusion impairment. Diffusing capacity is found to be impaired at the time of diagnosis in most patients with IPF. The decrease in D_{LCO} is due to effacement of the alveolar capillary units and $\dot{V}/\dot{Q}$ mismatch. In some instances right-to-left shunting and cardiac dysfunction may also contribute to hypoxemia, but this is usually a late finding that occurs preterminally.

Alveolar dead space ventilation is also elevated in pulmonary interstitial diseases, leading to mismatch of ventilation and perfusion. Dead space ventilation does not decrease (the normal response) when exercise is undertaken. This is the result of an inability to increase tidal volume during exercise due to abnormally high elastic recoil of the fibrotic lungs. The pattern of breathing with restrictive interstitial diseases is one of rapid, shallow breathing, which increases the overall work of breathing.

Right ventricular dysfunction may occur with moderate degrees of interstitial lung disease or fibrosis, due to elevated pulmonary vascular resistance and pulmonary hypertension. The right ventricle initially hypertrophies in order to compensate for this increased workload, but if pulmonary artery pressure and vascular resistance continue to increase, right ventricular failure eventually occurs.

This failure is manifested clinically as cor pulmonale (right ventricular failure secondary to pulmonary hypertension). Adverse changes in the pulmonary circulation may be exacerbated by exercise, leading to more severe dyspnea with increased physical activity, as well as gas exchange abnormalities (primarily worsening of hypoxemia). Pulmonary circulation changes are commonly due to obliterative changes in the vascular bed as pulmonary architecture is remodeled with inflammation and fibrosis, as well as vascular (intimal) changes in some subsets of pulmonary parenchymal disease. Hypoxic pulmonary vasoconstriction, the primary mechanism of maintenance of ventilation and perfusion matching, may also contribute to pulmonary hypertension. Some authors have observed a rise in pulmonary artery pressure immediately preceding death in patients with severe pulmonary fibrosis.

DIAGNOSTIC & CLINICAL CONSIDERATIONS

When evaluating a patient with DPLD, it is important to realize that there are a vast number of possible etiologies for this presentation, and symptoms and signs are not sufficiently distinctive to clearly distinguish among all of the possibilities (Table 7–1). Particular attention should be paid to the nature, onset, duration, and progression of dyspnea. Associated symptoms, such as arthralgias or lower extremity edema, may provide clues to the cause or to developing complications (eg, collagen vascular disease, cor pulmonale, etc). Any history of environmental, drug, or toxic exposures should also be investigated. Those patients with acute interstitial pneumonia (AIP) usually present with a precipitous acute illness, with severe dyspnea and the rapid development of acute respiratory failure. When interstitial parenchymal inflammation and fibrosis occur, the common symptoms are gradually progressive dyspnea (usually over several months), often accompanied by a nonproductive cough. Fever and chest pain are generally not present. Patients with COP usually present with a subacute history of dyspnea and cough, generally lasting for a few weeks to a few months. This usually begins as an upper respiratory tract infection that does not resolve completely. The shorter duration of symptoms generally distinguishes this disorder from IPF. Symptoms usually persist despite one or more courses of antibiotics. The clinical presentation of sarcoidosis is highly variable and depends on the stage of the pulmonary disease. It may include constitutional symptoms (eg, fever, malaise, and weight loss), but gradually progressive dyspnea and cough may also be a presenting feature.

Physical signs are not likely to point to the specific cause of the DPLD, but they may be helpful in determining the extent of the disease and/or the presence of complicating features. Joint swelling or tight skin may suggest a collagen vascular disease. Physical findings may include fine end-inspiratory crackles ("Velcro" rales) and/or digital clubbing. In late stages, hypoxemia, cyanosis, elevated central venous pressure, and pedal edema may signal the development of right ventricular failure (cor pulmonale).

Chest x-ray results are abnormal in the majority of patients with DPLDs at presentation, but up to 15% of patients with IPF may have x-rays without apparent abnormalities. Common changes are reticular, nodular, or reticulonodular

Table 7–1. Classification of idiopathic diffuse parenchymal lung diseases

Histologic pattern	Abbreviation	Clinical diagnosis	Abbreviation	Synonyms
Usual interstitial pneumonitis	UIP	Idiopathic pulmonary fibrosis	IPF	Cryptogenic fibrosing alveolitis, idiopathic interstitial pneumonia
Nonspecific interstitial pneumonia	NSIP	Nonspecific interstitial pneumonia	NSIP	
Diffuse alveolar damage	DAD	Acute interstitial pneumonia	AIP	Hamman-Rich syndrome
Lymphoid interstitial pneumonia	LIP	Lymphoid interstitial pneumonia	LIP	
Desquamative interstitial pneumonia	DIP	Desquamative interstitial pneumonia	DIP	
Respiratory bronchiolitis interstitial lung disease	RBILD	Respiratory bronchiolitis disease	RBILD	
Organizing pneumonia	OP	Cryptogenic organizing pneumonia	COP	Idiopathic bronchiolitis obliterans organizing pneumonia

opacities usually diffuse in location, often with lower lobe predominance (Figure 7–10). Small (<1 cm) cystic changes may occur (known as honeycomb lung), usually signifying irreversible end-stage fibrosis with accompanying lung destruction. A ground-glass pattern of homogenous infiltration signifying alveolar filling may also occur. ARDS and AIP generally present with diffuse alveolar filling characteristic of pulmonary edema. As this is due to a capillary injury and leak rather than left ventricular failure, common signs of heart failure, such as cardiac enlargement, pulmonary vascular engorgement, and pleural effusions, are usually absent. Some diseases may mimic these radiographic patterns (Table 7–2), but are not true DPLDs. Depending on the cause of the interstitial process, adenopathy or pleural disease may be accompanying features. These latter signs are unusual in IPF. Tuberculosis or sarcoidosis may have accompanying adenopathy, but this is a nonspecific sign.

The role of high-resolution computed tomography (HRCT) is to separate patients with UIP/IPF from those with non-UIP lesions. HRCT may suggest

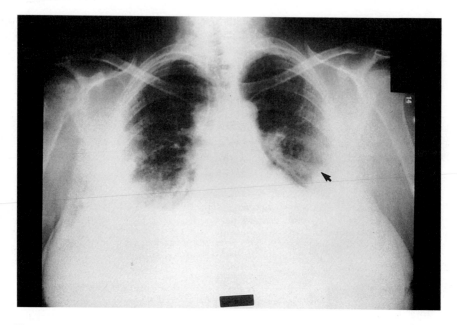

Figure 7–10. Chest x-ray of a patient with IPF. Note the relatively small lung volumes and the diffuse reticulonodular infiltrates, most apparent in the lung bases (arrow).

Table 7–2. Mimics of diffuse parenchymal lung disease

Pulmonary edema
Chronic bronchitis with prominent pulmonary vasculature
Bronchiectasis
Diffuse infectious pneumonia (nongranulomatous; ie, viral, *Pneumocystis jiroveci*, and
 atypicals)

other diagnoses of DPLDs such as sarcoid, hypersensitivity pneumonitis, lymphangioleiomyomatosis (LAM), and Langerhans cell histiocytosis or another idiopathic interstitial pneumonia. A confident radiologic diagnosis of UIP is based on classic findings of a bilateral, subpleural, basal-predominant, reticular pattern associated with subpleural cysts (honeycombing), and traction bronchiectasis. When based on these findings, a radiologic diagnosis of UIP is correct in more than 90% of cases. HRCT may help guide the location of biopsy to increase the yield. Ideally multiple lung biopsies should be obtained from more than one lobe of the lung and should include the full spectrum of the gross disease appearance.

 Based on the specificity of the clinical evaluation and the HRCT findings, the American Thoracic Society and the European Respiratory Society have developed criteria for the diagnosis of IPF without a surgical biopsy. Unfortunately, although the HRCT findings are specific they are not sensitive, and atypical HRCT findings may reveal UIP on biopsy. Therefore, if the cause of the interstitial process remains unknown after the clinical evaluation and HRCT, a lung biopsy should be considered to confirm the diagnosis. Transbronchial biopsies obtained via fiber optic bronchoscopy most often do not yield enough tissue to diagnose the histologic patterns of idiopathic interstitial pneumonias, but have an excellent yield in cases of infectious diseases or granulomatous processes.

MANAGEMENT PRINCIPLES

It is difficult to generalize a discussion of therapy for the myriad disorders that may result in DPLDs. However, given that the lung has only a limited number of ways that it can respond to infectious or inflammatory insult, there are some general principles of management. If the primary problem has an infectious cause, the mainstay of therapy will be the specific antimicrobial agent or agents to which the organism is sensitive. In the absence of an infectious pathogen, damage to the lung is often due to an overexuberant inflammatory response. For that reason, anti-inflammatory therapies are employed in an attempt to arrest the process and limit the damage. It is of utmost importance to exclude an infectious agent prior to initiation of anti-inflammatory therapy, due to the propensity of these drugs to mitigate host defenses and allow the infectious process to progress in the absence of specific antimicrobial therapy. For this reason a lung biopsy (or other diagnostic procedure such as bronchoalveolar lavage) should be undertaken to search for infectious agents. As a general principle and specifically in RB-ILD and DLCH, smoking cessation has been shown to improve lung function and should be the cornerstone of management. The most commonly used drugs are corticosteroids, but adjunctive agents are sometimes used, including cyclophosphamide, azathioprine, n-acetylcysteine, or mycophenolate. These drugs have anti-inflammatory properties without the side effects of steroids. However, some carry a potential for hematologic and gastrointestinal toxicities, and patients on therapy should be monitored closely and maintained on the lowest effective dose. Randomized trials to evaluate the most effective therapy are either lacking or disappointing. Therefore, therapeutic guidelines are largely empiric in nature. The issue is confounded by the fact that in certain diseases, such as sarcoidosis, spontaneous remissions can occur which may erroneously be attributed to the therapeutic regimen. Some subsets of DPLDs have a large fraction of affected patients who responds to anti-inflammatory therapy, including COP, in which approximately 60%–70% of patients may be expected to have a beneficial response to steroid therapy. In contrast, in patients with IPF, only 20%–25% will have a detectable response to a therapeutic trial of anti-inflammatory agents. Once a therapeutic trial is embarked upon, objective goals should be sought, and in the absence of a beneficial response, therapy should be adjusted or withdrawn accordingly. Attempts have been made to correlate prognosis of DPLDs with derangements in pulmonary function. While the plethora of causes make generalizations risky, in general it has been established that the more cellular and less fibrotic changes there are in the lung, the greater the likelihood for a response to therapy and the better the overall prognosis. Many factors may contribute to worsening symptoms in patients with DPLDs, including disease progression, adverse effects of therapy, or complications

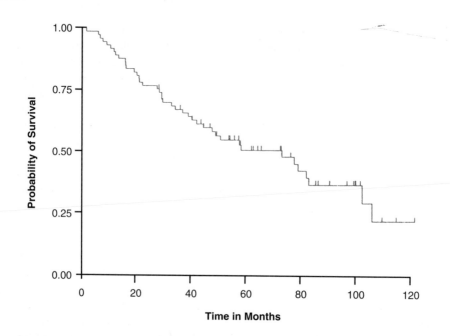

Figure 7–11. Survival curve from a series of 74 patients with IPF from onset of respiratory symptoms. (Reproduced with permission from Schwartz DA, Helmers RA, Galvin JR, et al: Determinants of survival in idiopathic pulmonary fibrosis. *Am J Respir Crit Care Med.* 1994;149:450.)

related to the disease. When patients succumb to IPF, death is most often caused by respiratory failure. Cor pulmonale, bronchogenic carcinoma, atherosclerotic heart disease, pulmonary emboli, or infectious complications (eg, pneumonia) are frequently associated with death in this group of patients. Approximately 50% of patients with IPF succumb to this illness within 5 years of the time of diagnosis (Figure 7–11). Newer modalities of therapy are currently under investigation, and lung transplantation may provide prolonged survival for patients with IPF as well as certain subsets of patients with other DPLDs.

CLINICAL SCENARIOS

Case 1

A 55-year-old man with a 50–pack-year smoking history presents with complaints of slowly worsening shortness of breath over the past year. This problem progressed to the point that he had to quit his job as a shopping mall security officer 2 months ago due to excessive fatigue at the end of his usual 8-hour shift. Currently he can walk two blocks prior to having to stop due to dyspnea. He has no fever but reports an occasional cough that is nonproductive. He remembers nothing unusual about the onset of this problem and has had no occupational or toxic exposures that he can recall. He has no significant past medical history and has been healthy except for the present problem.

Physical Examination: On physical examination he is well developed and mildly dyspneic on exertion, he is afebrile, and vital signs are normal. On pulse oximetry, his room air saturation is 95% at rest. Pertinent findings on physical examination are normal estimated jugular venous pressure, fine end-inspiratory "Velcro" crackles at the lung bases, normal cardiovascular findings, and clubbing of his fingers. A chest x-ray reveals normal cardiac size and silhouette, diffuse reticulonodular opacities more prominent in subpleural areas and lung bases with no evidence of pleural disease, and no signs of adenopathy. Pulmonary function testing reveals a restrictive pattern with a reduced diffusion capacity (DLCO) and no evidence of airway obstruction. A HRCT of the chest demonstrated a bilateral, subpleural, basal-predominant, reticular pattern associated with honeycombing and minimal ground-glass opacities. A transbronchial biopsy ruled out sarcoid and any infectious etiology.

Discussion: The patient's presentation including his history and the physical findings, as well as radiographic and pulmonary function testing results are consistent with a diagnosis of an idiopathic usual interstitial pneumonia. Given the chronicity and progression of symptoms, the apparent lack of occupational and/or toxic exposures or other concurrent illnesses, and classic findings on HRCT of the chest, a highly probable diagnosis of IPF can be made without an open lung biopsy.

Although no pharmacologic therapy to date has proven to alter or reverse the inflammatory process of IPF, the ATS/ERS recommend a trial of anti-inflammatory therapy for patients who have no relative contraindications to therapy (eg, obesity, diabetes mellitus, etc). Features consistent with a more favorable outcome include young age, female gender, short symptomatic period, and predominant ground-glass opacities on HRCT. In this patient, a therapeutic course of corticosteroids should be initiated along with azathioprine or cyclophosphamide. After 3 months, an objective response to therapy should be assessed clinically and by pulmonary function tests. If no significant improvement is noted then, these agents should be discontinued because of their potentially significant side effects. Newer drug trials are under investigation but data are preliminary. Finally, lung transplantation should be considered in suitable candidates at the time of diagnosis.

CLINICAL PEARLS

- IPF presents with chronic progressive dyspnea and other nonspecific symptoms. In the absence of intercurrent illness or occupational, environmental, and/or toxic exposures, the combination of clinical restrictive pulmonary function abnormalities and typical HRCT findings makes diagnosis reasonably accurate even without obtaining a lung biopsy.
- The presence of a predominant honeycombing and fibrotic pattern on HRCT indicates irreversible end-stage lung destruction and makes a response to medical therapy unlikely.

Case 2

A 58-year-old man with no previous medical problems presents complaining of persistent fever, cough, malaise, and dyspnea for the past month despite completing a course of oral antibiotics for pneumonia. The patient has no occupational exposure history and the remainder of his review of systems is unremarkable.

Physical Examination: His physical exam reveals bilateral crackles but is otherwise normal. Routine lab tests are normal. The chest radiograph reveals bilateral peripheral air space disease. Pulmonary function tests reveal a mild restrictive ventilatory defect, with a decreased D$_{LCO}$ and hypoxemia. Transbronchial biopsies are obtained and the patient is started on oral corticosteroids with improvement of his symptoms.

Discussion: The transbronchial biopsies revealed an organizing pneumonia pattern with bronchiolitis and intraluminal polyps. This pattern of injury may be seen with many other diseases, but when the etiology of this pattern is unknown and is secondary to the clinical scenario described above, the syndrome is called COP. COP, formerly known as idiopathic BOOP (bronchiolitis obliterans with organizing pneumonia), is a syndrome characterized by fever, dyspnea, malaise, weight loss, and cough, usually of short duration (less than 3 months). The most common radiographic findings include peripheral patchy air space disease, although multiple and single nodules may also be seen in some cases. A majority of patients recover completely after receiving corticosteroids. Relapse may occur if the steroids are weaned too early. A few patients may develop a progressive fatal form of the disorder.

CLINICAL PEARLS

- COP is characterized by respiratory symptoms that are of unknown etiology occurring for less than 3 months with organizing pneumonia with or without intraluminal polyps on biopsy.
- COP usually quickly responds to corticosteroids and has a good prognosis.

KEY CONCEPTS

1 Diffuse parenchymal lung diseases (DPLDs) are a heterogeneous group of nonneoplastic disorders resulting from damage to the lung parenchyma by varying patterns of inflammation and fibrosis.

2 Signs and symptoms of these disorders are nonspecific, but the underlying clinical scenario and a high-resolution CT scan may be helpful in reaching the diagnosis. Open lung biopsy may be needed at times to confirm the specific diagnosis.

STUDY QUESTIONS

7–1. A patient with idiopathic pulmonary fibrosis diagnosed 1 year ago returns to the office with worsening dyspnea on exertion and new onset of lower extremity edema. The physical examination reveals a new right ventricular parasternal *heave and 1+ pitting pretibial edema. Regarding the pulmonary hypertension that develops in patients with progressive idiopathic pulmonary fibrosis:*

a. *It is one of the initial findings characterizing this disease.*

b. *It is due to venous thromboemboli that invariably complicate pulmonary fibrosis.*

c. *Pulmonary vascular resistance is mildly elevated for most of the course of the disease, but a severe elevation may occur preterminally.*

d. *It is purely accounted for by the hypoxia accompanying pulmonary fibrosis.*

7–2. *Pulmonary function testing of patients with pulmonary fibrosis typically shows restrictive abnormalities, with reductions in the total lung capacity, the vital capacity, and the forced expiratory volume in 1 second (FEV1, which is reduced proportionately to the forced vital capacity, FVC), so that the FEV1:FVC ratio is normal. Diffusing capacity and static pulmonary compliance are also reduced. All of the following may contribute to the decreased static lung compliance EXCEPT:*

a. *increased elastic recoil as parenchymal fibrosis occurs;*

b. *loss of alveolar units as parenchymal inflammation and fibrosis progress;*

c. *destruction of alveolar units by excessive protease activity, as occurs in emphysema;*

d. *increase in surface tension with resulting reduced alveolar size due to surfactant abnormalities.*

SUGGESTED READINGS

American Thoracic Society/European Respiratory Society International Multidisciplinary Consensus classification of idiopathic interstitial pneumonias. *Am J Respir Crit Care Med.* 2002;**165**:227–304.

Phan SH, Thrall RS. *Pulmonary Fibrosis: Lung Biology in Health and Disease.* Vol. 80. New York: Marcel Dekker; 1995:1–864.

Pulmonary Vascular Disease | 8

Suma Jain & Bennett P. deBoisblanc

OBJECTIVES

- ▶ *Identify the components of the pulmonary vasculature and discuss the pathophysiology and causes of hypoxemia and its relation to pulmonary hypertension.*
- ▶ *Evaluate the other causes of pulmonary hypertension.*
- ▶ *Review the clinical implications and management of venous thromboembolic disease and pulmonary embolism.*

INTRODUCTION

Unlike most of the other organs in the body, the lung has dual circulation. It receives blood flow from both the pulmonary and systemic circulations. The pulmonary arteries and arterioles carry mixed-venous blood from the right ventricle and distribute it over the pulmonary capillary-alveolar membrane, where gas exchange takes place. Oxygenated blood is then returned to the left atrium via the pulmonary venules and veins. The nutrient requirements of respiratory bronchioles and the elastic components of the lung are met by the pulmonary circulation, while their oxygen requirements are principally satisfied directly by alveolar ventilation. In contrast, the bronchial circulation arises from the aorta and supplies the tracheobronchial tree with oxygen and nutrients to the level of the terminal bronchioles. The pulmonary circulation is normally a high-compliance, low-resistance, low-pressure system that receives the entire output of the right ventricle, approximately 3.5 L/min/M². In contrast, the bronchial circulation is a low-compliance, high-resistance system with a blood flow of approximately 70 mL/min/M² and a pressure equal to aortic pressure. The bronchial circulation can have important clinical implications as discussed later in this chapter.

In health, the pulmonary vascular bed is a thin-walled, high-compliance, low-resistance system with a resting mean pulmonary artery pressure of approximately 12–14 mm Hg, a pulmonary capillary pressure of 6–8 mm Hg, and a pulmonary venous pressure of 5–7 mm Hg. During conditions in which pulmonary blood flow is transiently increased, such as exercise, the ability to recruit and distend pulmonary vessels permits up to a sevenfold increase in cardiac output with less than a doubling of mean pulmonary artery pressure. Elevation of hydrostatic pressures beyond this normal range will produce distinct clinical syndromes depending on whether the pressure elevation is precapillary (arteries and arterioles) or postcapillary (venules, veins, or left side of the heart).

The primary determinants of mean pulmonary artery pressure under normal circumstances are left atrial pressure, pulmonary blood flow, and pulmonary vascular resistance. The clinical causes related to these determinates are outlined (Table 8–1).

Table 8–1. Pathophysiological classification & causes of pulmonary hypertension

---

I. Diseases associated with chronic increases in pulmonary blood flow
  A. Congenital left-to-right shunts
    1. Intracardiac
      a. Atrial septal defects
      b. Ventricular septal defects
    2. Extracardiac
      a. Patent ductus arteriosus
II. Diseases that increase pulmonary vascular resistance
  A. Increased resistance primarily in precapillary arteries and arterioles
    1. Increased resistance caused by hypoxic vasoconstriction
      a. Cause of hypoxemia low inspired partial pressure of oxygen
        i. Chronic residence at high altitude
      b. Cause of hypoxemia chronic or recurrent alveolar hypoventilation
        i. Morbid obesity
        ii. Neuromuscular weakness
        iii. Severe kyphoscoliosis
        iv. Obstructive sleep apnea
      c. Cause of hypoxemia primarily ventilation-perfusion mismatch
        i. Chronic obstructive pulmonary disease
        ii. Chronic bronchitis
        iii. Asthma
        iv. Emphysema
        v. Bronchiectasis
        vi. Chronic interstitial lung diseases
    2. Increase in resistance caused by intraluminal obstruction, fibrosis, or destruction of arteries or arterioles
      a. Pulmonary embolism
      b. Schistosomiasis
      c. Sickle cell disease
      d. Pulmonary fibrosis
      e. Pulmonary vasculitis
      f. Toxins
        i. Anoretic drugs
        ii. Cocaine
        iii. Intravenous drugs
      g. Human immunodeficiency virus (HIV)
      h. Cirrhosis with portal hypertension
        i. Primary pulmonary hypertension
  B. Increase in resistance primarily in postcapillary venules and veins
    1. Pulmonary venoocclusive disease
    2. Sclerosing mediastinitis
    3. Anomalous venous return

(continued)

Table 8–1. Classification of causes of pulmonary hypertension *(continued)*

III. Diseases that increase left atrial pressure
   A. Left ventricular systolic dysfunction
   B. Left ventricular diastolic dysfunction
      1. Hypertrophic cardiomyopathy
      2. Constrictive pericarditis
   C. Valvular heart disease
      1. Mitral stenosis
      2. Mitral regurgitation
   D. Miscellaneous
      1. Left atrial myxoma

PRECAPILLARY PULMONARY HYPERTENSION

Pathophysiology

Pulmonary arterial hypertension (PAH) is the term used to describe the remodeling of pulmonary vessels in a fashion that leads to an increase in vascular resistance and pulmonary artery pressure. For epidemiologic purposes, pulmonary hypertension is defined as a mean pulmonary artery pressure greater than 25 mm Hg at rest or greater than 30 mm Hg during exercise. Both genetic and epigenetic risk factors for PAH have been identified in patients with PAH.

A majority of patients with familial PAH have mutations in the bone morphogenic protein receptor-2 (BMPR2) gene that codes for type II receptors in the TGF-ß superfamily. These mutations increase the propensity for unregulated growth and proliferation of smooth muscle cells and fibroblasts in vessel walls. Many of these mutations are inherited in a Mendelian dominant fashion and demonstrate incomplete penetrance and genetic anticipation. Incomplete penetrance means that not all individuals with the mutation will be affected. Genetic anticipation means that subsequent generations often develop the symptoms of the disease at an earlier age than previous generations.

In contrast to gene mutations, epigenetic factors represent injuries, insults, or pathophysiologic states that can influence the expression of even normal genes in a way that can lead to disease. In the case of PAH, these insults can initiate the process of vascular remodeling that leads to pulmonary hypertension. Some of these epigenetic risk factors are well known, such as congenital left-to-right shunts, connective tissue diseases, use of selected anorectic drugs, portal hypertension, and infection with the human immunodeficiency virus (HIV).

Regardless of the etiology of PAH, the endothelium from pulmonary arteries of patients with PAH produces fewer naturally occurring vasodilators and growth inhibitors such as prostacyclin and nitric oxide, and more vasoconstrictors and growth stimulators such as thromboxane and endothelin-1. This imbalance in the controllers of vascular tone and vascular remodeling in the lung is thought to be an important pathogenic mechanism in the development of PAH.

Atrial septal defects, ventricular septal defects, patent ductus arteriosus, and other congenital heart diseases associated with shunting of blood from the systemic to the pulmonary circulation can create a condition of chronic overcirculation and overdistension of the pulmonary vascular bed. When significant left-to-right shunts are not diagnosed and corrected in early childhood, the resultant chronic vascular wall stress induces the process of remodeling. Remodeling is characterized histologically by medial hypertrophy, intimal thickening, and adventitial fibrosis of pulmonary arteries and arterioles. These changes further increase pulmonary vascular resistance and eventually become irreversible. In such cases, pulmonary hypertension may continue to worsen after shunt correction. Late in the disease process, right-sided pressures can exceed systemic pressures, causing a reversal of the shunt. In such cases, termed Eisenmenger's complex, poorly oxygenated mixed-venous blood bypasses the lungs and enters the systemic circulation, causing severe hypoxemia.

Fibrosing lung diseases may also cause precapillary pulmonary hypertension by destroying small arterioles and alveolar capillaries. When the destruction is severe enough and the cross-sectional area of the pulmonary vascular bed is significantly reduced, pulmonary vascular resistance rises. Although connective tissue diseases can cause pulmonary fibrosis, they often cause pulmonary hypertension that is out of proportion to the severity of either the fibrosis or the resultant hypoxemia. This is particularly characteristic of limited scleroderma, a disease in which up to 40%–90% of patients will develop PAH. In scleroderma, deposition of collagen in the walls of small arterioles occurs in the lung as well as in other organs, contributing to the increase in pulmonary vascular resistance.

Hypoxemia is the term used to describe a decrease in the partial pressure of oxygen in the systemic arterial blood. It can contribute to the development of precapillary pulmonary hypertension by inducing hypoxic vasoconstriction in pulmonary arterioles. Hypoxemia is one of the most common manifestations of cardiopulmonary disease and results from one of six pathophysiologic mechanisms:

1. decreased atmospheric pressure
2. decreased inspired fraction of oxygen
3. alveolar hypoventilation
4. ventilation-perfusion mismatch
5. shunt
6. diffusion abnormalities

In the United States the most common disease associated with hypoxemia is chronic obstructive pulmonary disease (COPD). In patients with COPD, the severity of pulmonary hypertension is generally modest with mean pulmonary artery pressures rarely exceeding 30 mm Hg. Chronic alveolar hypoventilation, also often seen in COPD, can exaggerate the hypoxic vasoconstrictor response. Pulmonary hypertension occurs in association with other causes of significant hypoxemia and alveolar hypoventilation, such as morbid obesity with obstructive sleep apnea or kyphoscoliosis (Table 8–1). In hypoxemic patients, enhanced erythropoietin production can raise the blood hematocrit and viscosity, further aggravating the pulmonary hypertension and increased right ventricular workload. When hypoxemia is chronic, vascular remodeling occurs, leading to persistent pulmonary hypertension. Supplemental oxygen in this setting may not completely resolve the pulmonary hypertension.

Pulmonary embolism is an important and reversible cause of precapillary pulmonary hypertension. *Venous thromboembolism* is a term used to describe the spectrum of clinical presentations of deep vein thrombosis and pulmonary embolism. Venous thromboembolism remains an important cause of mortality in the United States. It has been estimated that there are 5 million cases of deep vein thrombosis that result in 500,000 cases of symptomatic pulmonary embolism each year. Approximately 10% of cases of pulmonary embolism are fatal, accounting for up to 35% of all hospital deaths. It has been estimated that over 70% of patients who die of pulmonary embolism are diagnosed with pulmonary embolism for the first time at autopsy. Late complications of venous thromboembolism include 500,000 new cases of venous stasis ulcers each year in the United States. This diagnosis will be dealt with in more detail later in the chapter.

Some diseases do not fit well into any of the above categories, such as hemoglobin SS, schistosomiasis, and sarcoidosis. The pathogenesis of pulmonary hypertension in these diseases is variable. For example, in schistosomiasis there is obstruction of pulmonary vessels both from the schistosomes themselves and from the intense perivascular inflammation that accompanies the parasitic infestation, while in sarcoidosis, noncaseating granulomatous inflammation may be present.

Diagnostic & Clinical Considerations

HISTORY

The most common presenting symptoms in patients with precapillary pulmonary hypertension are chronic dyspnea on exertion, fatigue, angina pectoris (precordial pressure-like chest pain), and occasionally syncope. Hoarseness due to compression of the recurrent laryngeal nerve by an enlarged main pulmonary artery is an uncommon but unique manifestation of pulmonary hypertension not seen in other cardiopulmonary diseases. Symptoms of hypoxemia depend on its severity and range from headache, confusion, and somnolence to clouding of the consciousness. Cardiovascular decompensation can occur with brady- or tachyarrhythmias (see Chapter 13 on respiratory failure).

PHYSICAL EXAMINATION

The initial adaptive response to a chronic elevation in pulmonary artery pressure is right ventricular hypertrophy, which can reduce diastolic compliance of the right ventricle. Chronic pressure overload eventually results in reduced systolic performance as well. When cardiac output begins to fall, maladaptive compensatory mechanisms increase sodium and water reabsorption under the influences of aldosterone and antidiuretic hormone. Sodium and water retention results in volume overload, which is manifested as distended neck veins, ascites, and leg edema. This syndrome of right ventricular failure is termed *cor pulmonale* when the pulmonary hypertension results from lung disease or hypoxemia. If the right atrium contracts against a poorly compliant right ventricle, intraatrial pressure will rise sharply, producing a prominent "a" wave visible in the jugular veins at the base of the neck. Palpation of the precordium may reveal a parasternal lift, which is caused by contraction of the hypertrophied, dilated right ventricle just below the sternum. On auscultation, the pulmonic component of the second heart sound (P_2) is often accentuated and split from the aortic component during both inspiration and expiration. Persistent splitting of the second heart sound is due to slower right ventricular ejection against increased load that results in delayed closure of the pulmonic valve. Dilation of the right ventricle and pressure overload may cause the tricuspid valve to become incompetent during systole, creating a systolic murmur heard best over the right lower sternal border. Severe tricuspid regurgitation briskly elevates central venous (CV) pressure, producing a prominent cv wave that can be visible in the jugular veins or can be palpable in the liver.

When hypoxemia is severe (partial arterial oxygen pressure [P_{AO_2}] <40 mm Hg), central cyanosis, a bluish-gray discoloration of the skin and mucous membranes, may be present. Cyanosis confined to the fingers and toes is usually indicative of poor peripheral blood flow rather than of hypoxemia. Because the symptoms and physical signs of hypoxemia are insensitive and nonspecific, arterial blood gas analysis is usually performed if the suspicion of hypoxemia is high. Pulse oximeters can estimate the percentage of oxygenated hemoglobin in the systemic capillary bed by comparing the transcutaneous absorption of various wavelengths of light that are specific for oxygenated and deoxygenated hemoglobin. The oxyhemoglobin saturation estimated by a pulse oximeter may be erroneous in heavily pigmented patients or in patients with methemoglobinemia, peripheral vascular disease, or shock.

IMAGING

Chest x-rays often provide clues to the cause of pulmonary hypertension (Figure 8–1). Prominence of the main pulmonary arteries is seen in many patients with pulmonary hypertension, regardless of the cause (Figure 8–2). The contour of the cardiac silhouette may suggest either isolated right ventricular enlargement or biventricular enlargement if left ventricular dysfunction is the cause of pulmonary hypertension.

Echocardiographic studies are now used almost routinely in the evaluation of suspected or proven pulmonary hypertension, since they provide both diagnostic and prognostic information. Enlarged intracavitary dimensions, increased wall thickness, and decreased systolic function of the right ventricle often provide the first suspicion of pulmonary hypertension in patients being evaluated for dyspnea of undetermined origin (Figure 8–3). The flow velocity of the tricuspid regurgitation jet from the right ventricle into the right atrium can be measured by Doppler ultrasound technique. Because the regurgitant flow velocity increases as pulmonary artery pressure increases, this measurement can be used to estimate pulmonary artery pressure. Intracardiac shunts that cannot be visualized by standard echocardiographic techniques may be identified after the intravenous injection of micronized bubbles of air suspended in saline solution. Mixing of the echogenic bubbles with a stream of sonolucent blood can identify the site of shunting.

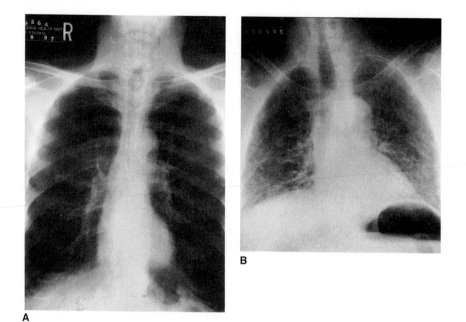

A

B

Figure 8–1. The chest x-ray in the differential diagnosis of pulmonary hypertension. **A.** Chest x-ray of a 60-year-old man with severe chronic obstructive pulmonary disease (COPD) due to smoking-related emphysema. Note the increased lung volume with hyperlucent lung parenchyma. **B.** Chest x-ray of a 55-year-old man with idiopathic pulmonary fibrosis. The lung volumes are much smaller and the lung parenchyma has increased linear densities, which represent areas of scarring. Both patients had mean pulmonary artery pressures of approximately 30 mm Hg.

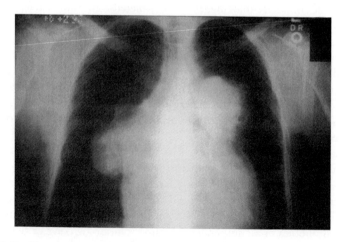

Figure 8–2. Chest x-ray showing large pulmonary arteries.

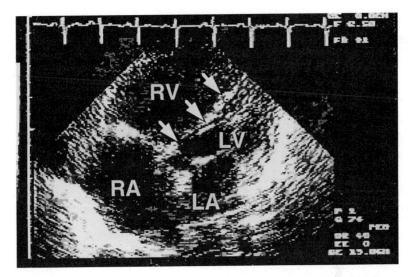

Figure 8–3. Echocardiogram in the assessment of pulmonary hypertension. This transthoracic echocardiogram from a 40-year-old woman with pulmonary hypertension due to pulmonary venoocclusive disease shows enlargement of the right atrium (RA) and right ventricle (RV) with displacement of the interventricular septum to the left (arrows), compromising filling of the left ventricle (LV). The left atrium (LA) is normal in size. Her mean pulmonary artery pressure was 60 mm Hg.

LABORATORY EVALUATION

When the cause of precapillary pulmonary hypertension remains obscure, measurement of selected autoantibodies may be warranted. In cases of pulmonary hypertension due to scleroderma, anticentromere antibodies or antitopoisomerase I (Scl-70) antibodies are usually present. Similarly, when the antiphospholipid syndrome is associated with pulmonary hypertension, high titers of antiphospholipid antibodies may be present. These antibodies can cause small thrombi to develop in pulmonary arterioles. Serological testing for other autoimmune disorders may be helpful also.

RIGHT HEART CATHETERIZATION

Direct measurement of pulmonary artery pressure with a balloon-tipped pulmonary artery catheter is used to definitively diagnose pulmonary hypertension and to assess responses to treatment when noninvasive measures are technically inadequate. The catheter is passed from a peripheral or central venous access site across the tricuspid and pulmonic valves into a proximal pulmonary artery. Advancement of the catheter into the wedge position with the balloon inflated is used to estimate left atrial pressure (Figure 8–4). When pulmonary embolism is suspected but cannot be proven by scintillation lung scanning, pulmonary angiography is performed by injecting iodinated contrast through a properly positioned catheter (see below for a more detailed description of venous thromboembolism). Table 8–2 summarizes

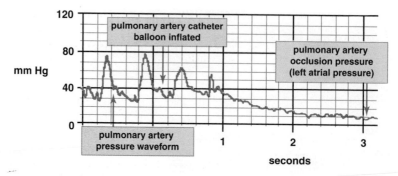

Figure 8–4. Use of a pulmonary artery catheter in the assessment of pulmonary hypertension. A balloon-tipped catheter can be introduced into a central vein and flow directed through the right atrium, across the tricuspid valve, through the right ventricle, across the pulmonic valve, and into the main pulmonary artery. The catheter can be advanced until it occludes a segmental pulmonary artery. After occlusion, the pulmonary artery pressure falls until it is equal to the back pressure of the left atrium. This 55-year-old woman had primary pulmonary hypertension. Her pulmonary artery pressure was very high (80/30 mm Hg), but her occlusion (left atrial) pressure was normal (10 mm Hg).

the diagnostic tests that may be useful in the differential diagnoses for pulmonary hypertension.

PULMONARY FUNCTION TESTING

Pulmonary function testing is used to identify obstructive ventilatory defects characteristic of COPD. An increase in the functional residual capacity, indicative of air trapping in alveoli with long time constants for emptying, is also typical. Interstitial lung diseases, such as sarcoidosis, pneumoconioses, and the connective tissue diseases are associated with restrictive ventilatory defects identified by a reduction in static lung volumes. The diffusing capacity for carbon monoxide (D$_{CO}$), a measure of the integrity of the alveolar-capillary membrane, may be variably affected in COPD but is almost always decreased in severe interstitial lung diseases. Neuromuscular diseases may reduce inspiratory and/or expiratory muscle strength. When the reduction is severe enough to cause significant hypoxemia and hypercapnia, the vital capacity is significantly reduced. With neuromuscular disease, the functional residual capacity may be normal or slightly reduced due to basilar atelectasis. The obesity-hypoventilation syndrome is associated with a reduced vital capacity and functional residual capacity. Neuromuscular disease may be differentiated from the obesity-hypoventilation syndrome by measurement of inspiratory muscle forces. D$_{CO}$ is preserved in both of these disorders which helps to differentiate them from interstitial lung diseases.

POLYSOMNOGRAPHY

Patients with the sleep apnea syndrome may have profound nocturnal hypoxemia that is undetected by an arterial blood gas determination made while awake.

Table 8–2. Diagnostic tests and findings that may be useful in the differential diagnosis of pulmonary hypertension

---

I. Tests that help identify pulmonary parenchymal diseases, airways diseases, or impairment of ventilatory pump
   A. Chest x-ray
      1. Hyperinflation in chronic obstructive pulmonary disease (COPD) or interstitial infiltrates in pulmonary fibrosis
      2. Kerley B lines or other signs of pulmonary edema in diseases with high left atrial pressure
   B. Pulmonary function tests including spirometric studies, lung volume determination, measurement of diffusing capacity, and determination of inspiratory/expiratory pressures
      1. Obstructive defects and air trapping in COPD
      2. Restrictive defects and reduced diffusing capacity in interstitial lung diseases
      3. Reduced inspiratory/expiratory pressures in neuromuscular diseases
   C. Arterial blood gas analysis
      1. Awake hypoxemia
      2. Hypercapnia
   D. Serologic studies
      1. Vary with specific connective tissue disease or pulmonary vasculitis
II. Tests that can identify hypoxemia confined to sleep
   A. Polysomnography
      1. Oxyhemoglobin desaturation during apneas
III. Tests that help identify occult cardiac disease
   A. Pulmonary artery catheterization
      1. Elevated wedge pressure indicative of left atrial hypertension
      2. Step-up in oxyhemoglobin saturation while transiting from the vena cava to the pulmonary artery characteristic of left-to-right shunts
   B. Echocardiography
      1. Abnormal right and/or left ventricular systolic diastolic function
      2. Congenital heart disease, including atrial septal and ventricular septal defects
      3. Valvular dysfunction
IV. Tests that can diagnose pulmonary embolism
   A. Ventilation-perfusion lung scan
      1. Segmental perfusion defects in areas of normal ventilation
   B. Pulmonary angiogram
      1. Intraluminal clot
V. Tests that can quantify the severity of pulmonary hypertension
   A. Echocardiography
      1. Estimates pulmonary artery pressure by measuring flow velocity of tricuspid regurgitation jet
   B. Pulmonary artery catheterization
      1. Directly measures pulmonary artery pressure and cardiac output

---

Repetitive nocturnal oxyhemoglobin desaturations may induce hypoxic pulmonary vasoconstriction that persists during wakefulness. Polysomnographic studies measure various physiologic parameters during sleep, including ventilation and oxyhemoglobin saturation via inductance plethysmographic and pulse oximetric measurements, respectively (see Chapter 12 on respiratory abnormalities with sleep disorders).

Management Principles

OXYGEN

Administration of supplemental oxygen is usually the initial management step while attempts are made to reverse the underlying cause of hypoxemia. Oxygen may be administered by nasal cannula, face mask, transtracheal catheter, or endotracheal tube. Because the nasopharynx is a relatively small gas reservoir, a nasal cannula cannot reliably provide a level of inspired oxygen (FIO_2) above 0.40. This is usually adequate for hypoxemia due to ventilation-perfusion mismatch, as is seen in asthma and COPD. Transtracheal oxygen catheters and oxygen masks with reservoir bags can usually achieve an FIO_2 of 0.80. When a large intrapulmonary or intracardiac shunt is present, supplemental oxygen administration usually has only a modest effect on hypoxemia, since the oxygen content of the shunted blood is not affected. When alveolar derecruitment is the cause of the shunt, mechanical ventilation with positive end-expiratory pressure (PEEP) may help open and stabilize collapsed alveoli.

PHARMACOTHERAPY

Relatively selective pulmonary vasodilators may be useful, especially prostanoids, phosphodiesterase-5 inhibitors, and endothelin receptor antagonists. Diuretics may be administered to help control ascites and lower extremity edema formation that develops from right ventricular failure. Finally, long-term anticoagulation with warfarin is thought to confer benefit.

Prognosis

The outcome of patients is heavily influenced by the etiology of pulmonary hypertension. Some diseases, such as scleroderma or primary pulmonary hypertension, have a progressive course, which may be slowed but not arrested by treatment, while in other cases, such as congenital left-to-right shunts, progression can be prevented with early intervention. In a patient without significant comorbidities, exercise tolerance and the pulmonary hemodynamic profile are predictive of long-term outcome. Low cardiac output and high right atrial pressure are predictors of poor prognosis.

VENOUS THROMBOEMBOLISM

Pathophysiology

Systemic venous thromboses most commonly arise in the valve cusps of the deep veins of the lower extremity. Risk factors for deep vein thrombosis include conditions that cause venous stasis, hypercoagulation, or venous intimal damage. Venous stasis may result from bed rest, low cardiac output, or general anesthesia. The synthesis of clotting factors may be an adaptive response to surgical trauma or a paraneoplastic complication of cancer. Finally, venous intimal damage is a complication of direct venous trauma or prior deep vein thrombosis.

Once thrombi have developed, they can propagate proximally into the large veins of the thigh and pelvis. Freshly propagated clots are friable and may fragment and embolize to the pulmonary circulation where they are trapped. Pulmonary emboli may be small and asymptomatic or large enough to raise pulmonary vascular resistance. If the right ventricle can handle the increase in vascular resistance, cardiac output may be preserved. If the right ventricle cannot handle the increased afterload, it may fail leading to a fall in cardiac output and systemic hypotension. Hypotension in pulmonary embolism is a particularly ominous sign since coronary perfusion to the right ventricle is dependent on systemic blood pressure.

Diagnostic & Clinical Considerations

Many investigations have shown that the history and physical exam are inaccurate predictors of the presence of deep vein thrombosis. Symptoms are rare when the thrombosis is confined to the calf, and even when there is extensive iliofemoral thrombosis, patients are usually asymptomatic and have normal examination of the legs. The most sensitive objective sign of deep vein thrombosis, asymmetry in calf circumference, is found in less than half of patients with deep vein thrombosis, but is present in up to 40% of patients without deep vein thrombosis.

The signs and symptoms of pulmonary embolism are also nonspecific and insensitive. Accordingly, it would be prudent to view any cardiopulmonary symptoms or signs in a patient with significant risk factors with the suspicion that venous thromboembolism has occurred. Since the history, physical exam, and routine laboratory data alone cannot reliably exclude pulmonary embolism, additional testing must be performed when such suspicion exists.

When pulmonary embolism is extensive, tachypnea and tachycardia are present in almost all patients. Patients with massive pulmonary emboli or preexisting cardiopulmonary disease may experience the sudden onset of precordial pain, dyspnea, syncope, or shock. Distended neck veins, cyanosis, diaphoresis, precordial heave, loud pulmonic component of the second heart sound, right ventricular third heart sound, or a murmur of tricuspid regurgitation may also be present. The chest x-ray and the electrocardiogram are more useful in excluding competing diagnoses.

Noninvasive testing with compression ultrasonography of the lower extremities is the preferred initial test for the detection of clinically suspected deep vein thrombosis. Ultrasound has excellent sensitivity and specificity for proximal deep vein thrombosis in symptomatic patients, but is not as sensitive for detecting proximal thrombi in asymptomatic patients or thrombi that are confined to the calf. Since thrombi confined to the calf rarely cause pulmonary embolism, the absence of thrombus in a large proximal deep leg vein such as the popliteal or superficial femoral vein is reassuring that pulmonary embolism is not imminent. However, if a calf thrombus is detected, propagation into the popliteal or iliofemoral segments over the ensuing days must be excluded by serial ultrasound testing. If serial studies cannot be performed, treatment is indicated.

The process of thrombosis is regulated by the simultaneous processes of thrombolysis that results in the liberation of fibrinolytic products such as D-dimers into the systemic circulation. The quantitative measurement of D-dimer in the blood is a sensitive but nonspecific method of detecting deep vein thrombosis and pulmonary embolism. The poor specificity of D-dimers relates to their production in other thrombotic conditions, such as the normal postoperative state, trauma, and systemic infection.

The confirmatory tests most commonly used to document pulmonary embolism include the ventilation-perfusion (V/Q) lung scan, the computed tomographic angiogram (CTA), and the pulmonary arteriogram. A V/Q scan is a nuclear medicine scan that anatomically maps the distribution of ventilation and perfusion. The scan is performed by injecting macroaggregates of radiolabeled albumin into a systemic vein. These aggregates flow into normally perfused areas of the lung and stick in the capillaries of those well-perfused segments. Detection of normal amounts of isotope with a gamma camera over a lung segment is evidence of normal perfusion to that segment. Segmental ventilation is measured by having a patient inhale a gas or aerosol containing a different radioisotope and then rescanning the chest. The finding of two or more lung segments that have absent perfusion but preserved ventilation (V/Q mismatch) is highly suggestive of pulmonary embolism (Figure 8–5), while a V/Q scan that demonstrates normal perfusion throughout the lung excludes pulmonary embolism. V/Q scan patterns that have either subsegmental V/Q mismatches or matched defects are not specific

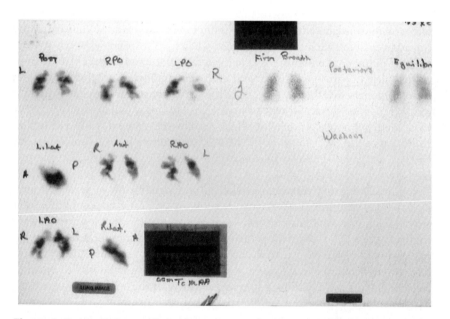

Figure 8–5. Ventilation-perfusion lung scan in pulmonary embolism. Radioactive macroaggregates of albumin are injected into a peripheral vein. These aggregates transiently embolize in the capillaries of perfused lung segments. Radioactive xenon gas is then inhaled into the lung from a reservoir. This 35-year-old woman experienced syncope and hemoptysis 14 days following a femur fracture. The lung scan shows multiple segmental perfusion defects representing occlusion of segmental pulmonary arteries by emboli (left). Ventilation is normal (right). She had a pulmonary artery pressure of 45 mm Hg.

for pulmonary embolism. Patients with suspected pulmonary embolism whose $\dot{V}/\dot{Q}$ scan falls into this last category require further testing.

CT angiography has gained popularity in recent years as a diagnostic test for pulmonary embolism because of its ease of use and its improved accuracy compared to the $\dot{V}/\dot{Q}$ scan. The CT images are acquired following the rapid intravenous injection of radiographic contrast. Pulmonary emboli are identified as intraluminal filling defects in otherwise opacified pulmonary arteries (Figure 8–6). CT angiography is generally more specific than the $\dot{V}/\dot{Q}$ scan, but because it cannot accurately visualize beyond fifth-generation pulmonary arteries, it should not be used to exclude pulmonary embolism in patients with a high likelihood of pulmonary embolism.

Pulmonary arteriography is performed by inserting a catheter into a central vein, threading it through the right atrium and right ventricle and out into a first- or second-generation pulmonary artery. Radiographic contrast is injected directly into the pulmonary circulation during rapid sequence x-ray cinematography. Unlike CTA, pulmonary arteriography can identify even very small intraluminal filling defects and is thus considered the gold standard for the diagnosis of pulmonary embolism.

Management Principles

Although occasionally patients will die of a single massive pulmonary embolism, most patients who die have recurrent emboli over days to weeks. The primary

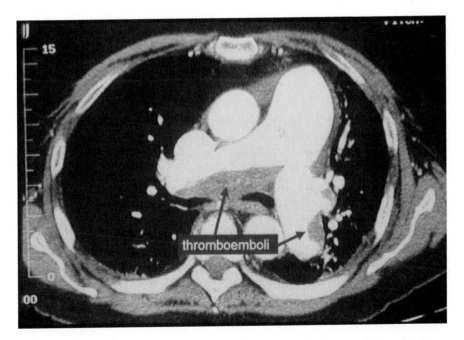

Figure 8–6. CT scan showing intraluminal filling defects highly suggestive of pulmonary emboli.

focus of treatment is the prevention of recurrence. In patients without a contrain-dication to the use of anticoagulants, full anticoagulation with unfractionated or low molecular weight heparin or a direct factor Xa inhibitor should be initiated as soon as the diagnosis is considered. Once the diagnosis is confirmed, anticoagula-tion should be continued with oral warfarin.

If treatment is started promptly, patients with normal cardiopulmonary reserve and small pulmonary emboli generally have good outcomes. When there is sig-nificant cardiopulmonary disease or a large embolism, respiratory failure and hypotension may develop. Vasopressors, oxygen, and mechanical ventilatory sup-port may be needed.

Despite the lack of data demonstrating better survival, the use of thrombolytic therapy is still recommended by many experts in patients with shock due to pulmo-nary embolism who do not have contraindications. However, the use of thrombolytics is associated with significantly more bleeding complications, including fatal intrac-erebral hemorrhage. Coagulation studies are not useful in either guiding the dosing or in predicting the complications of any of the currently approved thrombolytic agents, and monitoring is not recommended until after heparin therapy is initiated. There is no apparent advantage to intrapulmonary administration of thrombolytics over peripheral intravenous administration with regard to the rate of clot resolution.

The widespread use of thrombolytic therapy and improved strategies for sup-porting patients with massive pulmonary embolism has reduced the applicability of surgical embolectomy for acute pulmonary embolism to those patients who are on vasopressors with persistent shock and those who have absolute contraindica-tions to thrombolysis (eg, recent intracranial hemorrhage).

POSTCAPILLARY PULMONARY HYPERTENSION & PULMONARY EDEMA

Pathophysiology

The lung and the skin are the only organs that are continuously exposed simulta-neously to both the aqueous environment of the vital fluids and the gaseous envi-ronment of the atmosphere. The skin makes use of a tough, keratinized epithelium several cell layers thick to separate these media, whereas the lung accomplishes the same feat with a delicate gas-permeable membrane less than 1 mm thick. Because of its large surface area (approximately 70–120 m^2, or an area about the size of a tennis court) and delicate structure, the pulmonary capillary bed is a major site of fluid flux from the vascular compartment into the interstitial spaces of the lung. It is estimated that several hundred milliliters of fluid normally enter the pulmonary interstitium each day and are removed by evaporation in the alveoli, reabsorption into venules, or exportation via lung lymphatics. Lung lymph flow can increase more than 10-fold the normal rate during periods of high fluid flux such as occurs with normal exercise. When fluid flux into the lung interstitium exceeds the rate at which fluid can be removed by the lymphatics, extravascular lung water begins to accumulate, eventually leading to alveolar flooding. Symptoms of breathlessness may develop if the efficiency of ventilation and gas transfer is affected by the edema formation. As an inhomogeneous group, diseases that lead to pulmonary edema are among the most common causes of respiratory failure in intensive care unit patients (see Chapter 13).

Increased hydrostatic pressure in pulmonary capillaries is the primary determinant of pulmonary edema, but edema formation can be greatly magnified by increased permeability of the capillary endothelium (Figure 8–7). In a healthy lung, pulmonary capillary pressure must exceed approximately 25 mm Hg before lung lymphatic reserve is exhausted and pulmonary edema develops. However, in the setting of increased capillary endothelial permeability, such as that which occurs in the acute respiratory distress syndrome (ARDS), even small increases in capillary hydrostatic pressure within the physiologic range can cause significant lung water accumulation. The terms "hydrostatic pulmonary edema" and "permeability pulmonary edema" have been coined to describe the primary pathophysiologic mechanism driving edema formation. In clinical practice, hydrostatic pulmonary edema is more common than permeability pulmonary edema.

High pulmonary capillary hydrostatic pressure is most commonly observed in patients with left heart disease, such as left ventricular systolic dysfunction, left ventricular diastolic dysfunction, and mitral or aortic valve disease. Hydrostatic pulmonary edema may also be observed in patients who are volume overloaded due to renal failure.

A less common cause of pulmonary edema is an acute elevation in pulmonary artery pressure. When pulmonary artery pressure is chronically elevated,

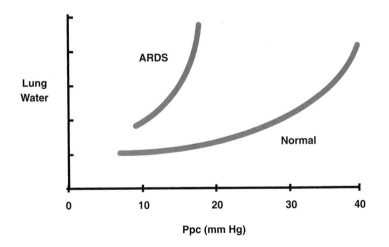

Figure 8–7. Relationship between pulmonary capillary hydrostatic pressure (Ppc) and pulmonary edema formation. Because fluid flux is less than the lymphatic drainage capacity, extravascular water does not begin to accumulate in the normal lung until pulmonary capillary hydrostatic pressures exceed 25 mm Hg. However, in the setting of increased permeability of the capillary endothelium, as occurs in acute respiratory distress syndrome (ARDS), flux out of the capillaries is greater at any given capillary hydrostatic pressure. Lymphatic capacity is easily exceeded at low capillary pressures, leading to pulmonary edema.

increased pulmonary arterial resistance generally protects the pulmonary capillary bed from the high hydrostatic pressures. However, if pulmonary artery pressure rises suddenly, such as during generalized tonic-clonic seizures or unacclimatized high-altitude exposure, or following narcotic drug overdose, significant pulmonary edema may result.

Rarely, pulmonary venous resistance may be selectively increased due to sclerosis or thrombosis of pulmonary veins, a condition known as pulmonary veno-occlusive disease. Pulmonary veno-occlusive disease may be observed following chemotherapy, bone marrow transplantation, or may occur idiopathically.

Permeability pulmonary edema results from injury to the alveolar-capillary membrane. Injury may initially begin either on the endothelial side or on the epithelial side of the membrane. Endothelial injury most commonly occurs as a result of the systemic inflammatory response syndrome (SIRS), the body's hypermetabolic response to life-threatening infection, major trauma, pancreatitis, or massive transfusion. Epithelial injury can result from toxic gas inhalation or gastric acid aspiration. Once injured, the alveolar-capillary membrane becomes more porous to both fluid and proteins, resulting in alveolar flooding at normal hydrostatic pressures.

Plasma oncotic pressure is usually slightly higher than interstitial oncotic pressure. This oncotic pressure gradient helps to draw fluid from the lung interstitium back into the vascular compartment. Low plasma oncotic pressure, as is seen in protein losing states such as nephrotic syndrome, is never the sole cause of pulmonary edema. This is likely due to the observation that such protein losing states also lower the interstitial oncotic pressure to an equal degree. However, an acute fall in the plasma oncotic pressure out of proportion to that in the tissue compartment may aggravate preexisting permeability or hydrostatic edema formation. This situation may occur during massive resuscitation with intravenous crystalloid solutions.

Relatively little is known about the control of lung lymph flow in health or disease. Rarely, impaired drainage due to cancer obstructing lung or mediastinal lymph nodes may lead to congestion of the lung parenchyma.

Diagnostic & Clinical Considerations

The accumulation of extravascular lung water reduces static lung compliance and deranges gas exchange, both of which lead to a reflex increase in respiratory drive. Regardless of the cause of pulmonary edema, shortness of breath is a universal symptom. In patients with pulmonary edema, breathlessness is usually aggravated by assumption of the supine position (orthopnea), since this position is associated with higher hydrostatic pressures in the lung compared to those in the upright position. On physical examination, the respiratory rate is usually markedly elevated and respiratory excursions may be reduced. Inspiratory crackles may be audible over the chest. In patients with left heart disease as the cause of pulmonary venous hypertension and pulmonary edema, the cardiac silhouette on the chest radiograph is usually enlarged and the lung parenchyma opacified by patchy infiltrates (Figure 8–8A). The accumulation of extravascular lung water within interlobular septae can be visualized as Kerley B lines on chest radiograph (Figure 8–8B).

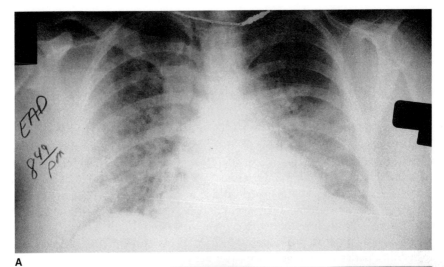

A

Figure 8–8. Use of the chest x-ray in the diagnosis of pulmonary edema. **A.** A 45-year-old man with left ventricular systolic dysfunction due to previous anteroseptal myocardial infarction. Bibasilar parenchymal infiltrates and cardiomegaly are seen. Bibasilar crackles were heard on auscultation. **B.** A 35-year-old man with mitral stenosis due to previous rheumatic fever (arrow). Pulmonary interstitial edema can thicken the interlobular septae, which are seen as horizontal white lines approximately 1 cm in length abutting the pleura. These are termed Kerley B lines.

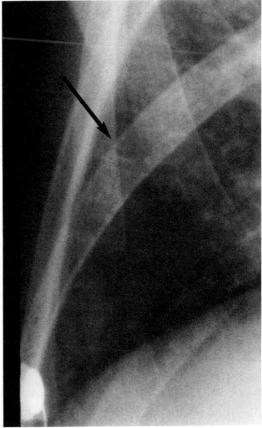

B

Echocardiography provides a reliable assessment of left ventricular performance and aortic and mitral valve function. In cases where transthoracic echocardiographic (TTE) studies are difficult, for example, patients with severe COPD or obesity, transesophageal echocardiographic (TEE) studies with a flexible transducer can provide excellent images.

Management Principles

Therapy of hydrostatic pulmonary edema is directed at lowering the pulmonary capillary pressure. If the cause is heart disease, treatment often involves the use of diuretics. Inotropic agents and/or vasodilators are usually employed to improve left ventricular function if it is depressed. Valvular heart disease is often amenable to surgical correction. Volume overload due to renal failure may require dialysis, while narcotic overdose, neurogenic pulmonary edema, and high-altitude pulmonary edema will often resolve with supportive measures only. Oxygen is always indicated in hypoxemic individuals. Mechanical ventilation is used in severe cases to stabilize patients while other therapies are explored. Use of PEEP in conjunction with mechanical ventilation helps recruit alveoli and improve oxygenation until the edema fluid is cleared.

PULMONARY VASCULITIS

General Considerations

Pulmonary vasculitis is a term used to describe a broad range of clinical entities that pathologically show inflammation and vascular destruction (Table 8–3). Lung involvement can be seen in all forms of vasculitis, but is more commonly present in the small vessel or antineutrophil-associated vasculitides. When pulmonary involvement is present, hypoxemia and hemoptysis can be life threatening.

Pathophysiology

Wegener granulomatosis is a small-medium vessel vasculitis characterized by necrotizing granulomatous inflammation. It is the most common of the antineutrophil cytoplasmic antibody (ANCA)-associated vasculitides. Involvement of the upper airway, lower respiratory tract, and kidney are common.

Churg-Strauss syndrome is another small-medium vessel, ANCA positive vasculitis, which occurs in the setting of asthma, hypereosinophilia, pulmonary infiltrates, and allergic rhinitis. The pathology reveals eosinophilic inflammation with granuloma formation. Manifestations of Churg-Strauss are protean and include

Table 8–3. Common pulmonary vasculitides

- Wegener granulomatosis
- Churg-Strauss syndrome
- Goodpasture syndrome
- Pauci-immune capillaritis

upper and lower respiratory tract, skin lesions, cardiovascular, neurologic, renal and gastrointestinal disease. Asthma usually precedes the vasculitis phase of the disease by many years.

Goodpasture syndrome is a pulmonary-renal syndrome that affects predominantly men between the ages of 18 and 60. While only a minority of patients with Goodpasture syndrome have histopathologic evidence of true vasculitis, the disease presents in fashion similar to other pulmonary vasulitides. Lung and kidney involvement may occur simultaneously or sequentially. Autoantibodies directed against the glomerular basement membrane in the kidney disrupt the integrity of capillaries in the glomerulus resulting in hematuria and acute kidney failure. These same autoantibodies cross-react with basement membranes in the lung causing diffuse alveolar hemorrhage.

Pauci-immune capillaritis of the lung mimics Goodpasture syndrome in that it causes diffuse alveolar hemorrhage. However, unlike Goodpasture, autoantibodies are not present and the kidney is not involved.

Diagnostic & Clinical Consideration

Multiple history and physical exam findings can alert practitioners to the diagnosis of systemic and/or pulmonary vasculitides. Symptoms are related to the organ systems involved and include sinusitis, subglottic stenosis, cough, chest pain, shortness of breath and hemoptysis, and a decreased hematocrit. Rapidly progressive glomerulonephritis, identified by hematuria, red blood cell casts, chest radiographs with nodular or cavitary disease, palpable purpura on skin exam, and mononeuritis multiplex should also raise suspicion for vasculitis.

A search for antiglomerular basement membrane antibodies, ANCA, and other autoantibodies is warranted in selected cases; however, surgical biopsy of involved organs is the gold standard for diagnosis.

Management Principles

Alveolar hemorrhage can be rapidly fatal. Death is usually not due to exsanguination but rather is due to drowning. Emergent management is focused on trying to optimize gas exchange and the airway clearance of blood. Intubation and mechanical ventilation may be necessary.

DISORDERS OF THE BRONCHIAL CIRCULATION

The bronchial circulation rarely becomes of concern to clinicians. However, chronic infectious and inflammatory or necrotizing diseases of the lung such as tuberculosis or bronchiectasis can lead to an increase in the size and number of bronchial arteries with intense neovascularization with resultant hemorrhage. Some of these arteries can form collaterals with intercostal arteries. Because bronchial arteries originate from the high-pressure systemic circulation, when necrosis of lung parenchyma involves these bronchial vessels, life-threatening hemoptysis can occur (see Chapter 3 for further details of pathophysiology in this context).

CLINICAL SCENARIOS

Case 1

A 49-year-old woman is referred to the rheumatology clinic with complaints of shortness of breath and blue fingers over the past 5 months. She also complains of dyspepsia, dry cough, and tightening of the skin around her mouth.

Physical Examination: Her examination is remarkable for distended neck veins, a loud pulmonic component of her second heart sound, and a right ventricular heave. Pulmonary function shows a forced vital capacity of 80% of predicted but a diffusing capacity of only 35% of predicted. Her oxyhemoglobin saturation is 93% on room air.

Her chest x-ray is normal except for cardiomegaly. On echocardiography her right atrium and ventricle are dilated and her pulmonary artery systolic pressure is estimated to be 85 mm Hg. She has a normal ventilation-perfusion lung scan. Pulmonary hypertension is confirmed by right heart catheterization.

Discussion: There are classic symptoms of scleroderma. Her shortness of breath could be due to parenchymal fibrosis and this would also explain her cough. Her cough could also be due to gastroesophageal reflux, since esophageal dysmotility is common in scleroderma. Respiratory symptoms such as shortness of breath associated with the skin changes, Raynaud's phenomenon, and acrocyanosis seen in this patient usually imply a connective tissue disorder. Pulmonary manifestations of scleroderma include fibrotic/interstitial lung disease (about 70% of patients) and pulmonary vascular disease (about 10% of patients) resulting in pulmonary hypertension. There is also an increased risk of lung cancer in these patients.

CLINICAL PEARL

A low diffusing capacity out of proportion to the forced vital capacity in a dyspneic patient with scleroderma is highly suggestive of pulmonary arterial hypertension.

Case 2

A 50-year-old woman develops acute shortness of breath 1 week after beginning chemotherapy for stage 4 breast cancer. As cancer is a major risk factor for venous thromboembolism, the diagnosis of acute pulmonary embolism is entertained. Her physical exam is normal except for tachypnea.

Physical Examination: Full anticoagulation with low molecular weight heparin is initiated in the emergency department before her work-up is begun, since early anticoagulation is the best way to prevent recurrence. She is sent for a $\dot{V}/\dot{Q}$ scan. Her scan shows several segmental $\dot{V}/\dot{Q}$ mismatches (normal ventilation with absent perfusion). This scan pattern in a high-risk patient confirms the diagnosis of pulmonary embolism. She is also started on warfarin and her low molecular weight heparin is continued for 5 more days because it takes 4–5 days to get the maximum anticoagulant effect of warfarin. She is discharged home with an International Normalized Ratio (INR) of 2.5 and followed up in the oncology clinic. Because her breast cancer is advanced she is considered to be at lifelong risk for recurrent pulmonary embolism. The decision is made to continue her warfarin for life with monthly monitoring of her INR.

Discussion: In this patient, based on clinical grounds, acute pulmonary embolism is suspected. Immediate anticoagulation should be initiated pending results of confirmatory tests. Both $\dot{V}/\dot{Q}$ scan and spiral CT with a pulmonary embolism protocol can be used to confirm this diagnosis. However, the pulmonary angiogram remains the gold standard diagnostic test. The duration of anticoagulation therapy in thromboembolic disease depends on the underlying conditions and risk stratification.

CLINICAL PEARL

Because the physical exam is insensitive and nonspecific for the diagnosis of venous thromboembolism, patients with risk factors for pulmonary embolism and unexplained chest pain or dyspnea should undergo formal testing.

KEY CONCEPTS

Pulmonary hypertension most commonly presents with dyspnea, chest pain, or syncope. In experienced hands Doppler echocardiography is a sensitive screening tool for pulmonary hypertension and can help exclude congenital heart disease. Primary pulmonary hypertension is a diagnosis of exclusion. A search for the etiology of pulmonary hypertension should include a careful history for prescription and illicit drug use, a thorough physical exam, liver function tests, imaging studies, arterial blood gas, full pulmonary function tests, a ventilation-perfusion lung scan, an echocardiogram, and appropriate serologies for collagen vascular diseases.

Pulmonary embolism should be strongly considered in any patient who has unexplained dyspnea and risk factors for venous thromboembolism. The physical exam and basic laboratory testing cannot exclude this diagnosis and other supplemental tests are required to rule out the diagnosis of venous thromboembolic disease.

STUDY QUESTIONS

8–1. *A 71-year-old man develops acute shortness of breath 5 days after a hip fracture that he sustained in a fall. He is tachypneic, has a blood pressure of 100/60 mm Hg, and has distended neck veins. He has a $\dot{V}/Q$ lung scan performed that shows three large segmental matched $\dot{V}/Q$ defects. An ultrasound of his lower extremities is negative. You would next*

    a. *perform a CT angiogram*

    b. *measure the D-dimer level*

    c. *treat with warfarin for 6 months*

    d. observe

    e. repeat the ultrasound of his lower extremities.

8–2.   A 30-year-old woman presents to your office complaining of 2 years of progressive dyspnea on exertion. Her physical exam is remarkable for central cyanosis, distended neck veins, ascites, and leg edema. Her second heart sound is split during both inspiration and expiration and the pulmonic component is accentuated. She has normal respiratory excursions and auscultation of her lungs is normal.

       The most likely cause of this patient's pulmonary hypertension is

    a. primary pulmonary hypertension

    b. chronic pulmonary embolism

    c. atrial septal defect

    d. asthma

    e. systolic left ventricular failure.

8–3.   A 65-year-old man is admitted to the intensive care unit with acute onset of severe shortness of breath while climbing stairs. He has a history of rheumatic fever as a child. His physical exam is remarkable for atrial fibrillation with a heart rate of 130 beats/min. He has diffuse crackles on auscultation of his lungs and a diastolic rumbling murmur over the lower left sternal border. His chest radiograph shows perihilar patchy infiltrates with thickened septal lines. Which of the following diagnostic tests would be most useful in determining the cause of his pulmonary edema?

    a. Measurement of plasma oncotic pressure

    b. Echocardiogram

    c. Measurement of pulmonary artery occlusion pressure

    d. Ventilation-perfusion lung scan

    e. Arterial blood gas.

8–4.   A 35-year-old man with sarcoidosis has had recurrent exacerbations of bronchiectasis over the past several years. Each event has been associated with copious purulent sputum production and low-grade fever. He has been coughing up blood for 6 hours and has now expectorated a total of 150 mL. His chest radiograph 6 hours ago was unchanged from the one obtained last month. The best way to identify the location of the bleeding vessel is to

    a. perform a bronchial arteriogram

    b. perform a pulmonary arteriogram

    c. measure the partial oxygen pressure of the expectorated blood

    d. repeat his chest radiograph

    e. ask the patient.

SUGGESTED READINGS

Dalen JE, ed. Venous thromboembolism. In: *Lung Biology in Health and Disease.* Vol. 180. Tucson: University of Arizona, Marcel Dekker; 2003.

Peacock AJ, Rubin LJ, eds. *Pulmonary Circulation.* London: Edward Arnold; 2004.

Occupational/Inhalational/Environmental Disease

9

Judd Shellito

OBJECTIVES

▶ *Identify the lung diseases caused by inhalation of foreign material from the environment or during the course of specific occupations.*

▶ *Identify the lung diseases related to adverse environmental conditions such as near drowning and ascent to high altitudes (mountain sickness).*

▶ *Understand the pathophysiology of pulmonary reactions to these insults.*

▶ *Describe the clinical presentation and treatment of the various disorders.*

GENERAL CONSIDERATIONS: FACTORS AFFECTING DEPOSITION OF INHALED MATERIAL

The site of deposition of material inhaled into the respiratory tract is dependent on water solubility for gases and particle size for solids. Highly soluble gases such as ammonia will be trapped in the moist mucus lining of the nose and oropharynx, while less soluble gases such as phosgene may cause damage to the large airways or the lung parenchyma. Particle size or aerodynamic diameter is of greatest importance in determining the level of deposition for inhaled particulates (Figure 9–1). Large particles (>10 μm) are efficiently filtered by the nose, although filtration efficiency decreases with exercise because of mouth breathing and increased airflow. Particles 3–10 μm in diameter are deposited preferentially in the trachea and large airways, while particles 0.1–3 μm in size reach the alveolar space. Very small particles (<0.1 μm) do not settle out from the air stream and are poorly deposited at any location in the respiratory tract, and many are exhaled. For inhaled fibers, deposition is based upon their aerodynamic diameter rather than length, which explains why very long asbestos fibers may penetrate deeply into lung tissue.

The likelihood that an inhaled gas or particle will cause pulmonary disease is dependent not just on deposition within the respiratory tract, but also on the total burden of inhaled material retained in the lungs over time. Tissue burden is not only influenced by particle size, but also by the concentration of material within

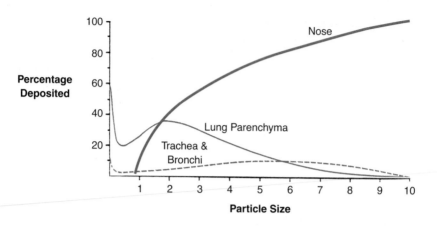

Figure 9–1. Where an inhaled particle deposits within the respiratory tract is dependent upon the size of the particle. (Based on data from Bates DV, Fish BR, et al: Deposition and retention models for internal dosimetry of the human respiratory tract. Task group on lung dynamics. *Health Phys.* 1966;12:173.)

the inhaled air stream, the duration of exposure, and the clearance mechanisms operative at various anatomic levels of the respiratory tract. Thus, both short-term but high-intensity and low-intensity but long-term exposures may cause pulmonary disease. Finally, host factors due to genetic differences or concomitant pulmonary disease such as emphysema significantly influence pulmonary reactions to inhaled materials.

OCCUPATIONAL ASTHMA

Occupational asthma is defined as sensitivity to inhaled materials in the workplace with development of asthmatic symptoms de novo. It should be distinguished from exacerbation of underlying asthma in the workplace environment related to fumes, dusts, cold air, and the like. Occupational asthma requires both exposure to a specific antigen and individual susceptibility. The mechanisms for this susceptibility are poorly understood, but it is well recognized that one worker may develop asthma while many coworkers with identical exposures remain asymptomatic.

Pathogenesis

Occupational asthma can be divided into two categories depending on the molecular weight of the implicated antigen. High molecular weight antigens are often organic in nature. Workers who develop asthma in relation to these antigens are often atopic and presumably more susceptible to asthma. For example, animal care workers may become sensitized to animal proteins, and bakers may develop asthma in response to inhalation of flour. Low molecular weight antigens may also induce an asthmatic response, but there is often no underlying atopy. Examples of such antigens include plicatic acid which is contained in red cedar wood and toluene diisocyanate which is contained in some paints and chemicals.

Occupational asthma requires the generation of an immune response to an inhaled antigen, the proliferation of antigen-specific T-lymphocyte clones, and the elaboration of specific antibodies (IgE and IgG) to the offending antigen. These antibodies may become fixed to mast cells in the airways. Inhalation of the antigen stimulates mast cell release of histamine and other proinflammatory substances. Chemoattractants are released for eosinophils and neutrophils, resulting in cellular infiltration of the airway walls, mucosal edema, and mucus secretion. Many of the mediators released also stimulate constriction of airway smooth muscle.

Pathophysiology

The end result of this sequence of events is airway obstruction and increased resistive work of breathing. Static lung compliance is unaltered, but airway obstruction reduces dynamic compliance. Thus, many alveoli have delayed emptying and may not empty fully at the end of exhalation. Retained air within these lung units will increase residual volume (RV) and functional residual capacity (FRC). Gas exchange is also compromised during an asthma attack, since mediator release interferes with hypoxic pulmonary vasoconstriction and poorly ventilated alveoli are perfused, causing hypoxemia. In severe asthma, the increased resistive work of breathing may precipitate acute respiratory failure with CO_2 retention and respiratory acidosis. However, asthma is a reversible disease. With treatment or cessation of exposure to the antigen, all of these pathophysiologic processes may resolve completely.

Diagnostic & Clinical Implications

SYMPTOMS & PHYSICAL FINDINGS

Because occupational asthma involves immunologic sensitization, there is often a delayed period from first exposure to the development of symptoms. This latent interval varies from weeks to years. Many workers with occupational asthma complain of chest tightness, wheezing, cough, and dyspnea within 10–20 minutes of exposure to a particular material. If they are examined immediately, it may be found that such workers have tachypnea and wheezing on auscultation of the chest. However, with removal from antigen exposure, the symptoms resolve and the findings on physical examination are often normal. Other workers may have a delayed or late onset of bronchoconstriction following exposure (see section on pulmonary function tests [PFTs] below). In these individuals, symptoms may not occur until 4–6 hours after exposure, which may make it difficult to relate the symptoms to a specific exposure.

IMAGING

Because asthma affects the airways and not the alveoli, the chest x-ray is usually normal. During an attack or with repeated attacks, hyperinflation may be visible on x-ray.

PULMONARY FUNCTION TESTS

Pulmonary function abnormalities in occupational asthma vary with time after antigen exposure. Twenty-four hours after exposure, pulmonary function may be normal. The hallmark of occupational asthma is a bronchoconstrictor response to the specific antigen implicated in the disease. This response can be duplicated in the laboratory with aerosolization of graded concentrations of the suspect antigen with repetitive pulmonary function testing. Such an inhalation challenge can be very helpful in identifying specific antigens responsible for symptoms so that work practices can be modified to decrease exposure. Patients with occupational asthma are hyperresponsive to specific antigens and show an exaggerated drop in forced expiratory volume in the first second (FEV_1) and in the FEV_1:FVC (forced vital capacity) ratio with the causal antigen, and no change in FEV_1 with irrelevant antigens. Two patterns are seen in response to aerosolized antigen. Early or immediate-onset reactions may be seen within 10–20 minutes and last for about 2 hours. These reactions generally reflect IgE-mediated responses. In other patients, reactions are delayed (late onset) for 4–6 hours following exposure and may last for up to 24 hours. These reactions may reflect IgG-mediated responses. Combination, or dual-onset, responses are also seen.

Management Principles

Therapy for occupational asthma revolves around identifying the causal antigen and modifying work practices to eliminate further exposure. Bronchodilators and corticosteroids may help treat symptomatic workers but will eventually fail if antigen exposure continues.

LUNG DISEASE FOLLOWING INHALATION OF INORGANIC DUSTS: PNEUMOCONIOSES

Pneumoconioses are fibrotic lung diseases of the pulmonary parenchyma following chronic inhalation of inorganic dusts, typically during work exposures such as mining. The three pneumoconioses discussed here are silicosis, coal worker's pneumoconiosis (CWP), and asbestosis.

Silicosis follows the inhalation of airborne silica fibers. High-risk occupations include hard rock miner, stone cutter, foundry worker, sandblaster, and ceramic worker. Acute and accelerated forms of silicosis have been described, but most cases occur in workers with long-term exposure (more than 15 years).

CWP is caused by the inhalation of coal dust during mining or processing of coal. Similar conditions may occasionally be seen in graphite miners. Coal dust is not a uniform material but contains variable amounts of carbon and mineral contaminants, including clay and quartz. In many coal miners, lung disease is caused by quartz contained in the coal and is more accurately termed silicosis than CWP.

Asbestosis follows the inhalation of asbestos fibers. Asbestos is a group of fibrous silicates with widespread application in industry. High-risk occupations include asbestos miner, asbestos textile worker, sheet metal and insulation worker, boilermaker, and pipefitter.

Pathogenesis

Retention of inhaled inorganic particles stimulates fibrosis within the lung interstitium. Lung tissue from workers with silicosis shows fibrotic nodules preferentially involving the upper lobes. Microscopically, these nodules can be seen to contain silica fibers in the center surrounded by whorls of collagen and a cellular capsule containing fibroblasts. Silicotic nodules are initially localized around respiratory bronchioles and arterioles and in paraseptal and subpleural locations. With advanced disease, the surrounding fibrosis destroys lung tissue, and nodules may become confluent. Nodules may also be found in hilar lymph nodes, which often show peripheral, or "eggshell," calcification. In CWP, the principal pathologic lesion is the coal macule, a pigmented lesion containing dust-laden macrophages surrounding respiratory bronchioles. In contrast to silicotic nodules, coal macules contain little collagen and there is no surrounding fibrosis. Lungs of workers with asbestosis show peribronchiolar fibrosis characteristically involving the lower lobes. Alveolar spaces may be filled with inflammatory cells, and asbestos bodies (asbestos fibers or other mineral particles such as glass, iron, or talc coated with hemosiderin, generically called ferruginous bodies) are usually seen with special stains.

Pathophysiology

The consequence of parenchymal fibrosis in silicosis and asbestosis is decreased lung compliance due to increased elastic recoil. Since affected individuals must therefore generate a greater transpulmonary pressure to inflate the lungs to the same volume, the work of breathing is increased, initially with exercise, and with advanced disease at rest. In asbestosis, although airways may be destroyed, pulmonary resistance is usually normal. In silicosis, involvement of small airways may contribute to airflow obstruction and emphysema. In CWP, the absence of fibrosis means that both lung compliance and resistance are normal unless there is concomitant silicosis or smoking-related obstructive disease.

Besides parenchymal fibrosis, inhaled asbestos fibers also migrate to reach the parietal pleura, where they commonly stimulate the formation of fibrous plaques with calcification. Extensive pleural plaques may cause increased tissue resistance (decreased chest wall compliance) and increased work of breathing. Pleural plaques are also seen to a lesser extent in silicosis. Pleural reactions are not seen in CWP.

Work exposures to both asbestos and silica are associated with increased risk of intrathoracic malignancy. By itself, CWP does not alter individual cancer risk. The signal neoplasm associated with asbestos exposure is malignant mesothelioma. This rare and usually fatal tumor may involve the pleural or peritoneal space. Approximately three quarters of patients with malignant mesothelioma have a significant work or environmental exposure to asbestos. Asbestos workers are also at increased risk for all types of lung cancer, particularly if they also smoke cigarettes. The increased risk of lung cancer appears to be restricted to those workers who have developed parenchymal fibrosis or asbestosis. Emerging epidemiologic evidence supports a similar relationship between silicosis and lung cancer.

Diagnostic & Clinical Implications

SYMPTOMS & PHYSICAL FINDINGS

Symptoms are caused by increased work of breathing as well as through stimulation of nerves in the interstitial space (J receptors). Exertional dyspnea is slowly progressive over many years. A productive or nonproductive cough may also be present. In

CWP, symptoms usually reflect tobacco-related disease rather than the pneumoconiosis itself. Physical findings include inspiratory crackles on auscultation of the chest. Digital clubbing may be present in asbestosis but not in silicosis or CWP.

IMAGING

Most individuals with these disorders exhibit abnormal findings on chest x-ray, but in as many as 10%, the x-ray findings may be normal. In silicosis the chest x-ray pattern is one of small nodular opacities involving mainly the upper lung fields. The reasons for this upper lung zone pattern are unknown. Calcification of the hilar lymph nodes may be seen with an eggshell pattern. In a complicated form of silicosis called progressive massive fibrosis (PMF), the nodular opacities coalesce to form large conglomerate shadows in the upper lobes and perihilar regions. In CWP, opacities are also seen preferentially in the upper lung zones and also have a nodular or rounded appearance. PMF may be seen due to coexisting silicosis. In asbestosis, irregular and linear rather than nodular opacities are the rule, preferentially involving the lower lung fields. Pleural plaques, often with calcification, may be seen involving the hemidiaphragms or the lateral portions of the chest wall. Pleural adhesions described as rounded atelectasis have been described which may mimic mass lesions on the x-ray. It is important to distinguish asbestos-related pleural plaques from the disease process asbestosis which implies a clinical and physiological derangement of lung parenchyma with radiographic and/or pathologic confirmation in a patient with asbestos exposure (Table 9–1).

PULMONARY FUNCTION TESTS

PFTs depend on the type of pneumoconiosis and the severity of the disease. Because many patients with pneumoconioses also smoke cigarettes, the presence of cigarette-related emphysema or chronic bronchitis will also influence the results of PFTs. In simple silicosis of mild intensity, silicotic nodules in lung parenchyma have little discernible influence on pulmonary function. However, with more advanced disease and particularly with PMF, lung compliance decreases and restrictive changes may be seen on spirometric testing (decreased FVC and FEV_1, and normal FEV_1:FVC ratio) and measurement of static lung volumes (decreased total lung capacity [TLC], FRC, and RV). The diffusing capacity (D_{LCO}) may also be decreased due to interstitial fibrosis. In some patients with silicosis, involvement of the small airways may produce an obstructive defect on pulmonary function testing. Because of the absence of fibrosis, CWP usually exhibits no abnormality on PFTs. On the other hand, asbestosis may produce severe restrictive defects with decreased FVC, TLC, and D_{LCO}.

Management Principles

There is no specific treatment for any of the pneumoconioses. Affected workers should be removed or precluded from further exposure to dust. Oxygen is indicated in the presence of hypoxemia, along with bronchodilators if there is obstructive disease. Smokers should be encouraged to stop smoking cigarettes. Silicosis is associated with a unique predisposition to infection with *Mycobacterium tuberculosis*. The reasons for this are not fully understood but may be related to altered

Table 9-1. Imaging features of various lung disorders caused by inhalation of foreign materials

	Silicosis	CWP	Asbestosis
Exposure	Airborne silica	Coal dust clay/quartz	Asbestos fibers
Occupation	Stone cutters and blasting/ceramics	Coal mining/graphite miners	Asbestos miners/sheet metals/insulation/pipefitter
Pathophysiology	Pulmonary fibrosis/nodules restriction	Coal macules but no fibrosis	Peribronchial fibrosis/pleural plaques/asbestos bodies/restriction
Radiographic	Small nodular opacities in the upper zone; egg-shell calcified lymph nodes; PMF	Nodules in the upper zones	Linear and irregular opacities in the lower zones; pleural plaques; rounded atelectasis
Risks	Malignancy; TB		Mesothelioma, intrapulmonary malignancy

host defense function of alveolar macrophages due to internalized silica fibers. All workers with silicosis should receive skin testing for tuberculosis, and acute or latent tuberculosis should be ruled out.

LUNG DISEASE FOLLOWING INHALATION OF ORGANIC DUSTS: HYPERSENSITIVITY PNEUMONITIS

Repetitive inhalation of antigenic material (usually organic in nature) may stimulate an inflammatory reaction in the pulmonary alveolar and interstitial spaces. The generic term for this disease process is *hypersensitivity pneumonitis* (HP), although the condition has often been described in relationship to specific occupations, such as "farmer's lung" and "bird breeder's lung." The disorder has also been called extrinsic allergic alveolitis.

HP has been linked to a wide variety of antigen exposures (Table 9–2). The antigenic material must be inhaled repetitively to produce the disease. HP does not follow one-time or sporadic exposures.

The antigens responsible for HP can be grouped into four categories:

1. *Fungal:* The most common cause of HP and the cause of farmer's lung, particularly the thermophilic actinomycetes.
2. *Animal:* Exposure to avian proteins in bird droppings or feathers may result in bird breeder's lung.
3. *Bacterial:* Exposure to *Bacillus subtilis* in detergent workers.
4. *Inorganic:* Some exposures to toluene diisocyanate, trimellitic anhydride, or nitrofurantoin.

Table 9–2. Causes of hypersensitivity pneumonitis

Causes	Condition	Antigen
Fungal	Farmer's lung	Thermophilic actinomycetes
	Air conditioner lung	Thermophilic actinomycetes
	Bagassosis	Thermophilic actinomycetes
	Mushroom worker's lung	Thermophilic actinomycetes
	Malt worker's lung	*Aspergillus clavatus*
	Cheese washer's lung	*Penicillium casei*
	Maple bark stripper's disease	*Cryptostroma corticale*
	Sequoiosis	*Aureobasidium pullulans*
	Woodworker's disease	*Cryptostroma corticale*
	Suberosis	*Penicillium frequentans*
	Paprika splitter's lung	*Mucor* spp
	Dry rot lung	*Merulius lacrymans*
	"Dog house disease"	*Aspergillus versicolor*
	Lycoperdonosis	*Lycoperdon* spp
Animal	Bird breeder's lung	Avian protein, bloom
	Rat handler's lung	Rat protein
	Wheat weevil disease	Wheat Weevil
	Furrier's lung	Animal fur
	Pituitary snuff taker's lung	Ox and pork protein
Chemical	Isocyanate lung	TDI, MDI, HDI
	Pauli's reagent lung	Pauli's reagent
	Vineyard sprayer's lung	Bordeaux mixture
	Hard metal disease	Cobalt
	Cromolyn sodium lung	Cromolyn sodium
Bacterial	Washing powder lung	*B subtilis* enzymes
	Bacillus subtilis alveolitis	*B subtilis*
	Bacillus cereus alveolitis	*B cereus*
Uncertain	Sauna lung	Lake water (?)
	New Guinea lung	Hut thatch (?)
	Ramin lung	Ramin wood (?)
	Insecticide lung	Pyrethrum (?)

Note: HDI, hexamethylene diisocyanate; MDI, methylene bisphenyl isocyanate; TDI, toluene diisocyanate.
Source: Reproduced with permission from Morgan WK, Seaton A. *Occupational Lung Diseases.* 3rd ed. Philadelphia: Saunders; 1995:526.

Pathogenesis

The pathogenesis of HP probably involves a combination of type III (immune complex) and type IV (cell-mediated) immune responses to an inhaled antigen. Presumably these immune reactions to inhaled antigens are somehow unregulated and cause tissue injury. Because most workers exposed to inhaled antigens never develop HP, it has been proposed that those workers who do develop disease may have an immunoregulatory defect. HP is not type I or IgE mediated and does not characteristically involve the airways. Lung tissue from patients with HP shows interstitial and alveolar infiltrates of mononuclear cells and plasma cells with noncaseating sarcoid-like granulomata. In advanced cases, there may be few granulomata and varying degrees of collagenous fibrosis.

Pathophysiology

Infiltration of inflammatory cells into the alveoli and pulmonary interstitium along with edema fluid decreases lung compliance, causing increased work of breathing. Hypoxemia is often present due to ventilation-perfusion mismatch. The inflammatory process may trigger systemic symptoms of fever and anorexia. Initially these physiologic abnormalities are transient, occurring 4–12 hours after antigen exposure and then slowly resolving. This latent interval is believed to represent the time necessary for inflammatory cells to be recruited into lung tissue. With continued exposure and with the advent of pulmonary fibrosis, physiologic derangement becomes permanent.

Diagnostic & Clinical Implications

SYMPTOMS & PHYSICAL FINDINGS

Clinically, HP may have an acute or a chronic presentation. In the acute syndrome, fever, chills, cough, and dyspnea are experienced 4–12 hours after antigen exposure. Crackles may be present on physical examination, but wheezing is usually not present. In the chronic syndrome, there are insidious dyspnea, cough, and weight loss with little relationship to antigen exposure or avoidance. Fever is usually not present. Inspiratory crackles may be heard in the chest.

IMAGING

In the acute syndrome, bilateral alveolar infiltrates with nodular character may be seen anywhere in the lung. Pleural effusion and hilar adenopathy are uncommon. These changes may be mistaken for an infectious pneumonia. In the chronic syndrome, increased interstitial markings representing interstitial fibrosis are seen mainly in the upper lobes. There may be hilar retraction and honeycombing. High-resolution CT (HRCT) scan is more sensitive to detect "ground-glass" radiographic changes.

PULMONARY FUNCTION TESTS

Pulmonary function abnormalities may or may not be present, depending on the time elapsed since the last exposure to antigen. When pulmonary function is abnormal, the pattern is restrictive (decreased vital capacity and normal to increased FEV_1:FVC ratio) because of decreased lung compliance. Both the TLC and D_{LCO} may be decreased below the normal range. Hypoxemia is often present, initially with exercise, and then later at rest. There is no hypercapnia because ventilatory drive is unchanged and because CO_2 is much more soluble than oxygen.

SPECIAL STUDIES

The peripheral white blood cell count is often elevated (20,000–30,000 per mL). Most of these cells are neutrophils; eosinophilia is not a common finding. Serum immunoglobulin levels may be elevated, and rheumatoid factor test results may be positive. Serum precipitating IgG antibodies to the specific antigen responsible are found in most patients. However, clinical disease can occur in the absence of such antibodies, and antibodies are found in a higher percentage of exposed workers than the percentage that actually have disease. Thus, precipitating antibodies are a marker of antigen exposure rather than disease. However, their presence can help with establishing a diagnosis of HP.

In cases in which the diagnosis is unclear, it may be helpful to rechallenge a patient with the suspect antigen. One way to do this is to return the patient to the work or hobby that resulted in the exposure and follow symptoms and lung function. In other cases the work or exposure experience can be recreated in the pulmonary function laboratory with close monitoring of symptoms, temperature, spirometric data, and DLCO. Aerosolized antigen can also be inhaled, but this is potentially dangerous (possibly causing fever or hypoxemia) and so is restricted to research centers and experienced physicians.

Management Principles

The cornerstone of treatment for patients with HP is antigen avoidance. The work or hobby experience must be modified to decrease antigen exposure and the patient followed carefully. If this is not possible, patients must change their job or hobby to avoid further exposure and progression of disease. Acute pneumonitis should resolve completely within a few weeks. Respiratory protection is of limited benefit because sensitized patients react to minute quantities of aerosolized antigen. Steroids may be helpful in acute disease but are of no proven benefit in chronic disease. In chronic disease, there may be irreversible fibrosis, making treatment largely symptomatic.

LUNG DISEASE FOLLOWING INHALATION OF TOXIC FUMES & GASES

Inhalation of noxious gases may cause a variety of pulmonary reactions. Exposure may occur in the ambient environment, as in a chemical spill; in the course of specific occupations, as in the chemical industry; or in the home, as in smoke inhalation. Accidental inhalation of smoke from fires involves complex exposures to a variety of toxic materials, including carbon monoxide, particulates, and chemical fumes.

Pathogenesis

In high concentrations some materials may displace oxygen from the inspired air, leading to asphyxia without direct pulmonary pathology. Clinical consequences are the result of hypoxemia and decreased oxygen delivery to the brain and other vital organs. Examples of such inhaled substances include carbon dioxide and methane. Pathologic reactions to inhaled materials are dependent on the type of inhaled material, its water solubility, and the presence or absence of particulate matter. Inhaled materials with irritant qualities may cause direct injury to the airways or alveoli. Highly water-soluble gases such as chlorine are dissolved in the moist membranes of the nose and oropharynx, while less soluble gases such as phosgene may cause damage to the lower respiratory tract. Airway reflexes, such as laryngeal spasm, coughing, and bronchoconstriction are often triggered upon inhalation. Damage to either the upper or lower airways may cause mucosal ulceration and bleeding.

Pathophysiology

Irritant injury to the alveoli alters alveolar capillary permeability, which if severe can lead to pulmonary edema, ventilation-perfusion imbalance, hypoxemia, and altered lung compliance. Even without an initial pulmonary edema response, inflammatory reactions in the airways following an irritant exposure may cause asthma or bronchiolitis obliterans with increased airway resistance and enhanced bronchospasm following an airway insult.

Diagnostic & Clinical Implications

SYMPTOMS & PHYSICAL FINDINGS

With asphyxiant exposures, consciousness may be lost with few other symptoms. Headache may be prominent with exposures to carbon dioxide, due to cerebral vasodilation. With irritant exposures, patients complain of profuse tearing, sore throat, skin irritation, chest tightness, and dyspnea. Physical examination reveals irritation of exposed mucous membranes and wheezing may be heard on auscultation of the chest. Intense exposures may precipitate acute pulmonary edema and acute respiratory failure with cyanosis, tachypnea, and crackles on physical examination. Inhalation exposures from fires may be complicated by burn injury to the upper airway with potential upper airway obstruction and stridor.

IMAGING

The chest x-ray is a poor indicator of either the type or the severity of toxic exposures. With asphyxiants, the chest x-ray is often normal. In irritant-induced lung injury, the chest x-ray may be normal or may show abnormalities ranging from alveolar infiltrates to diffuse pulmonary edema.

Management Principles

The immediate goal for any suspected toxic inhalation is to prevent further exposure. This usually means evacuating the patient to the outside environment. Oxygen is generally administered at 100% concentration. Intubation and mechanical ventilation may be necessary. Hyperbaric oxygen should be considered for carbon monoxide exposures if a facility is available. Most patients should be admitted to a hospital and observed for delayed effects even if the initial x-ray is normal.

NEAR DROWNING

Drowning is defined as death following submersion in a liquid. Near drowning, on the other hand, requires survival at least temporarily following a submersion episode. Drowning and near drowning affect all age groups, although most cases occur in children. In addition to adverse effects from hypoxemia and lung injury, near-drowning victims commonly suffer from hypothermia.

Pathogenesis

Following submersion, small amounts of water may be aspirated. This triggers laryngospasm to protect the airway. Ensuing hypoxemia precipitates a panic reaction in the victim. At this point, one of two pathophysiologic sequences occurs. In 85% of cases, reflex laryngospasm will resolve, allowing water to enter the trachea and distal respiratory tract. Copious amounts of water can be recovered from these victims. In an estimated 15% of cases, laryngospasm persists, and the victim experiences asphyxia and worsening hypoxemia and hypercapnia. Resuscitation or autopsy of these victims reveals no water in the lungs. In cases in which water enters the lungs, subsequent injury is determined at least in part by the tonicity of the aspirated water. Aspirated fresh water has a low tonicity and is rapidly absorbed from the alveolar space into the pulmonary capillaries. Aspirated salt water, however, is hypertonic and draws fluid into the alveoli. Thus, salt water drowning is associated with more extravascular lung water than is fresh water drowning.

Pathophysiology

If water reaches the alveolar space, both fresh and salt water can disrupt surfactant function and damage alveolar epithelial cells. This predisposes the victim to alveolar collapse and alveolar edema. Ventilation-perfusion matching is disrupted, and severe hypoxemia occurs. In many cases, this initial alveolar injury precipitates a generalized loss of alveolar capillary permeability, causing what is recognized clinically as the acute respiratory distress syndrome (ARDS).

Diagnostic & Clinical Implications

Near-drowning victims may present with cyanosis and either tachypnea or apnea. A cough may be present, often productive of frothy sputum. Abdominal distention and vomiting of swallowed water also occur. Tachycardia and hypotension are common.

Management Principles

Resuscitation of near-drowning victims should focus on reversal of hypoxemia. An airway should be secured and the victim intubated if necessary. Supplemental oxygen should be provided at the highest concentration possible. Because water in the alveoli promotes alveolar collapse, the application of positive end-expiratory pressure (PEEP) is usually indicated. The PEEP raises FRC and prevents collapse of unstable lung units, thus improving ventilation-perfusion matching and hypoxemia. All near-drowning victims should be monitored closely for 24 hours for the development of ARDS.

MOUNTAIN SICKNESS & HIGH-ALTITUDE PULMONARY EDEMA

Multiple health risks exist for travelers to high altitude. For the purposes of this discussion, high altitude is considered elevations in excess of 10,000 feet above sea level. The major pulmonary problem associated with altitude is pulmonary edema. Pulmonary edema is probably a severe manifestation of acute mountain sickness (AMS), which is also described here.

Pathogenesis

Pathologic reactions to altitude all relate to ambient hypoxia. As barometric pressure decreases with ascent, inspired oxygen tension drops significantly. This compromises tissue delivery of oxygen and sets in motion a variety of compensatory responses. Ventilatory responses to acute hypoxia may be divided into three stages. First, ascent to high altitude produces a fall in arterial oxygen tension. This stimulates peripheral chemoreceptors in the carotid and aortic bodies to increase tidal volume and respiratory rate. The resultant increased minute ventilation attenuates tissue hypoxia but is modulated by the effects of increased ventilation on acid–base homeostasis. Hypoxia-driven hypocapnia induces a respiratory alkalosis, which inhibits ventilation through actions at the central chemoreceptors. Thus, alveolar partial oxygen pressure (PAO_2) is partially corrected at the expense of respiratory alkalosis. Over several days, the next stage of acclimatization ensues as the kidneys compensate for the alkalosis by renal excretion of bicarbonate. This normalizes arterial pH (and the pH of the cerebrospinal fluid) and allows further increases in ventilation, with corresponding increases in PAO_2. The final ventilatory response to hypoxia is seen in residents at high altitude and is characterized by a fall in minute ventilation and a loss of the normal ventilatory drive to hypoxia. The reasons for this "hypoxic desensitization" are not known, but may involve long-term effects of hypoxemia on the central respiratory center.

In addition to causing ventilatory changes, high altitude also influences pulmonary hemodynamics, gas exchange, and blood volume. Pulmonary arterial pressure is increased at high altitude, presumably due to hypoxic pulmonary vasoconstriction. This local response is generally assumed to decrease perfusion to small segments of the lung with relatively poor ventilation. However, in the setting of ambient hypoxia, this vasoconstrictor reflex extends to the entire pulmonary arterial circulation, raising pulmonary arterial pressure and compromising ventilation-perfusion matching. Gas exchange is also altered at high altitude. Because of the low PAO_2 at high altitude, oxygen transfer from the alveolus to the capillary blood actually becomes the rate-limiting step for oxygen transport with exercise (ie, oxygen transfer becomes diffusion limited instead of perfusion limited). In addition, with increased cardiac output during exercise, rapid transit time across the alveolar capillaries may provide insufficient time for hemoglobin to load oxygen from the alveolus, and oxygen saturation of pulmonary venous blood will decline. Finally, polycythemia is a routine finding in residents at high altitude, due to stimulation of erythropoietin release by the kidney to increase oxygen delivery to the tissues.

Pathophysiology

AMS is a clinical syndrome believed to result from exaggeration of the mechanisms that compensate for high altitude. Headache, nausea, and insomnia are felt to be secondary to hypocapnia and cerebral vasodilation in response to hypoxemia. The syndrome is also aggravated by fluid shifts from the intravascular to the intracellular and interstitial spaces. Pulmonary edema is a potentially life-threatening form of mountain sickness. The pathophysiologic mechanisms of high-altitude pulmonary edema are unclear, but include alveolar capillary damage from very high pulmonary arterial pressures during exercise and increased alveolar capillary permeability due to hypoxia-mediated epithelial damage.

Diagnostic & Clinical Implications

AMS may be seen in association with a wide variety of outdoor activities. No longer restricted to mountaineers, mountain sickness is now seen in skiers, trekkers, and visitors to the Incan ruins in Peru. The syndrome is more likely to be seen in individuals who ascend rapidly to high altitude and is further aggravated by heavy exertion, alcohol consumption, and dehydration. Symptoms typically are delayed for several hours after reaching high altitude. Mild mountain sickness consists of headache, insomnia, lethargy, anorexia, and nausea. These symptoms may resolve during the first week. More severe symptoms include vomiting, confusion, ataxia, and coma. Pulmonary edema is characterized by dyspnea, cough, and cyanosis. Inspiratory crackles are audible on auscultation of the chest.

Management Principles

The treatment of AMS depends on its severity. In mild cases, rest is prescribed along with acetazolamide therapy. Acetazolamide is a carbonic anhydrase inhibitor that promotes renal loss of bicarbonate and accelerates the process of acclimatization. It may also decrease cerebral edema through diuresis. Other drugs have also shown some efficacy and have been used to prevent or reduce the symptoms of AMS. In severe cases of mountain sickness, supplemental oxygen is indicated along with the descent from high altitude. When mountain sickness is complicated by high-altitude pulmonary edema, the mortality rate is high, mandating prompt descent (if possible) along with supplemental oxygen.

CLINICAL SCENARIOS

Case 1

A 65-year-old man is seen in consultation for shortness of breath. He states that his shortness of breath has been present for many years but is getting slowly worse. He now becomes dyspneic after climbing one flight of stairs. He has had a morning cough for many years that produces scanty sputum. He has a 60–pack-year cigarette smoking history, and he continues to smoke. He has seen other physicians and has been told he has chronic obstructive pulmonary disease (COPD). Bronchodilator medications have been of little benefit.

His past medical history is negative for other forms of lung disease. There is no history of heart disease. Occupational history shows that he was a boilermaker working in a local shipyard for 30 years until his retirement 10 years ago, when his breathing problems prevented him from working.

Physical Examination: Physical examination reveals a pleasant male in no acute distress. His blood pressure is 156/78 mm Hg, his heart rate is 82 beats/min and regular, and his respiratory rate is 28 breaths/min. There is no jugular venous distention. Clubbing of the fingernails is present. Auscultation of the chest reveals bibasilar inspiratory crackles. There are no audible wheezes. Examination of the heart yields normal findings.

An office chest x-ray shows that the lungs are decreased in size, with irregular interstitial opacities throughout both lower lung fields. The cardiac silhouette is normal. Calcified pleural plaques are present over both hemidiaphragms.

Office spirometric testing is performed, showing a FVC of 2.12 L (52% of predicted), an FEV_1 of 1.48 L (45% of predicted), and an FEV_1:FVC ratio of 70%. More complete pulmonary function testing is performed at a local hospital, where it is determined that the TLC is 3.83 L (66% of predicted) and the D_{LCO} is 16.4 (58% of predicted).

Discussion: Not all smokers with shortness of breath have COPD. On pulmonary function testing, COPD would exhibit obstructive rather than restrictive changes and would not be associated with crackles on auscultation, digital clubbing, or interstitial opacities on chest x-ray as seen in this case. This patient has the clinical, radiographic, and pulmonary function evidence of asbestosis. The calcified pleural plaques seen on the x-ray are a marker of exposure to asbestos and do not by themselves indicate asbestosis.

CLINICAL PEARL

Pneumoconiosis may progress even after exposure to the offending material has ceased. Presumably this is due to retained mineral fibers in lung tissue, and it underscores the importance of a complete occupational history in the work-up of patients who are short of breath.

Case 2

A 42-year-old woman is seen in consultation for recurrent pneumonia. Earlier in the year she had been treated in a hospital for fever and shortness of breath. A chest x-ray had shown bilateral alveolar infiltrates. The peripheral white blood cell count was elevated. She was treated for bacterial pneumonia with antibiotics, she had a good clinical response, and the x-ray returned to normal. Now, 2 weeks after hospital discharge, she is again admitted to the hospital for recurrent fever, shortness of breath, and cough. She is a nonsmoker and gives no history of previous lung disease. She lives on a farm, where she helps her husband take care of his racing pigeons. She has noticed that she feels feverish on occasion after working in the pigeon coop.

Physical Examination: On physical examination her temperature is 38.8°C (102°F) measured orally. Her oxygen saturation on room air is 88%. Physical examination shows bibasilar inspiratory crackles. The peripheral leukocyte count is elevated at 24,000 per mL. The differential cell count is normal. The chest x-ray shows new alveolar infiltrates.

Discussion: The working diagnosis is HP, which can be confirmed by a panel of serum antibodies to antigens associated with HP. The patient recovers after a few days in the hospital and is discharged. She is instructed to avoid further exposure to birds. Two weeks later, antibodies to avian proteins are detected in the patient's serum. She experiences no further symptoms after giving up her work in the pigeon coop.

CLINICAL PEARL

HP may mimic viral or atypical pneumonia. The key to the diagnosis is the occupational history. One should be particularly suspicious of jobs or hobbies that bring a patient into contact with animal or vegetable material.

KEY CONCEPTS

 Fibrotic lung disease and increased work of breathing may follow long-term inhalation of inorganic dusts.

 Pulmonary immune responses to inhaled organic materials may be excessive and cause damage to lung tissue resulting in hypersensitivity pneumonitis.

 Workers may become sensitized to occupational antigens and develop asthma. Occupational asthma is common and underrecognized by clinicians.

STUDY QUESTIONS

9–1. A 62-year-old man with known silicosis presents to the office with a 2-month history of fever, weight loss, shortness of breath, and intermittent hemoptysis. He has a long history of work as a sandblaster along with a 40–pack-year cigarette-smoking history. Silicosis was diagnosed on a chest x-ray 20 years previously. In the office, he is an anxious-appearing man with a respiratory rate of 32 breaths/min, blood pressure of 145/85 mm Hg, and oral temperature of 38.5°C (101.4°F). Auscultation of the chest shows inspiratory crackles throughout all lung fields. There is no wheezing. A chest x-ray shows bilateral nodules that are unchanged from a previous x-ray as well as a new cavitary lesion in the right upper lung zone. An arterial blood gas analysis on room air reveals a pH of 7.42, Pco_2 of 41, Po_2 of 75, and arterial oxygen saturation of 92%. Which test or treatment would you perform first?

a. Administer supplemental oxygen at 2 L/min

b. Prescribe aerosolized bronchodilators

c. Obtain a sputum sample for tuberculosis culture

d. Administer glucocorticoids.

9–2. *A 19-year-old man is pulled unconscious from a swimming pool. He is resuscitated at the scene, with return of breathing and blood pressure, and brought to the emergency room. In the emergency room he is somnolent but arousable, with an oral temperature of 38.6°C (97.9°F), a blood pressure of 155/70 mm Hg, heart rate of 110 beats/min, and respiratory rate of 50 breaths/min. He is using his accessory muscles of ventilation. Auscultation of the chest shows basilar crackles. A chest x-ray shows bilateral alveolar infiltrates. The heart is of normal size. Arterial blood gas measurements are pH 7.50, P_{CO_2} 30, and P_{O_2} 45. The most likely cause of this man's hypoxemia is*

   a. *hypoventilation*

   b. *ventilation-perfusion mismatch*

   c. *heart failure with low mixed venous P_{O_2}.*

   d. *diffusion abnormality.*

9–3. *The clinician is evaluating a 45-year-old male for HP. He is a bird breeder with complaints of intermittent fever and shortness of breath. Chest x-rays have shown migratory infiltrates. Pulmonary function testing has been normal. Precipitating antibodies to bird proteins are present in his serum. The clinician advises him that he probably has HP and recommends that he stop his exposure to the birds. He returns to the office 6 weeks later with continued symptoms. He does not feel that he can stop working with his pigeons and asks for advice. Which of the following would you recommend?*

   a. *Hold your breath when you are in the pigeon coop.*

   b. *Build up your tolerance to the birds by spending 1 hour per day with them for 2 weeks, then 2 hours per day for 2 weeks, and so forth.*

   c. *Stop exposure to birds.*

   d. *Wear a surgical-type mask when around the birds.*

SUGGESTED READINGS

Glazer CS, Newman LS. Occupational interstitial lung disease. *Clin Chest Med.* 2004;25(3):467–478.

Selman M. Hypersensitivity pneumonitis: a multifaceted deceiving disorder. *Clin Chest Med.* 2004;25(3):531–534.

Stream JO, Grissom CK. Update on high-altitude pulmonary edema: pathogenesis, prevention, and treatment. *Wilderness Environ Med.* 2008;19(4):293–303.

Tarlo SM, Balmes J, Balkissoon R, et al. Diagnosis and management of work-related asthma: American College of Chest Physicians Consensus Statement. *Chest.* 2008;134(3 Suppl):1S–41S.

Respiratory Infections

10

Carol M. Mason & Warren R. Summer

OBJECTIVES

▶ Describe the major defensive mechanisms used by the host to remain free of respiratory tract infections.
▶ Recognize important pathogens in lower respiratory tract infections.
▶ Identify various risk factors for and clinical features of lower respiratory tract infections.
▶ Understand the principles of management for these infections.

GENERAL CONSIDERATIONS

The respiratory tract is constantly exposed to a vast number of potentially harmful agents. As efficient as our pulmonary clearance mechanisms are, infectious agents still do deposit in the airways. Thus, in spite of the availability of potent antibiotics and great advances in supportive care, respiratory tract infections remain a major cause of disease, death, and health care costs. Pneumonia is the seventh leading cause of death in the United States and the most common cause of death due to an infection.

PATHOGENESIS: LUNG HOST DEFENSE MECHANISMS

The defense system is distributed throughout the respiratory tract, from the nares to the alveolar surface (Table 10–1 and Figure 10–1). Infectious agents may gain access to the tract through inhalation of airborne droplets or aspiration of oral secretions. Smaller droplets (approximately 1–5 μm in size) remain airborne for long periods and may penetrate to the alveoli or be exhaled. Larger particles cannot remain airborne or are intercepted by anatomic barriers such as the nasal hair and turbinates, the epiglottis, and the larynx. The multiple branches of the tracheobronchial tree also serve a filtration function by causing deflection of the air stream, inducing airborne particles to impact and deposit on mucosal surfaces. The epithelium of the upper airway consists primarily of ciliated columnar epithelium covered by a mucus blanket. The cilia beat back and forth in a highly coordinated manner and interact with the mucus blanket to eventually deliver trapped

Table 10–1. Lung host defenses

Host defenses	Defect	Potential infection and sequelae
Nasopharynx		
Ciliated epithelium in nasopharynx	Poor nutrition, chronic illness, smoking, viral infection	Colonization with pathogenic bacteria
Conducting airways		
Mechanical barriers	Bypassing barriers with an endotracheal tube or tracheostomy	Colonization with pathogenic bacteria
Mucociliary clearance	Structural defects in cilia	Stagnant secretions and bronchiectasis
Cough	Depressed cough reflex	Failure to clear secretions
Bronchoconstriction	Hyperactive airways/asthma	Failure to clear secretions
	Mucus hypersecretion	ABPA/ABPM
Local immunoglobulin secretory IgA	Use of corticosteroids IgA deficiency Functional deficiency from breakdown by bacterial IgA and proteases	Sinopulmonary infections Abnormal colonization
Alveoli		
Opsonic IgG	Acquired hypogammaglobulinemia; IgG_4, IgG_2 deficiency	Pneumonia with encapsulated bacteria
Iron-containing proteins (transferrin and lactoferrin)	Iron deficiency	May not inhibit certain bacteria (*Pseudomonas spp, Escherichia coli, Legionella* spp)
Alternate complement pathway activation	C3 and C5 deficiency	Repeated bacterial infections
Surfactant	Decreased synthesis, acute lung injury	Loss of opsonization activity, pneumonia, atelectasis
Alveolar macrophages	Subtle effects from immunosuppression with inability to kill intracellular bacteria or augment antibacterial response	*Pneumocystis carinii (jiroveci) Legionella* spp *Mycobacterium* spp
PMNs	Bone marrow suppression; intrinsic defect in motility or lack of chemotactic stimulus	Poor inflammatory response, propensity for gram-negative bacillary and *Aspergillus* spp infections

Note: ABPA, allergic bronchopulmonary aspergillosis; ABPM, allergic bronchopulmonary mycosis; PMN, polymorphonuclear neutrophil.

Source: Adapted with permission from Reynolds HY: Normal and defective host defense. In: Pennington JE, ed. *Respiratory Infections: Diagnosis and Management.* 3rd ed. New York, Raven Press, 1994, pp 1–21. Chaudary M, SanPedro G: Respiratory infections. In: *Pulmonary Pathophysiology.* 1st ed. New York, McGraw-Hill, 1999, pp 115–140.

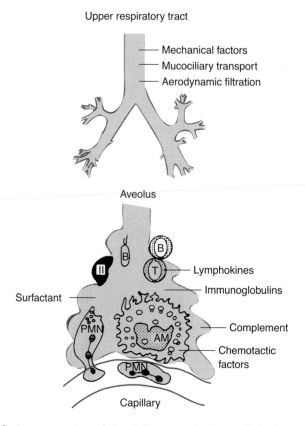

Upper respiratory tract

— Mechanical factors
— Mucociliary transport
— Aerodynamic filtration

Aveolus

— Lymphokines
— Immunoglobulins
Surfactant —
— Complement
— Chemotactic factors

Capillary

Figure 10–1. Representation of the defense mechanisms of the lung. (Reproduced with permission from Reynolds HY: Pulmonary defense mechanisms against infection. In: Fishman AP, ed. *Pulmonary Diseases and Disorders.* 2nd ed. New York, McGraw-Hill, 1988, pp 265–274.)

particles to the oropharynx (the "mucociliary escalator"), where they are coughed out or swallowed. In distal bronchioles and alveoli, other factors are brought to bear: surfactant, iron-containing proteins, such as transferrin, IgG opsonins, and complement pathway activation are other defenses that serve as barriers against inhaled particles or microorganisms.

Alveolar macrophages are the principal phagocytic cells of innate immunity in the distal air spaces. They are ultimately responsible for engulfing and destroying material that evades upper airway clearance. The macrophage may present antigens to other effector cells through a series of complex interactions involving mediators also known as cytokines, initiating a specific adaptive immune response. Assisting the macrophages are other components of the humoral immune system and various lipoproteins and glycoproteins represented in the alveolar lining fluid. Should these local defenses prove inadequate, an inflammatory reaction can be initiated, unleashing potent polymorphonuclear neutrophils, complement factors, vasome-diators, and other humoral immune elements from systemic sources. These mecha-nisms are highly efficient, rendering the lower respiratory tract sterile under normal conditions. The naso- and oropharynx are densely colonized by a complex mixture of aerobic, anaerobic, and microaerophilic bacteria. Normal oral flora may include *Streptococcus* spp including *S pneumoniae, Neisseria* spp, *Candida* spp, *Fusobacterium* spp, anaerobic streptococci, and certain *Bacteroides* spp. These organisms serve a protective function by competing with bacteria for adherence sites.

Normally sterile respiratory tract sites include the paranasal sinuses and the lower tract (arbitrarily defined as that portion of the tract distal to the vocal cords). *Haemophilus influenzae* and *Haemophilus parainfluenzae* are commonly recovered from tracheobronchial secretions of smokers, even when there is no evidence of acute infection. In patients with chronic bronchitis, tra-cheobronchial colonization is common and may include *H influenzae, H parain-fluenzae, Moraxella catarrhalis, S pneumoniae,* and occasionally gram-negative bacteria. Colonization with the last becomes particularly common in patients with ciliary dysfunction (including cystic fibrosis and bronchiectasis), patients on corticosteroid therapy, and those with immunodeficiency, prior antibiotic therapy, previous viral infection, malnutrition, or endotracheal intubation.

Thus, normal hosts with their normal flora intact are resistant to coloniza-tion by many pathogenic bacteria, even when exposed to large quantities of the organisms. In contrast, ill individuals may have their indigenous bacterial flora replaced by the more virulent pathogens. The likelihood that a given individual will have upper airway colonization by these pathogenic bacteria is directly related to the severity and duration of illness. In patients with altered consciousness with swallowing difficulty and impaired host defenses, infectious secretions may be aspirated into the airways and cause disease. Risk factors for upper airway coloni-zation include alcoholism, endotracheal intubation, neutropenia, prior antibiotic use, azotemia, coma, hypotension, smoking, surgery, prior viral illness, immuno-suppression, and malnutrition.

The humoral immune system also plays an important role in keeping the air-ways clear of potential pathogens. The immunoglobulin IgA, which accounts for up to 10% of the total protein in nasal secretions, has specific antibacterial and antiviral activity. Patients with selective IgA deficiency are at risk for recurrent upper respiratory tract infections and gram-negative lower respiratory tract infec-tions. IgG is the predominant immunoglobulin in lower airway secretions and functions as an opsonin there.

Several kinds of infectious agents are responsible for respiratory disease in humans (Tables 10–2 & 10–3).

BACTERIAL PNEUMONIA

Pneumonia, or infection of the lung parenchyma, occurs in as many as 6 million Americans annually. It can be caused by organisms acquired in the community or from the hospital. The annual incidence of community-acquired pneumonia (CAP) in the United States is estimated to range from 2 to 4 million cases. Approximately

Table 10–2. Common pathogens for upper respiratory tract infections

Pharyngitis	Group A streptococci
	Adenoviruses
	Enteroviruses
	Influenza viruses
	Epstein-Barr virus
	Herpesvirus hominis
Laryngitis	Viruses
	Chlamydia pneumoniae
Common cold	Rhinovirus
	Adenovirus
	Coronavirus
Sinusitis	*Haemophilus influenzae*
	Streptococcus pneumoniae
	Anaerobes
	Rhinovirus
Epiglottitis	*H influenzae*
	Haemophilus parainfluenzae
	Staphylococcus aureus
	Group A *Streptococcus*
Croup	Parainfluenza virus
	Respiratory syncytial virus
	Adenovirus
	Mycoplasma pneumoniae

Source: Reproduced with permission from Niederman SN, Sarosi GA: Respiratory tract infections. In: George RB, Light RW, Matthay MA, et al, eds. *Chest Medicine: Essentials of Pulmonary & Critical Care Medicine*. Baltimore, Williams & Wilkins, 1995, pp 377–429.

900,000 of these individuals require hospitalization, accounting for 3% of all patients hospitalized. Mortality among hospitalized patients with CAP is reported to be between 10% and 15% but approaches 35% among those treated in intensive care units (ICUs). However, the vast majority of CAP patients are treated as outpatients. While mortality for this group is low (less than 5%), CAP is estimated to result in 53 million days of reduced productivity. The incidence of CAP and its course vary within the population. It is most common at the extremes of life, among the very young and the very old, and during the winter months. The risk of death increases with age, and when there is significant coexisting illness (eg, chronic obstructive pulmonary disease, renal failure, congestive heart failure, or immunosuppression). The severity and modality of illness is also related to the virulence of the offending pathogen (eg, resistant gram-negative organisms or *Legionella* spp).

Hospitalized patients are exposed to a different set of bacterial flora. Many patients receive ventilator support. Hospital-acquired (or nosocomial) pneumonia (HAP), or health care–associated pneumonia (HCAP) or ventilator-associated pneumonia (VAP), is often due to resistant pathogens and has a high incidence of mortality. Pneumonia is the second most common cause of nosocomial infection, but the first leading cause of death in hospitalized adult patients in the ICU. The estimated annual incidence of HAP in the United

Table 10–3. Common pathogens for lower respiratory tract infections

Bronchitis	*Haemophilus influenzae*
	Streptococcus pneumoniae
	Moraxella catarrhalis
	Mycoplasma pneumoniae
	Adenoviruses
	Influenza
	Rhinovirus
	Respiratory syncytial virus
Bronchiolitis	Respiratory syncytial virus
	Parainfluenza virus
	Adenoviruses
	Rhinovirus
Community-acquired pneumonia (CAP)	*Streptococcus pneumoniae*
	Legionella pneumophila
	M pneumoniae
	H influenzae
	Anaerobes
	Staphylococcus aureus
	Enteric gram-negative aerobes
	Influenza virus
	Respiratory syncytial virus
	Adenovirus
	Chlamydia pneumoniae
	Pneumocystis carinii (jiroveci)
Bronchiectasis	*Pseudomonas aeruginosa*
	S aureus
	Mucoid Escherichia coli
	H influenzae

Source: Reproduced with permission from Niederman SN, Sarosi GA: Respiratory tract infections. In: George RB, Light RW, Matthay MA, et al, eds. *Chest Medicine: Essentials of Pulmonary & Critical Care Medicine*. Baltimore, Williams & Wilkins, 1995, pp 377–429.

States ranges from 130,000 to 300,000 cases. HAP also causes higher hospital costs and longer hospital stays. The mortality attributable to HAP is estimated at 27% to 33%. In patients receiving mechanical ventilation, the mortality rates may be as high as 70%. Several factors have been associated with a greater mortality rate, including *Staphylococcus aureus* and *Pseudomonas aeruginosa* as pathogens, severity of underlying illness, inappropriate antibiotic therapy, age, shock, prior antibiotic therapy, and duration of prior hospitalization and drug resistance strains.

Pathophysiology

The onset of infection and proliferation of microorganisms within the alveolar space elicits an acute inflammatory response. Local effects of the cellular influx, cytokine production, and increased alveolar capillary permeability results in impaired ventilation and decreased lung compliance. Major ventilation-perfusion mismatch occurs with increased right-to-left shunting as consolidation progresses.

Hypoxia, seen in severe pneumonia, produces pulmonary vasoconstriction which often attenuates the right-to-left shunt.

The reduced pulmonary compliance increases the work of breathing and with associated inflammation produces dyspnea. The local inflammatory response results in the production of a number of cytokines that migrate out of the lung and produce fever, leukocytosis, and a number of metabolic and vascular changes. Severe pneumonia may result in bacteremia, systemic inflammatory response syndrome (SIRS), septic shock, and multiorgan dysfunction syndrome. The most common cause of acute respiratory distress syndrome (ARDS) is sepsis secondary to pneumonia (see Chapter 13).

Clinical Implications

Two thirds of patients with CAP have a low mortality risk and could be managed on an outpatient basis (Table 10–4). The clinical presentation of individuals with bacterial pneumonia has traditionally been divided into typical and atypical pneumonia but recent evidence suggests that the diagnostic utility of this classification is doubtful (Figure 10–2A and B).

Management Principles

Management of individual cases of pneumonia is usually determined by the agent or agents suspected of causing the pneumonia. However, the spectrum of potential pathogens responsible for pneumonia is large, and use of traditional clinical, radiographic, and laboratory features or diagnostic tests is limited by problems with sensitivity and specificity, side effects, and expense. Even when diagnostic testing is used, most patients initially receive an empiric regimen and there are a number of guidelines for empiric therapy. Any delay in administration of an appropriate antibiotic can be associated with worse outcome, and a goal for therapy is to begin antibiotics within 4 hours of presentation (Table 10–5).

Table 10–4. Empiric outpatient treatment regimens for community-acquired pneumonia

Patients < 65 years of age without coexisting disease:
   Antimicrobial therapy: an oral macrolide or oral doxycycline
Patients > 65 years of age and/or coexisting disease
   Antimicrobial therapy: second-generation cephalosporin, a β-lactam/β-lactamase inhibitor combination, or trimethoprim-sulfamethoxazole with or without a macrolide or new-generation fluoroquinolone

Note: Coexisting diseases include diabetes mellitus, congestive heart failure, and chronic renal and hepatic insufficiency.

Source: Adapted with permission from Niederman MS, Bass JB, Campbell GD, et al. Guidelines for the initial management of adults with community-acquired pneumonia: Diagnosis, assessment of severity, and initial antimicrobial therapy. American Thoracic Society. Medical Section of the American Lung Association. *Am Rev Respir Dis.* 1993;148:1418.

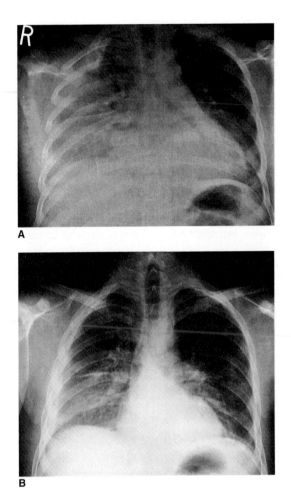

Figure 10–2. A series of films from a patient with acute bacterial pneumonia. **A.** This is a 56-year-old man who presented to the emergency department with a 4-day history of fever, shaking chills, cough productive of purulent sputum, and pleuritic right-sided chest pain. On examination, he had decreased breath sounds over the right lower lung field posteriorly with crackles noted over the right lateral and anterior chest and scattered crackles over the left lower lung field posteriorly. His chest x-ray shows the loss of the right heart border ("silhouette sign") and visible small bronchi in the right base ("air bronchograms") consistent with a right middle lobe pneumonia. Moreover, there is an increased density over the entire right lower and midlung, haziness of the right hemidiaphragm, and a thick pleural stripe extending from the right midlung almost to the apex, consistent with a large parapneumonic effusion. He was admitted and begun on empiric broad-spectrum antibiotics. Both pleural fluid cultures and blood cultures grew *Streptococcus pneumoniae*. He received 7 days of intravenous antibiotics and was discharged on oral penicillin. **B.** His discharge chest x-ray shows a return of the right heart border and right hemidiaphragm and resolution of most of the pleural effusion. He was seen in follow-up in the medical clinic with a normal chest x-ray 3 weeks after discharge.

The choice of an initial empiric antimicrobial regimen can be simplified by identifying factors that narrow the spectrum of potential pathogens. The time of year and geographic location are associated with an increased likelihood of certain viral agents and endemic fungi, as well as unusual bacterial pathogens. Some easily identifiable host characteristics that influence the spectrum of potential pathogens are age, presence of coexisting illness, immunosuppression, place of residence (such as a nursing home), and severity of illness and incidence of drug resistance patterns in the community at the time of presentation. These factors allow rational choices for initial empiric therapy for either CAP, HAP, or HCAP. It should be kept in mind that these are guidelines only; additional studies may suggest other approaches (Tables 10–6 and 10–7).

Table 10–5. Empiric inpatient treatment regimens for community-acquired pneumonia

Patients requiring hospitalization but not intensive care unit admission:
   Antimicrobial therapy: second- or third-generation cephalosporin or a β-lactam/β-lactamase inhibitor combination with a macrolide, or an advanced fluoroquinolone
Severe CAP generally requiring intensive care unit admission:
   Antimicrobial therapy:β-lactam inhibitor plus either an azilide/macrolide or an advanced fluoroquinolone (one from each group); consider adding vancomycin if methicillin-resistant *S aureus* is suspected until culture results are in

Source: Adapted with permission from Niederman MS, Bass JB, Campbell GD, et al. Guidelines for the initial management of adults with community-acquired pneumonia: Diagnosis, assessment of severity, and initial antimicrobial therapy. American Thoracic Society. Medical Section of the American Lung Association. *Am Rev Respir Dis.* 1993;148:1418.

Table 10–6. Factors used to determine severity of pneumonia

Indicator	Higher severity[a]
Age	>65 years
Gender	Male
Comorbidities	Multiple or clinically significant[b]
Presence of fever	<35°C or >40°C
Cardiovascular instability	Heart rate >125/min
Respiratory rate	>30 breaths/min
Arterial oxygen pressure	<60 mm Hg
Saturation	<90%
Metabolic derangement	Blood urea nitrogen ≥ 30 mEq/L Sodium 130 mEq/L Glucose >250 mg/L pH <7.35

[a] High severity index: Hospital or ICU admission usually required.
[b] Significant comorbidities include malignancies, congestive heart failure, and renal or liver disease.

Table 10–7. Empiric treatment regimens for hospital-acquired pneumonia

---

Group 1: mild to moderate HAP or severe HAP with early < 5 days) onset
    Core pathogens: enteric gram-negative bacilli, *Escherichia coli, Klebsiella* spp,
        Proteus spp, *Serratia marcescens, Haemophilus influenzae*, methicillin-sensitive
        Staphylococcus, and *Streptococcus pneumoniae*
    Antimicrobial therapy: second-generation or nonpseudomonal third-generation
        cephalosporin, or a β-lactam/β-lactamase inhibitor combination; if penicillin-aller-
        gic, a fluoroquinolone or clindamycin plus aztreonam
Group 2: mild to moderate HAP with risk factors for specific organisms
    Core pathogens (same as above) and
    Anaerobes (recent abdominal surgery or witnessed aspiration)
    Staphylococcus aureus (coma, head trauma, diabetes mellitus, or renal failure)
    Legionella spp (high-dose steroids)
    Antimicrobial therapy: core antimicrobials (same as above) plus
        Clindamycin or a β-lactam/β-lactamase inhibitor combination (the latter alone)
        Vancomycin (until methicillin-resistant *S aureus* is ruled out)
        Erythromycin or azithromycin with or without rifampin (the latter if *Legionella* infec-
        tion is documented)
Group 3: severe HAP with risk factors or severe HAP with late (> 5 days) onset
    Core pathogens (same as above) and *Pseudomonas aeruginosa, Acinetobacter* spp, or
        methicillin-resistant *S aureus*
    Antimicrobial therapy: a fluoroquinolone or an aminoglycoside plus one of the
        following:
        Antipseudomonal penicillin
        β-Lactam/β-lactamase inhibitor combination
        Antipseudomonal third-generation cephalosporin[a]
        Carbepenem (imipenem or meropenem)
        Vancomycin (until methicillin-resistant *S aureus* is ruled out)

---

[a] Avoid if there is a high prevalence of resistant enteric gram-negative bacilli.

Source: Adapted with permission from Campbell GD Jr, Neiderman MS, Broughton WA, et al. ATS Consensus Committee. Hospital-acquired pneumonia in adults: Diagnosis, assessment of severity, initial antimicrobial therapy, and preventive strategies. *Am J Respir Crit Care Med.* 1996;153:1711–1725.

VIRAL PNEUMONIA

Viruses cause most pneumonia in infants and children but are relatively uncommon in adults. However, viral pneumonias have the potential for resulting in devastating respiratory failure and death, even among previously healthy adults. Many factors influence the incidence and epidemiologic characteristics of viral pneumonias. Age, season of the year, presence of influenza in the community, such host factors as smoking or immunodeficiency, and transmission within closed populations lead to increased incidence and recognition of viral pneumonias.

Pathogenesis

Viral exposure does not ensure that infection occurs. Viruses are obligate intracellular pathogens, and humans have developed a variety of mechanisms to prevent respiratory virus infections. Nonspecific defenses include many of the mechanisms already mentioned: the nasal turbinates and highly branched airways, the muco-ciliary escalator, the epithelial barrier, surfactant, complement, and alveolar mac-rophages. Once a cell is infected, spread of viruses to adjacent cells may be limited by elaboration of cytokines from virally infected cells and destruction of infected cells by natural killer lymphocytes. Helper T cells and macrophages elaborate a variety of cytokines and interferons that prevent viral replication, stimulate other host defenses, and attract more phagocytic cells. Specific defenses include B and T lymphocytes. Antibodies block further infection and promote viral killing through opsonization, neutralization, complement activation, and antibody-dependent cel-lular cytotoxicity. Cytotoxic T cells are important for recovery, and their activity is restricted by recognition of viral antigens expressed on the infected cell's surface.

Pathophysiology

During viral replication there is a loss of respiratory epithelial cells, and with the release of cytokines a systemic response in the form of fever and myalgias ensues. Local inflammation and cellular and cytokine influx are the major reasons for severe cough. Depressed tracheobronchial clearance and impaired pulmonary host defense mechanisms result in tracheobronchitis. Influenza and other viruses may infect alveolar lining cells and macrophages, leading to increased susceptibil-ity to secondary bacterial pneumonia, especially *S aureus*. Severe infection may lead to diffuse alveolar damage, hemorrhage, ARDS, and death (see Chapter 7).

Clinical Implications

A high degree of suspicion of viral infection is the most important key to the diag-nosis of viral pneumonia. Because the etiologic diagnosis of pneumonia is made in only about half of all cases, it is evident that the potential for a viral pathogen as a direct or contributing cause of pneumonia is large.

Clinical findings associated with viral infections are often nonspecific and include fever, cough, tachypnea, and hypoxemia. Influenza is characterized by the abrupt onset of fever, myalgias, headache, severe malaise, and nonproductive cough. Chest x-rays frequently show alveolar or interstitial infiltrates. Although symptoms are not helpful in distinguishing viral pulmonary infections, failure to respond to an appropriate antimicrobial regimen after several days of therapy should raise the possibility of viral infection. Furthermore, epidemiologic factors are helpful when a viral cause of pneumonia is being considered. During an influenza epidemic 15% of individuals may become infected and clinically ill if not vaccinated. Household infection may reach 100%. Awareness of the time of year and of the presence of community-wide epidemics is important because viral epidemics due to influenza or respiratory syncytial virus (RSV) often occur seasonally and are frequently asso-ciated with an increase in visits to physician offices and hospitals.

Management Principles

Until recently, making a diagnosis of viral pneumonia was important only for epide-miologic purposes. However, with the advent of antiviral therapy, some viral pneumo-nias may be treated effectively. The keys in making the diagnosis include the clinician's awareness of the potential for viral pneumonia and the pathogens commonly involved, followed by appropriate testing to achieve a rapid and accurate diagnosis.

Viral cultures are the means for diagnosing viral involvement. Unfortunately, specimens may be inadequate or may not be obtained at all. Viral serologic tests have also been employed. However, both cultures and serologic tests often require days to weeks before they can be interpreted, limiting their value. Newer tests that can rapidly detect the presence of viral antigens in nasal and pharyngeal secretions are commercially available.

The mainstay of treatment for viral infections is supportive: supplemental oxygen (and mechanical ventilation when necessary) and adjunctive use of antimicrobial agents to treat bacterial superinfections. With the introduction of specific antiviral agents, antiviral therapy was shown to hasten recovery, especially when viral infection was identified early and therapy was immediately initiated. The viral replication membrane blockers and the neuraminidase inhibitors are very effective in early treatment and prophylaxis of influenza A and B infection (Figure 10–3).

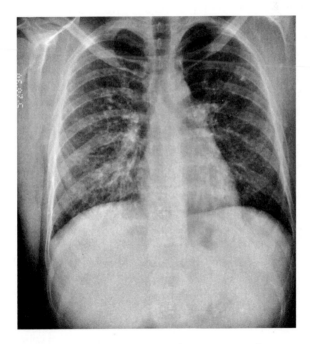

Figure 10–3. This 26-year-old man was seen in the emergency department with a diffuse rash of varying characteristics. The rashes on his extremities were largely erythematous macules with scattered vesicles, and those on his trunk were vesicular with many already crusting. He noted that his 4-year-old daughter had "chickenpox" 3 weeks ago and that he did not recall ever having had it himself. He was complaining of dyspnea and pleuritic midchest pains; on examination he had diffuse wheezing. His chest x-ray showed diffuse nodules consistent with varicella-zoster pneumonia. He was placed in strict isolation and received intravenous acyclovir, inhaled bronchodilators, and supplemental oxygen. He was discharged home in 10 days when his skin lesions were resolving.

In addition to treating the individual patient with viral pneumonia, it is important to try to prevent primary infection and spread to others. Strategies include vaccination programs and avoidance measures to prevent contact with infectious patients. When there is a good match between the vaccine and the circulating virus strains, vaccination is 70%–80% effective in healthy individuals under 65 years of age. This efficacy diminishes in elderly patients.

MYCOBACTERIAL DISEASES

Mycobacterial organisms are ubiquitous in the environment; many different species may be found in soil and water samples. Most do not cause human disease, but one important respiratory disease produced by this group is tuberculosis, caused by *Mycobacterium tuberculosis* (Mtb). However, other mycobacteria differentiated from Mtb by biochemical molecular and microbiologic criteria, and referred to as atypical or nontuberculous mycobacteria (NTM), may produce disease. While Mtb infection may be passed from human to human, the NTM infections are not transmitted in this manner, but are acquired from environmental sources. Thus, tuberculosis is a worldwide infectious disease problem and remains a significant public health hazard in the United States.

Tuberculosis

PATHOGENESIS

Mycobacterium tuberculosis is carried by infectious aerosols between 1 and 5 μm in size. These aerosols settle in the distal airways beyond the terminal bronchiole. The mycobacteria then multiply and are taken up by macrophages. They may continue to multiply in the macrophage or remain dormant for several years. Some organisms are also carried to the hilar and mediastinal lymph nodes and to other organs, including the liver, spleen, meninges, and kidneys. The upper lung zones are favored sites; the precise cause of this remains unclear, but the organisms are postulated to thrive in a high-oxygen environment. The macrophages process and present the mycobacterial antigens to lymphocytes. The host usually mounts a (lymphocyte) cellular immune response in 4–9 weeks, with organisms phagocytized and cleared into regional lymph nodes, where the infection is usually contained. The combination of one or more hilar nodes and a tuberculous focus in the lung periphery has been called a Ghon complex (Figure 10–4). Memory T cells persist in the body long after the initial infection; these T cells divide and release lymphokines when the individual is rechallenged with Mtb or antigens derived from the cell wall. Small granulomatous foci in the lung parenchyma or regional lymph nodes may be calcified over time and may appear as small (less than 1 cm) smooth calcifications on chest radiographs.

PATHOPHYSIOLOGY

The initial infection is known as primary tuberculosis. In many individuals, the primary infection is completely asymptomatic, but up to 10% may go on to develop clinical disease after the initial infection. Secondary tuberculosis (also known as "reactivation") may develop several years later. *M tuberculosis* organisms

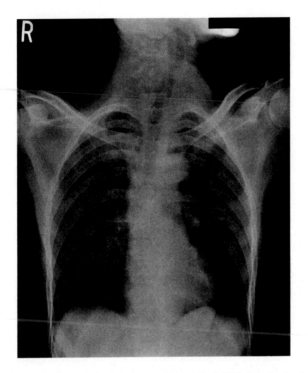

Figure 10–4. Mr. J. is a 69-year-old man in the medical clinic for continuing care for his hypertension and adult-onset diabetes. He recalls that as a child he had a "sickly" uncle living with his family who was eventually taken to a tuberculosis sanatorium. Mr. J.'s chest x-ray shows scattered, densely calcified granulomas over both hila, including a 1.5-cm calcified granuloma ("tuberculoma") in the left midlung field and densely calcified hilar nodes. A review of his old films shows that these findings have not changed in 5 years.

that have been dormant in macrophages, lymphatics, and other parts of the reticuloendothelial system multiply and can cause severe disease (including death) in these individuals. In this type, tuberculosis primarily occurs as fibrocavitary lesions in the upper lung zones. The pathophysiologic derangement is initially similar to that seen in any pneumonia with its sequelae (see the description in the section on bacterial pneumonia above). However, cavitary lesions resulting from caseation necrosis and endobronchial injury may result in vascular erosions causing hemoptysis. As architectural distortion, fibrosis, and scarring occurs, a restrictive ventilatory defect with increased work of breathing and hypoxemia ensues, and in the most severe cases, patients may develop respiratory failure.

CLINICAL IMPLICATIONS

Healthy immunocompetent individuals usually limit their infection after the initial exposure and develop latent TB infection (LTBI). The tuberculin skin test (TST) will be positive in those with latent infection. About 5%–10% of infected persons develop active disease. Risk factors that lead from infection to active disease include extremes of age, immunodeficient states such as HIV infection, malnutrition, alcoholism, malabsorption, gastrectomy, chronic treatment with high-dose glucocorticoids, and administration of cytotoxic chemotherapy. Patients with other lung conditions such as silicosis are also at increased risk. Crowded living conditions and lack of adequate ventilation increase the risk for transmission of disease.

The patients generally have constitutional symptoms, including weight loss, malaise, fever, night sweats, and poor appetite; they may also have cough and blood-tinged sputum, and in some cases progressive hematogenous spread (as in miliary TB) may result in a fulminant course. Local lung signs are dependent on the presence of pneumonia, cavitations, or pleural effusion.

Diagnosis is usually based on clinical and radiologic features and is supported by skin testing. It is confirmed by testing sputum for acid-fast bacilli (AFB) and finally by growth of AFB in culture media.

The cellular immune reaction to Mtb forms the basis for the purified protein derivative (PPD) skin test for tuberculosis. PPD is derived from filtrates of heat-sterilized cultures of Mtb; a delayed hypersensitivity reaction occurs in individuals previously exposed to Mtb and possessing viable clones of the memory T cells. Skin testing for tuberculosis is a valuable public health tool in the United States.

MANAGEMENT PRINCIPLES

Administering, reading, and interpreting TST results correctly are crucial in the screening of high risk populations and determining the need for treatment of LTBI. When AFB are seen on a sputum specimen, four drug therapy is initiated for active TB if the clinical suspicion is high. The diagnosis is confirmed only when Mtb grows in culture several weeks later. Various techniques using polymerase chain reactions and gene probes are now available to diagnose Mtb more rapidly.

Therapy for HIV-positive patients with a delayed response and for those who are late converters to culture negativity should be prolonged. Management of drug-resistant TB is complex and the treatment regimen must be customized according to the local resistance pattern. All cases of TB disease are reported to the health department.

Atypical or Nontuberculous Mycobacteria

Atypical or NTM such as *Mycobacterium avium complex* (MAC) or *Mycobacterium kansasii* are generally found in the environment, but usually cause disease only in elderly individuals with damaged lungs or in those with some form of immunosuppression. These organisms rarely cause lung disease by themselves but can coexist with chronic lung conditions such as bullous emphysema and old fibro-cavitary lung disease (Figures 10–5 & 10–6). However, NTM infection is now more common than Mtb in many communities. Various clinical scenarios related to MAC infection have been described in immunocompetent individuals along with disseminated infection seen in HIV-infected individuals.

FUNGAL INFECTIONS

Fungi are an important but uncommon cause of respiratory disease. Some fungal diseases, including histoplasmosis, blastomycosis, and coccidioidomycosis, are

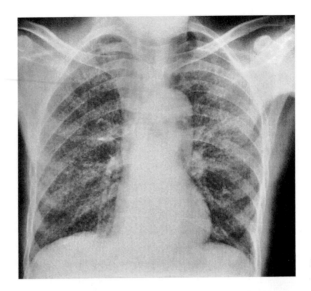

Figure 10–5. This image is of a 47-year-old man with HIV disease who was complaining about a week of progressively worsening generalized weakness, dyspnea, a nonproductive cough, and fever. The chest x-ray showed a diffuse lacy pattern. He was presumed to have *Pneumocystis carinii* pneumonia and was empirically treated with intravenous trimethoprim-sulfamethoxazole. However, he continued to deteriorate and he was transferred to a tertiary care hospital for continuing care. Shortly after his arrival to the second hospital, he experienced respiratory arrest requiring endotracheal intubation and mechanical ventilation. Tracheal aspirates were reported as showing acid-fast bacilli; Gram's, fungal, and silver stains showed no organisms. He was judged to have miliary tuberculosis and begun on four-drug therapy. However, his deterioration continued despite aggressive supportive therapy and he expired 4 days later.

endemic in certain regions of the United States. Histoplasmosis and blastomycosis are endemic in central United States along the Ohio and Mississippi River valleys; blastomycosis also occurs farther northward into Wisconsin, Minnesota, and Canada. Coccidioidomycosis is common in the arid southwestern region, including Arizona, southern California, and adjoining areas in Mexico. The other important fungi that cause lung infection are *Cryptococcus neoformans* and *Aspergillus* spp.

Pathogenesis

Fungal disease is rare in individuals with intact immune systems. Most people in the regions known for endemic mycoses are exposed and subsequently acquire immunity. Progressive infection requiring treatment usually occurs in persons with the acquired immunodeficiency syndrome (AIDS), individuals receiving glucocorticoids and other immunosuppressive agents, and patients on cancer chemotherapy. The organisms are inhaled as infectious aerosols. People who live in moist, wooded environments with exposure to bird droppings are at increased risk

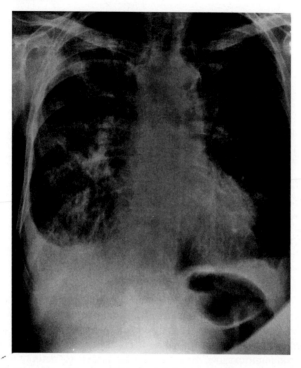

Figure 10–6. Mr. R. is a 67-year-old man with known severe chronic obstructive pulmonary disease. A chest x-ray 2 years ago showed a persistent infiltrate over the right mid- and lower-lung fields; no response was seen to several courses of oral antibiotics. Mr. R. noted little change in his dyspnea at rest or to his continued cough and sputum production. Multiple sputum samples were obtained but were unrevealing. He continued to deteriorate over the next year, with progression of his infiltrates; finally, two sputum samples were reported as growing *Mycobacterium kansasii*. He was seen in the pulmonary clinic with the chest x-ray shown here. His entire right lung is fibrotic with suggestion of cavities in the right upper lung zone. The pleura appears to be involved, with thickening and blunting of the right costophrenic angle (a subsequent right lateral decubitus view showed no free-flowing fluid). He was begun on three drugs: isoniazid, rifampin, and ethambutol, with a plan of continuing these for at least 18 months. Sputum samples continued to have acid-fast organisms seen on smears for 6 months; cultures remained positive for *M kansasii* for 4 months before finally becoming persistently negative. He began feeling slightly better, with improvement of his general well-being and his cough. He remains quite dyspneic and is on continuous supplemental oxygen.

of infection. Two kinds of immune defects are generally recognized in infected individuals:

1. T-cell dysfunction, as seen in HIV infection, predisposes patients to histoplasmosis, blastomycosis, and coccidioidomycosis. These organisms cannot be destroyed by phagocytes alone and need an intact cell-mediated immune system. In immunocompromised individuals, the organism is able to multiply and cause disease.

2. Neutropenia, as seen in patients receiving cancer chemotherapy, predisposes to *Aspergillus* and cryptococcal infection. These agents can be contained by phagocytes; in prolonged states of neutropenia, the organism causes disease. Since many patients with impaired cellular immunity are also neutropenic, cryptococcal infection commonly occurs in individuals with advanced HIV infection.

Pathophysiology

Endemic fungi may produce an acute pneumonia and may disseminate systemically. Hypoxemia and significant reduction in pulmonary compliance are uncommon. Chronic infection usually results in fibrocavitary or granulomatous changes with progressive pulmonary destruction. Long-term significant pathophysiologic impediments are uncommon, but radiographic changes may mimic those of TB.

Clinical Implications

Individuals from endemic areas who are also immunocompromised are at high risk for infection. In the immunocompetent individual, a large number of inhaled organisms can cause symptomatic infection with histoplasmosis, blastomycosis, and coccidioidomycosis. Rarely cryptococcal infection may also occur in a normal host. The clinical presentation of the endemic mycoses is similar to that of an atypical community-acquired infection. Most patients have cough, fever, and infiltrates on chest x-ray. Cavitary lesions can be seen in coccidioidomycosis and chronic histoplasmosis; disseminated histoplasmosis in the lung may have the radiologic appearance of miliary tuberculosis. Many patients with blastomycosis have a dense infiltrate that may bear radiologic resemblance to lobar bacterial pneumonia or a lung neoplasm. *Aspergillus* can colonize old tuberculous cavities or cause severe necrotizing lung and/or systemic infection.

Diagnosis depends on a high index of clinical suspicion. Most patients are brought to a specialist's attention because they have an infiltrate that has not resolved despite therapy; it is appropriate to exclude tuberculous infection. Fungi can often be seen in potassium hydroxide–treated sputum. Serologic testing is quite helpful in histoplasmosis, coccidioidomycosis, and to a lesser extent in blastomycosis. Often transbronchial lung biopsy and bronchoalveolar lavage with tissue and fluid cultures may be required to establish the diagnosis. Open-lung biopsy may be used as a last resort, but most clinicians would probably start empirical antifungal therapy in the appropriate clinical setting.

Management Principles

Antifungal therapy must be carefully monitored for side effects. Patients with AIDS need chronic maintenance therapy to prevent relapse (Figure 10–7A and B). With the availability of the new antifungal agents such as the azoles (the triazoles; eg, fluconazole, itraconazole, and voriconazole) and the glucan synthesis inhibitor caspofungin, the therapeutic options have increased and side effects of antifungal therapy are now relatively reduced.

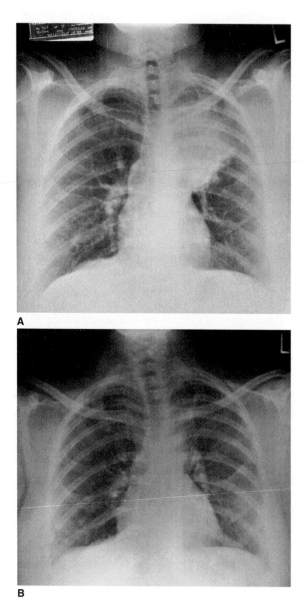

Figure 10–7. Mrs. S. was referred for a presumed left upper lobe lung tumor when a chest x-ray (**A**) showed a large density in the left upper lobe. Fortunately, sputum samples demonstrated the presence of broad-necked budding yeasts characteristic of *Blastomyces dermatitidis*. After 4 weeks of treatment with antifungal agents, her chest x-ray (**B**) showed almost total resolution of the density.

CLINICAL SCENARIOS

Case 1

A 65-year-old man with a long history of alcohol and tobacco abuse presents to the emergency department with a 4-day history of fever, cough that is productive of thick, foul-smelling sputum, and left-sided pleuritic chest pain.

Physical Examination: On examination, he has a temperature of 38.8°C (101.8°F). He has dullness to percussion over the posterior left lower lung zone; bronchial breath sounds and crackles are noted over the same area. His chest x-ray shows dense consolidation of his left lower lobe. He is admitted to the hospital with CAP.

Discussion: Ideally, rapid identification of the specific etiologic agent or agents, with therapy directed at those agents, should result in reduced risk of morbidity and mortality. However, currently available culture techniques take time and are often unable to isolate the specific organism. Guidelines for empiric management of CAP use easily identified clinical factors that allow categorization of patients into specific groups, which has important implications for the probable etiologic pathogens, and therefore on the recommended empiric antibiotic therapy. For each group of patients common pathogens may be identified. Major pathogens are those found in approximately 5% or more of the total number of cases of CAP; "miscellaneous" pathogens are less common (less than 1% of cases), but are significant in certain settings or are frequently not sought during routine work-up. The organisms likely to be found in each group and the recommended empiric therapies are presented in Tables 10–4 and 10–5. In the patient presented in this case, one should consider *S pneumoniae, H influenzae,* aerobic gram-negative bacilli, *M catarrhalis, Legionella* spp, and anaerobes.

CLINICAL PEARL

Current guidelines for management of CAP allow categorization of patients into stratified groups based on severity of disease and focus on empiric antibiotic treatment.

Case 2

A 53-year-old man presents to the emergency room with a complaint of coughing up blood several times over the last few days. He is coughing up dark yellow sputum streaked with blood. Further questioning reveals that he has been feeling poorly for a month and has lost 10 lb during that time. He has not taken his temperature, but has felt feverish during this time. He is a smoker and has been homeless after losing his job 6 months ago.

Physical Examination: On examination, he is a thin male appearing chronically ill. His temperature is 37°C (98.6°F), his pulse is 110 beats/min, but other vital signs are within normal limits. His cardiac exam reveals tachycardia and his lung exam is unremarkable. However, his chest x-ray demonstrates bilateral fibrocavitary infiltrates in the apices of both lungs with cephalad retraction of the hila. He is placed in respiratory isolation and further studies are ordered.

Discussion: All the information presented above is consistent with the possibility that this patient has developed an infection with *M tuberculosis.* He is immediately placed in respiratory isolation until the diagnosis can be confirmed. This will be accomplished with sputum studies for AFB in smears and cultures. If those studies are not confirmatory, a bronchoscopy for bronchial washings, bronchoalveolar lavage, and transbronchial lung biopsy will be done, all of which will also be examined with stains for AFB and mycobacterial cultures. A TST may add supportive information, but confirmatory studies will be required. However, appropriate four-drug empiric therapy should be initiated immediately with INH, RIF, PZA, and ETH for presumptive active tuberculosis while all studies are being submitted. If the studies procured are confirmatory, the four-drug regimen is continued until organism susceptibility tests are available, after which time (generally 8 weeks, assuming the organism is susceptible to all agents) the INH and RIF can be continued to complete a 6-month course (this may be extended in instances of delayed responses, including delayed sputum conversion to AFB-smear–negative). Arrangements must be made to administer the therapy under an office of public health directly observed therapy (DOT) program, in order to assure that it is completed as prescribed. The patient should be tested for HIV infection, as recommended for all new cases of tuberculosis due to the high rates of TB among HIV-infected hosts.

Additionally, though the patient most likely has active tuberculosis, one of the most common causes of hemoptysis is bronchitis, so he should be given a course of an antibiotic which would cover the most likely organisms (eg, doxycycline or a macrolide) concurrently. Social services evaluation is also in order to render assistance with his living situation.

CLINICAL PEARL

Where there is a high index of suspicion for active TB, appropriate four-drug therapy under a DOT program must be initiated while all studies are submitted and results of culture and sensitivity awaited.

KEY CONCEPTS

1. Though lower respiratory tract infections are among the leading causes of death in the United States, it is only through the breakdown and failure of the normal, intricate respiratory defense system that the normally sterile lower tract is breached by pathogenic microbes.

2. Pneumonia is a potentially fatal disease, and it is important to begin appropriate therapy as quickly as possible after the diagnosis is made. By necessity, early therapy (prior to return of confirmatory studies) must be empiric, so targeting of the most likely pathogen given the clinical presentation is necessary. Once confirmatory studies are received (within 24–48 hours), the initial therapy can be focused or adjusted as necessary, based on those studies and the initial response of the patient to the empiric therapy.

10–1. *A 40-year-old man is admitted via the emergency department with a 2-day history of right-sided pleuritic chest pain, low-grade fever, dyspnea, and a cough intermittently productive of blood-streaked sputum. His initial examination reveals a temperature of 38.2°C (100.7°F), tachypnea (respiratory rate 24 breaths/min), and point tenderness over the lateral and anterior chest with crackles over the same area. His extremities show no cyanosis or edema. His chest x-ray (Figure 10–8A) shows an infiltrate in the right upper and lower lobes extending to the pleura. Laboratory tests upon admission show hypoxemia with a partial pressure of arterial oxygen (Pao$_2$) of 66 mm Hg on room air, and a slight leukocytosis (total 10,600 per mL, with 60% granulocytes, 35% lymphocytes, and 4% monocytes). He is started on empiric antibiotics (a third-generation cephalosporin and a macrolide) and supplemental oxygen. Two days after admission, he is no better and continues to complain of dyspnea on exertion, with concomitant oxygen desaturation as determined by pulse oximetry. A second chest x-ray is obtained (Figure 10–8B). What interventions are appropriate at this point?*

   a. *Add another antibiotic with coverage for anaerobes.*

   b. *Begin empiric antifungal therapy.*

   c. *Begin empiric four-drug antituberculous therapy.*

   d. *Discontinue all antibiotics to eliminate the possibility of drug fever.*

   e. *Consider other noninfectious causes, such as pulmonary embolism.*

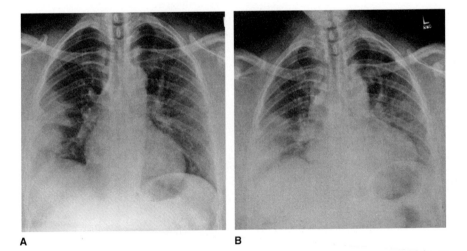

A B

Figure 10–8. *Case 1.* **A.** *Chest x-ray on admission.* **B.** *Chest x-ray on day 2.*

10–2. *A 29-year-old man, a recent immigrant from Pakistan, presents to his local public health department. He has been referred because of a TST with 14 mm of induration. The patient has no signs or symptoms of tuberculosis. He received BCG (bacille Calmette Guérin) vaccination as an infant. A chest x-ray is normal, with no* calcified granulomas or hilar nodes. What is the most appropriate interpretation of the skin test and suitable management for this patient?

a. The skin test result should be considered positive, indicating previous infection in his native country, and no therapy is necessary.

b. The skin test result should be considered positive, and he should receive INH prophylaxis.

c. The skin test result should be considered positive, and he should receive four-drug therapy (INH, RIF, ETH, and PZA).

d. The skin test result should be considered a false-positive (due to his previous BCG vaccination), and no therapy is necessary.

e. The skin test result should be considered negative, since it does not exceed 15 mm, and he should simply be followed with annual skin testing and chest x-rays.

SUGGESTED READINGS

Griffith DE, Aksamit T, Brown-Elliott B, et al. An official ATS\IDSA statement: Diagnosis, treatment and prevention of nontuberculous mycobacterial diseases. *Am J Respire Care Med.* 2007;175:367–416.

Mandell LA, Wunderink RG, Anzueto A, et al. Infectious Diseases Society of America/American Thoracic Society Consensus Guidelines on the Management of Community-Acquired Pneumonia in Adults. *Clin Infect Dis.* 2007;44:527–572.

Diseases of the Pleura

Susan Gunn & David Taylor

GENERAL CONSIDERATIONS

The term *pleura* refers to the membranous covering that overlies the organs within the thoracic cavity. It is divided into the nonpulmonary parietal and the pulmonary visceral pleura. Within the 10–20-μm distance between the pleural surfaces is the pleural fluid—a low-protein ultrafiltrate derived from the pleural microcirculation. The pleura anatomically and physiologically couples the lungs to the chest wall; furthermore, it has a significant impact on respiratory physiology during health and in illness.

Anatomy & Histology

The parietal pleura covers the chest wall (costal pleura), diaphragm (diaphragmatic pleura), and mediastinum (mediastinal pleura). The visceral pleura covers the lung parenchyma and lobar fissures. The pleura is made up of two layers: mesothelium and connective tissue. Mesothelial cells are of variable sizes (6–12 μm) and contain microvilli on their surface. The microvilli are present over the entire pleural surface, but their density varies depending on their location. Although the function of the microvilli is not completely certain, it appears that they enmesh glycoproteins (such as hyaluronic acid) to reduce friction between the parietal and visceral surfaces. It is estimated that 0.1–0.2 mL/kg of low-protein fluid is normally present between layers. The cells present in normal pleural fluid are mainly macrophages, monocytes, and mesothelial cells, although lymphocytes and neutrophils may also be present. Pleural fluid typically contains fewer than 1000 cells/mL.

The connective tissue layer of both the parietal and visceral pleura contains lymphatics, nerves, and microvessels. The major histologic difference between the parietal and visceral pleura is that the lymphatics of the parietal pleura contain stomata. The stomata are in direct communication with the pleural space and subsequently drain into lymphatic lacunae, lymphatic ducts, and lymphatic channels. The lymphatic channels of the costal pleura drain ventrally to the nodes along the internal thoracic artery and dorsally to the internal intercostal lymph nodes. The tracheobronchial and mediastinal lymph nodes collect lymph from the mediastinal pleura, while the lymphatics of the diaphragmatic pleura drain into the parasternal, middle phrenic, and posterior mediastinal nodes. The intercostal nerves supply the diaphragmatic pleura (peripheral portion) and the chest wall, while the phrenic nerve supplies the central diaphragmatic pleura. The roots of the phrenic nerve (C3, C4, and C5) also receive sensory input from the brachial plexus. This explains why diaphragmatic inflammation or injury can present as pain referred to the shoulder. The blood supply to the parietal pleura comes from the intercostal, pericardiacophrenic, superior phrenic, and musculophrenic arteries. The venous drainage is primarily via the intercostal veins.

The connective tissue layer of the visceral pleura contributes to the elastic recoil of the lung. It is composed of a network of collagen and elastin that prevents hyperinflation of the lung. Since stomata are not present in the connective tissue layer of the visceral pleura, fluid reabsorption does not occur there. The microcirculation contained within this layer is supplied by the bronchial artery and drained via the pulmonary vein. Pleuritic pain indicates injury or inflammation of the parietal pleura as there is no innervation of the visceral pleura.

Pleural Physiology

PLEURAL FLUID FORMATION

In the healthy state, pleural fluid is an ultrafiltrate that originates from the microvasculature of both the visceral and the parietal pleura. Fluid enters the pleural space due to a pressure gradient that exists between the pleural interstitium and the pleural space at a rate of 0.01 mL/kg/h.

Pleural fluid formation is thought to be determined by Starling's hypothesis of transcapillary exchange:

$$Qf = Lp^* A \left[(P_{cap} - P_{pl}) - \sigma d(\pi_{cap} - \pi_{pl}) \right]$$

where Qf = liquid movement, Lp = filtration coefficient, A = surface area; P = hydrostatic pressure in the capillary (cap) or pleural space (pl), π = oncotic pressure in the capillary (cap) or pleural space (pl), and σd = solute reflection coefficient (the membrane's resistance to passage of large molecules). Figure 11–1 shows the various pressures involved in the movement of fluid.

Therefore, formation of pleural fluid is determined by the hydrostatic pressure gradient (vascular minus pleural) minus the oncotic pressure gradient (vascular minus pleural).

As depicted, the net balance of forces in the visceral pleura is zero. It is hypothesized that there is little contribution from the visceral pleura to the development of

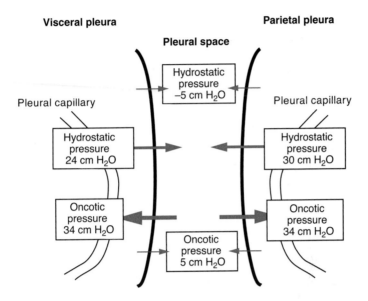

Figure 11–1. Pressures influencing pleural fluid formation. The net pressure across the visceral pleura is zero, whereas the net pressure across the parietal pleura is approximately 6 cm H_2O. Thus, the capillaries of the parietal pleura are the major source of pleural fluid formation. However, under certain conditions more fluid may come from the interstitium of the lungs across the visceral pleura.

pleural fluid; however, this has not definitively been demonstrated in human subjects. The filtration coefficient for the visceral pleura is less than that for the parietal pleura due to the greater distance between the visceral pleural capillaries and the pleural space. In the parietal pleura, the net balance favors pleural fluid formation.

THE PLEURA IN DISEASE STATES

Pleural Effusions

PATHOGENESIS

In the normal state, 0.5 mL of pleural fluid is formed every hour in human beings. To maintain a constant volume of fluid in the pleural space, fluid must be resorbed at the same rate it is formed. The parietal pleural lymphatics provide the pathway for drainage of the pleural fluid. Thus, formation of a pleural effusion results either from overproduction of pleural fluid or from inability of the lymphatic system to remove fluid as it is produced. Pleural fluid accumulates when intrapleural fluid loads are 30 times the normal steady state.

Pleural effusions due to increased fluid formation occur in the following settings:

1. increased interstitial fluid production (congestive heart failure, renal failure, pneumonia, or iatrogenic volume overload);
2. increased hydrostatic pressure in the pleural capillaries (left ventricular failure, pericardial effusion, or superior vena cava obstruction);

3. increased capillary permeability (pleural inflammation);
4. excessive peritoneal fluid (ascites or peritoneal dialysis in the presence of a diaphragmatic defect);
5. disruption of thoracic blood vessels or the thoracic duct (surgery, trauma, or malignancy);
6. decreased pleural pressure (bronchial obstruction).

Pleural effusions due to decreased pleural fluid absorption occur in the following settings:

1. elevation of systemic venous pressures (intravascular volume overload from any cause);
2. compression or dysfunction of pulmonary lymphatics (malignancy, lymphadenopathy, or a primary lymphatic disorder).

PATHOPHYSIOLOGY

The formation of pleural fluid can affect all organ systems adjacent to the pleura, especially the heart and lungs. The size of a pleural effusion generally correlates with the degree of physiologic abnormality, but is not always accompanied by dyspnea. The symptom of dyspnea is associated with a pleural effusion when there is underlying parenchymal lung disease, chest pain, splinting, or diaphragmatic dysfunction.

As pleural fluid accumulates, the shape and function of the diaphragm change. Initially the diaphragm remains domed and functions normally. However, with further increases in pleural fluid volume, the diaphragm becomes flattened and fixed. Continued accumulation eventually results in inversion of the diaphragm and subsequent dysfunction. These effects are more predominant on the left side of the chest because the presence of the liver on the right side prevents inversion.

Significant pleural effusions impose a restrictive ventilatory defect on the lungs. In animal and human models, a pleural effusion decreases total lung capacity and forced vital capacity by only 20%–30% of the effusion's size, so the remaining volume of the effusion must increase the size of the thoracic cavity. It is thought that this increase in cavity size contributes significantly to the sensation of dyspnea. Following thoracentesis, the length–tension relationship of the inspiratory muscles improves to create a more negative intrapleural pressure at any given lung volume.

In addition to affecting the lung and thoracic cavity, large pleural effusions can also alter cardiac function. In animal and human studies, the right and left ventricles have been reported to collapse as a result of pleural pressure elevation. The pressure elevation and cardiac collapse are reversible with therapeutic thoracentesis.

DIAGNOSTIC CONSIDERATIONS

Pleural effusions may initially be discovered by physical exam. Findings include absence of breath sounds on auscultation, decreased tactile fremitus, and dullness to percussion. Pleural effusions can then be confirmed by chest radiography. If a patient has a freely flowing effusion, it will settle into the most gravity-dependent portion of the chest. Thus the location and appearance will vary depending on the position of the patient and the amount of fluid present. For unclear reasons pleural fluid can accumulate between the inferior surface of the lung and the superior surface of the diaphragm (referred to as a subpulmonic effusion). If the fluid remains in this position it results in the appearance of an elevated or abnormally shaped hemidiaphragm (Figure 11–2). A left subpulmonic effusion may be seen as a large (>2 cm) separation between the gastric bubble and the hemidiaphragm.

When more than 75 mL accumulates, pleural fluid usually spills into the costophrenic sulcus resulting in blunting of the costophrenic angle on radiograph. It is the presence of fluid in this location that accounts for the meniscus sign that is the classic sign of a pleural effusion (Figure 11–3).

For patients in the supine position, pleural effusions can be especially difficult to diagnose as the meniscus sign is often absent. Fluid tends to layer posteriorly in the supine position and appears as a general opacification of the hemithorax. Pleural fluid opacifications are without air bronchograms and the pulmonary vasculature is visualized.

Some effusions are not free flowing and are referred to as *loculated*. This may result from inflammation or scarring of the pleural surface. Occasionally fluid can be trapped in an interlobar fissure, causing a mass-like opacity or pseudotumor (Figure 11–4).

Despite their widespread use to visualize pleural effusions, chest radiographs are relatively insensitive in determining pleural fluid accumulation. Computed tomography, on the other hand, is extremely sensitive and can determine the presence of as little as 2–10 mL of fluid (Figure 11–5).

Ultrasonography is becoming an important imaging tool for diagnosing pleural effusions. It is inexpensive and can be performed at the bedside to locate and

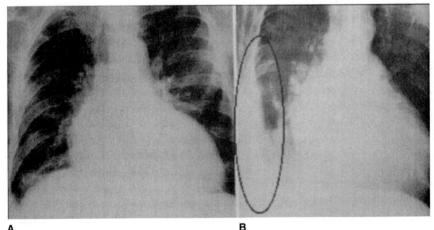

A   B

Figure 11–2. **A.** Subpulmonic effusion. The right hemidiaphragm is elevated and its apex displaced medially. **B.** Here the subpulmonic effusion is confirmed by a lateral decubitus view.

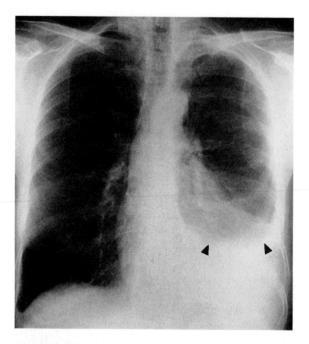

Figure 11–3. A free-flowing pleural effusion. This image shows a large left pleural effusion obliterating the heart border and hemidiaphragm. A meniscus can be seen in this upright x-ray (arrowheads). There is also a small effusion on the right, as manifested by blunting of the right costophrenic angle.

quantify effusion. Ultrasound can help rule out other etiologies of radiographic opacification including atelectasis, consolidation, mass or elevated hemidiaphragm. This is especially the case for critically ill patients who may be more difficult to move. Diagnostic thoracentesis should be performed simultaneously and ultrasound guidance results in fewer complications.

EVALUATING PLEURAL FLUID

Once a pleural effusion is recognized, a decision must be made regarding further evaluation of the fluid. Diagnostic examination is performed by a thoracentesis. This procedure should be performed with any clinically significant pleural effusion (at least 10 mm on a lateral decubitus film) that is unexplained. Effusions associated with fever, pain, or other atypical characteristics should be evaluated.

Initial assessment includes direct observation of the color, odor, and turbidity. Grossly bloody fluid should be tested for hemoglobin concentration; a value greater than 50% of the peripheral blood hematocrit indicates a hemothorax. Frank purulence indicates an empyema, and a putrid odor suggests the presence of anaerobic infection. Leukocytosis, cellular debris, or a high lipid level may cause turbidity. Milky, turbid, or purulent fluid should be centrifuged, since the supernatant of an empyema will clear whereas a chylothorax or pseudochylothorax will remain cloudy.

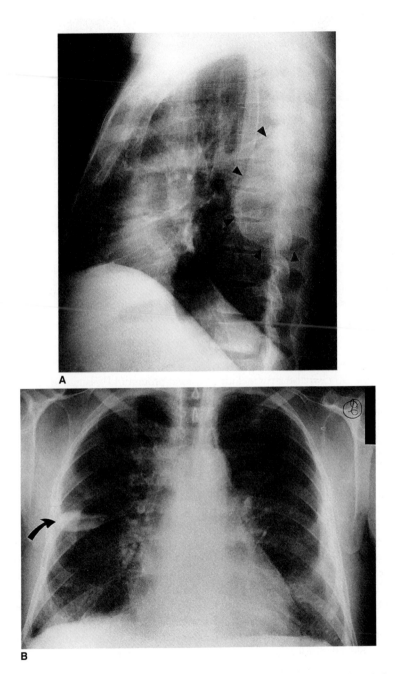

Figure 11–4. Pleural effusions that may be confused with masses. **A.** Loculated pleural effusion appearing as a well-demarcated density along the posterior chest wall (arrowheads). **B.** Collection of fluid in the minor fissure (arrow). This is called a pseudotumor because of its mass-like appearance.

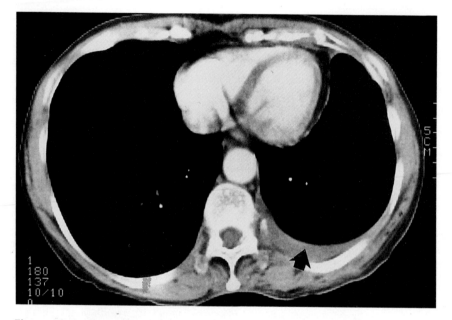

Figure 11–5. Pleural effusion as seen on CT scan (arrow). This effusion may be too small to see on a plain chest x-ray but is clearly evident on this CT scan.

Specific lab tests also may include pH, total protein (TP), lactate dehydrogenase (LDH), glucose, cell count, and differential. Pleural fluid pH should be performed with a blood gas analyzer. Normal pleural fluid pH is around 7.6. Pleural fluid acidosis may result from lactic acid production in the pleural space or tissues. A pH of less than 7.2 can be found in parapneumonic effusions, esophageal rupture, urinothorax, rheumatoid pleuritis, tuberculous pleuritis, hemothorax, systemic acidosis, lupus pleuritis, paragonimiasis, and malignancy. An elevation in LDH is a nonspecific marker of inflammation that is used along with TP to differentiate exudates from transudates (see below). Although the glucose level in the pleural fluid approximates the blood glucose, pleural fluid glucose levels less than 30 mg/dL are observed in tuberculosis, empyema, rheumatoid disease, or malignancy. The white blood cell count is fairly nonspecific, but the differential count may help in determining the diagnosis. Neutrophilic predominance generally indicates acute infection or pancreatitis. Lymphocyte predominance is more common in chronic diseases (such as TB) and malignancy. Pleural fluid adenosinedeaminase (ADA) level may be helpful in the diagnosis of TB. Eosinophils may indicate blood or air in the pleural space; additionally, pleural fluid eosinophils may be present in drug reactions, malignancy, benign asbestos pleural effusion, or parasitic infections. Depending on these initial findings, further testing may be warranted when an effusion proves to be exudative.

CLASSIFICATION OF TRANSUDATES VERSUS EXUDATES

The goal in evaluating pleural fluid is to determine the etiology of the effusion. In order to do this, the effusion is first classified as either a transudate or an exudate.

A transudative effusion results from a systemic process altering the Starling forces to favor fluid accumulation. The permeability of the pleural microvasculature is not changed in the formation of a transudative effusion. Congestive heart failure, nephrotic syndrome, and hepatic cirrhosis are all causes of transudates. In contrast, an exudative effusion results from a local process that alters the permeability of the pleural microvasculature, leading to pleural fluid formation.

Light's criteria are the most accepted for classifying effusions as exudates:

1. Pleural fluid:serum protein ratio > 0.5
2. Pleural fluid to serum LDH > 0.6
3. Pleural fluid LDH > two thirds the upper normal serum limit

If one or more of these criteria are fulfilled, there is a >95% sensitivity of the fluid being exudative. The specificity, however, is closer to 80%. Therefore, many transudates are mislabeled as exudates, or pseudoexudates. Serum to pleural fluid cholesterol ratio, pleural fluid cholesterol and albumin should then be measured to confirm an exudate. The pleural fluid cholesterol level is relatively specific for exudates (when the level is >60 mg/dL). Additionally, the serum–pleural fluid albumin difference can be used to determine the presence of an exudate; if the difference is less than 1.2, then an exudate is confirmed with over 90% specificity.

Pneumonia, malignancy, and tuberculosis are important causes of exudative effusions that may necessitate extensive testing to confirm the diagnosis. Exudative pleural effusions complicate approximately 40% of bacterial pneumonias. Parapneumonic effusions can range from acellular, protein rich fluid to a complicated effusion with bacteria present. Empyemas are the result of pus filling the pleural space. While nearly half of empyemas are the result of parapneumonic effusions, infection of the pleural space may also occur as a result of esophageal rupture or trauma. Pleural effusions associated with pneumonia should be evaluated with a gram stain of the pleural fluid in addition to the previously mentioned studies.

Malignant effusions are most commonly exudative, lymphocytic, and can be bloody in appearance. Cytology should be sent in all undiagnosed exudative effusions. Although 60%–90% of malignant effusions are positive for malignant cells, this number varies depending upon the extent of pleural involvement.

Tuberculous (TB) pleuritis is another important lymphocytic exudative effusion. It is often difficult to diagnose as acid-fast bacillus (AFB) stains are rarely positive and cultures grow only 60% of the time. ADA is released by lymphocytes activated by *Mycobacterium tuberculosis*. Pleural fluid ADA levels greater than 40 U/L supports the diagnosis of TB pleuritis when highly suspected clinically. Pleural biopsy is indicated when all other markers for disease are negative.

Management Principles

As previously mentioned, pleural fluid differentiation into exudates or transudates is important. Transudates are generally caused by an obvious systemic process and do not require further work-up. Treating the underlying illness usually results in reduction of the size of a transudative effusion (eg, CHF or cirrhosis). Exudative effusions on the other hand may require more detailed evaluation so that the specific cause may be identified and treated (Table 11–1). This is especially true for malignancy, tuberculosis, and empyema.

Regardless of the cause, effusions that compromise cardiac or pulmonary physiology require drainage via thoracentesis or chest thoracostomy. Recurrent effusions such as malignant effusions or chylothorax may require pleurodesis. Pleurodesis is a procedure that by chemical or mechanical means causes an inflammatory reaction in the pleural space. Successful pleurodesis results in adhesion of the visceral and parietal pleural surfaces and prevents significant pleural fluid accumulation.

Complicated parapneumonic effusions may require complete evacuation of the pleural space with either serial thoracentesis or chest tube drainage based on certain lab results. The most widely accepted indications for complete evacuation of the pleural space include Gram's stain of pleural fluid positive for organisms, LDH > 3 times the upper limit of normal for serum, loculated pleural fluid, pleural fluid glucose < 40 mg/dL, pleural fluid pH < 7.0 (Table 11–2).

Table 11–1. Causes of pleural effusions

Transudates		
Congestive heart failure[a]	Nephrotic syndrome	Peritoneal dialysis
Cirrhosis[a]	Atelectasis	Urinothorax

Exudates		
Infections	Collagen vascular disease	Drugs
Bacterial[a]	Rheumatoid disease	Bromocriptine
Tuberculous[a]	Systemic lupus erythematosus	Dantrolene
Fungal	Postoperative	Hydralazine[b]
Parasitic	Abdominal surgery	Methysergide
Viral[a]	Cardiac surgery	Methotrexate
Malignancy	Liver transplant	Nitrofurantoin[b]
Lung[a]	Lung transplant	Phenytoin[b]
Breast[a]	Gastrointestinal disease[a]	Procainamide[b]
Lymphoma[a]	Pancreatitis	Quinidine[b]
Mesothelioma	Abscess (hepatic, splenic, etc)	Iatrogenic
Other[a]	Esophageal perforation	Chylothorax/ pseudochylothorax
		Hemothorax
		Asbestos pleural effusions

Either transudates or exudates		
Sarcoidosis (E > T)	Myxedema	
Pulmonary embolism (E > T)	Malignancy (E > T)[c]	

Note: E > T, exudates more common than transudates.
[a] Most common causes.
[b] Associated with drug-induced lupus syndrome.
[c] Malignancy may cause bronchial obstruction and atelectasis, and effusions by this mechanism may be transudative. However, the vast majority of malignant effusions are exudates.

Table 11–2. Indications for chest tube drainage of parapneumonic effusions

Chest tube indicated	Chest tube may be necessary
Grossly purulent effusions (empyemas)	Pleural fluid pH < 7.20
Organisms seen on Gram's stain of pleural fluid	Pleural fluid LDH > 1000 IU/L
Pleural fluid glucose < 40 mg/dL	
Pleural fluid pH <7.00	

Note: Chest tubes are indicated if any of the listed criteria are present. For patients with pleural fluid pH between 7.00 and 7.20 or LDH ≥ 1000 IU/L, the decision to insert a chest tube must be made on an individual basis, depending on the condition of the patient. These criteria apply only to parapneumonic effusions and not to effusions with noninfectious causes such as rheumatoid or malignant effusions. LDH, lactate dehydrogenase.

Other Pleural Diseases

Although pleural effusion is the most commonly encountered pleural disease, many other diseases of the pleura exist. Trapped lung, fibrothorax, and pneumothorax can all significantly alter the physiology of the lungs and chest wall. These disorders will be discussed below.

TRAPPED LUNG

Pleural inflammation from various causes can result in the formation of a fibrous peel overlying the visceral pleura. The lung is subsequently trapped because this covering prevents the lung from expanding. This creates a net negative pleural pressure that results in decreased pleural fluid absorption and increased pleural fluid formation. The chronic pleural effusion that results will rapidly reaccumulate following attempted therapeutic thoracentesis.

Pathogenesis: Both malignant and nonmalignant pleural diseases can cause trapped lung. Malignant pleural effusions associated with trapped lung are most commonly seen in malignant mesothelioma and primary lung cancer. Nonmalignant causes of trapped lung include hemothorax, pneumonia, uremia, prior thoracic surgery, radiation therapy, and rheumatoid pleuritis. Additionally, long-standing transudative effusions have also been associated with the development of trapped lung.

Pathophysiology: Patients with trapped lung generally have a restrictive ventilatory dysfunction. In contrast to most other pleural effusions, the pleural pressures may fall by as much as 20 cm H_2O with removal of 1 L of fluid because the lung cannot expand to fill the space created by fluid removal. As mentioned previously, this results in rapid reaccumulation of the effusion.

Diagnosis of Trapped Lung: Diagnosis is suspected in patients who have a chronic pleural thickening or effusion and a history of pneumonia, uremia, or other prior pleural disease. In some cases the diagnosis is suggested when the size of the affected hemithorax is smaller than the unaffected side. A low pleural pressure (<5 cm H_2O) that falls precipitously upon the removal of 100–200 mL of fluid is also suggestive of the diagnosis. Definitive diagnosis is made by observing the expansion of the lung to fill the pleural space following decortication.

Management Principles: Surgical decortication is the only treatment for symptomatic patients with trapped lung; however, most patients have only modest degrees of entrapment and require no treatment.

FIBROTHORAX

The term *fibrothorax* refers to a condition that occurs when the visceral pleura is covered by a dense, thick, fibrous layer of connective tissue. This can result from either pleural or pulmonary disease; however, the clinical manifestations are similar to those of chest wall disorders such as severe scoliosis or pectus deformity. This may ultimately result in restrictive lung disease and chronic hypoventilation.

Pathogenesis: Fibrothorax can result as a consequence of intense pleural inflammation. The most common causes include hemothorax, tuberculous pleuritis, and parapneumonic effusion. Additionally, pancreatitis, uremia, and collagen vascular diseases can cause a fibrothorax. Less commonly, parenchymal diseases such as pulmonary tuberculosis, bronchiectasis, and lung abscess can result in fibrothorax. By the time fibrothorax develops, the symptoms of the precipitating disease have usually resolved.

Pathophysiology: With severe cases of fibrothorax, the chest wall, intercostal muscles, and ribs may become involved. This causes limited inspiratory excursion and may lead to scoliosis. Fibrothorax causes a moderate to severe restrictive ventilatory defect resulting in alveolar hypoventilation with subsequent hypercarbia and hypoxemia. Interestingly, pulmonary perfusion to the affected side is reduced out of proportion to the ventilatory decline. This results in increased dead space and wasted ventilation. In contrast to pleural effusions, the degree of functional impairment is typically out of proportion to the degree of pleural disease.

Diagnosis: Fibrothorax can be diagnosed radiographically when a "pleural peel" surrounds the lung. This is usually associated with a contracture of the ipsilateral hemithorax and narrowing of the ipsilateral intercostal spaces.

Management Principles: The only treatment for fibrothorax is surgical removal of the fibrous peel (decortication). Since patients with recent infection or hemothorax often improve spontaneously, decortication should only be considered in patients with related symptoms that have stable or worsening disease over a 6-month course. Treatment outcomes vary, but decortication of even long-standing fibrothorax may result in physiologic improvement. Ultimately the physiologic improvement following decortication depends on the condition of the underlying lung parenchyma.

PNEUMOTHORAX

 Pneumothorax is the presence of gas in the pleural space. When present, it indicates one of the following: gas-producing organisms in the pleural space, an abnormal communication between alveoli and the pleural space or an abnormal communication between the atmosphere and the pleural space.

Pneumothorax is classified as traumatic, iatrogenic, or spontaneous. Spontaneous pneumothorax is further divided into either primary or secondary.

Primary spontaneous pneumothorax occurs in patients who do not have clinically apparent lung disease. Conversely, secondary spontaneous pneumothorax occurs in patients with underlying lung disease.

Epidemiology: Most cases of primary spontaneous pneumothorax are sporadic although they typically occur in men and boys between the ages of 10 and 30 years. Risk factors include tall thin subjects who are current or former smokers. Some inherited conditions are also considered risk factors: they include Marfan syndrome, α-1 antitrypsin deficiency, cystic fibrosis, Ehlers-Danlos, tuberous sclerosis, and homocysteinuria. In contrast, secondary spontaneous pneumothorax occurs in patients of any demographic group who have significant underlying lung disease.

Pathogenesis: At end-expiration, the inherent tendency of the lung is to collapse, while the chest wall tends to expand. This contributes to the relative negative pleural pressure during the respiratory cycle. In health, the alveolar pressure is greater than the pleural pressure. When there is communication between the pleural space and alveolus, gas will flow into the pleural space.

Primary spontaneous pneumothorax typically results from rupture of apical subpleural bullae. These bullae have been demonstrated by computed tomography of the thorax, during thoracotomy, and at autopsy in patients without clinically apparent lung disease. The pathogenesis of bullae is either congenital or acquired secondary to airway inflammation (due to smoking).

Secondary spontaneous pneumothorax occurs in patients with underlying lung disease (Table 11–3). There are at least three mechanisms for pneumothorax

Table 11–3. Causes of pneumothorax

Spontaneous	Trauma	Iatrogenic
Primary	Penetrating chest trauma	Transthoracic needle biopsy
Secondary	Blunt trauma	Insertion of central venous catheter
COPD		
Pneumocystis carinii pneumonia		Mechanical ventilation
Pulmonary fibrosis (advanced)		Thoracentesis
Asthma		Transbronchial lung biopsy
Cystic fibrosis		Pleural biopsy
Catamenial pneumothorax		
Eosinophilic granuloma		
Pulmonary tissue necrosis[a]		

Note: COPD, chronic obstructive pulmonary disease.

[a] Pulmonary tissue necrosis refers to damage to lung parenchyma as a result of septic emboli, necrotizing pneumonia, and tuberculosis. It may also be the mechanism of pneumothorax in some patients requiring mechanical ventilation for acute respiratory distress syndrome.

in patients with underlying lung disease. Most commonly, rupture of bullae or blebs results in pneumothorax similar to the mechanism in primary spontaneous pneumothorax. In diseases associated with pulmonary necrosis such as *Pneumocystis carinii* pneumonia (PCP) or tuberculosis, alveoli may rupture and allow movement of air through the bronchovascular space into the mediastinum and then into the pleural space. Thus, any condition that results in alveolar pressure exceeding interstitial pressure can ultimately lead to pneumomediastinum and/or pneumothorax. Specific causes of pneumomediastinum are outlined in Table 11–4.

Pathophysiology: Given the natural tendency for the lung to collapse and the chest wall to expand, it is not surprising that the lung volume decreases when air separates the parietal from the visceral pleura. This results in a decrease in total lung capacity and vital capacity. Additionally, there is a drop in arterial oxygen tension and an increase in alveolar-arterial oxygen difference. The decreased arterial oxygen tension is due to both reduction of ventilation:perfusion ratios and shunting of blood in the collapsed lung. In healthy individuals, even moderate lung collapse is well tolerated. In patients with chronic lung disease, the collapse is often not well tolerated and may be life threatening.

Diagnosis: The history and physical examination is often adequate to diagnose pneumothorax, but chest radiography, ultrasonography, or computed tomography may be used for diagnostic confirmation. On the upright chest film, there is absence of lung markings on the affected hemithorax in addition to the presence of a visceral-pleural line (Figure 11–6). In the absence of prior pleural disease, air collects in an apicolateral location in an upright patient.

The position of the patient and the size of the pneumothorax will largely determine the appearance of the radiograph. In supine patients a deep sulcus sign may be seen due to the presence of air in the anteromedial pleural recess (Figure 11–7), even though a visceral-pleural line may not be detected.

Table 11–4. Causes of pneumomediastinum

Alveolar rupture	Ruptured esophagus	Tracheal/bronchial injury	Facial/oral injury
Mechanical ventilation	Vomiting	Penetrating trauma	Facial fractures
Blunt chest trauma	Iatrogenic (eg, during endoscopy)	Tracheostomy	Dental procedures
Valsalva			
During childbirth			
While smoking illicit drugs			
Asthma			
Coughing			
Laughing			

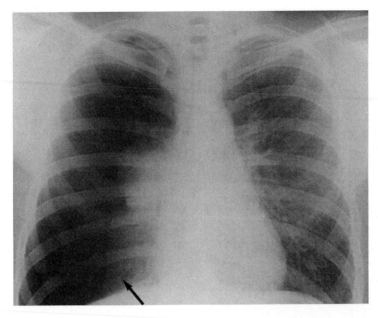

Figure 11–6. The arrow illustrates the collapsed right lung with a visceral-pleural line.

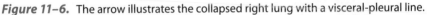

Tension pneumothorax results when the pressure in the pleural space exceeds atmospheric pressure. If untreated, this results in contralateral shift of the mediastinum, complete lung collapse, and cardiovascular compromise.

Management Principles: Because pneumothorax is a potentially life-threatening condition, early recognition and treatment is critical in preventing unfavorable outcomes. Treatment options depend on the size of the pneumothorax. In patients with a small pneumothorax (less than 2 cm between the lung and chest wall on radiograph) can be observed and placed on supplemental oxygen. Supplemental oxygen results in a lower partial pressure of nitrogen in the blood to favor nitrogen resorption from air in the pleural space, to cause more rapid reduction in the size of the pneumothorax. Patients refractory to treatment or who have recurrent disease may require tube thoracostomy. Tension pneumothorax necessitates emergent needle decompression followed by chest thoracostomy. Management of pneumomediastinum (Figure 11–8) depends upon the underlying cause and whether it is associated with a pneumothorax.

CLINICAL SCENARIOS

Case 1

A 40-year-old man with hepatitis C cirrhosis, human immunodeficiency virus (HIV) infection (CD4+ count 240), and prior miliary tuberculosis (TB) 14 years ago presents with a 4-month history of fevers to 102°F, 25-lb weight loss, and night sweats. Initial evaluation reveals him to be thin and chronically ill appearing.

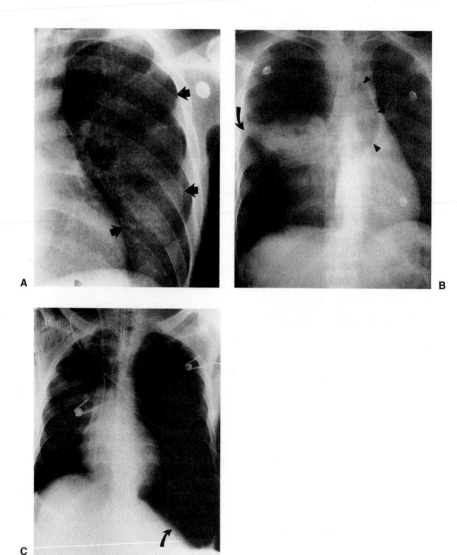

Figure 11–7. Pneumothorax. **A.** Left pneumothorax as seen on an upright chest x-ray. This patient has a pneumothorax that is manifested both medially and laterally as a hyper-lucent area demarcated by a thin white visceral pleural line (arrows). **B.** Tension pneumothorax. In this unusual manifestation of a tension pneumothorax, the right lung has been prevented from collapsing completely by a pleural adhesion (curved arrow). The heart and trachea are shifted into the left hemithorax, and air from the right pneumothorax can be seen herniating across the midline of the chest (arrowheads). **C.** Large left pneumothorax in a supine patient. The left hemidiaphragm is pushed down by this large pneumothorax (arrow). This is called a deep sulcus sign. Note that this is also a tension pneumothorax; the mediastinal structures are displaced toward the right hemithorax.

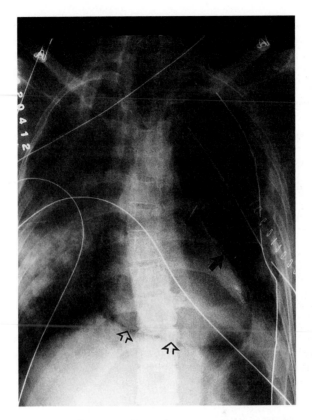

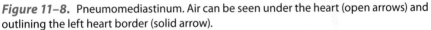

Figure 11–8. Pneumomediastinum. Air can be seen under the heart (open arrows) and outlining the left heart border (solid arrow).

Physical Examination: Vital signs include heart rate 105 beats/min, respiratory rate 26 breaths/min, temperature 102°F, and blood pressure 110/55 mm Hg. Chest examination reveals dullness to percussion halfway up the left chest with clear lung fields otherwise. Chest radiograph reveals a moderate-sized left pleural effusion, and tuberculous skin testing (TST) is negative. Thoracentesis demonstrated with the following results: LDH 220, protein 4.6 (serum 5.5), white blood cell count 5223, 92% lymphocytes on differential. Pleural fluid smears are negative for fungus, AFBs, and bacteria. Subsequent pleural biopsy reveals caseating granulomas. Special staining is positive for AFB that later proved to be *Mycobacterium tuberculosis* (see pathology below).

Discussion: Case 1 demonstrates the typical findings of tuberculous pleuritis. Pleural fluid analysis in tuberculous pleuritis typically yields a lymphocytic exudate, although a neutrophilic exudate is common early in the disease process. A high protein level (>5.0 g/dL) is also suggestive of tuberculosis. While pleural fluid culture is positive for tuberculosis in 40% of cases, diagnosis often requires pleural biopsy that increases the sensitivity to about 75%. The presence of granulomas on pleural biopsy is 90%–95% specific for the diagnosis of tuberculosis.

In HIV patients, the TST is positive in only 40%–60% of cases. Diagnosis is important because most untreated patients with tuberculous pleurisy develop active disease within the next 5 years.

CLINICAL PEARL

The diagnosis of tuberculous pleuritis must be strongly considered in patients with lymphocytic exudates and clinical risk for tuberculosis. A negative TST does not rule out infection with *M tuberculosis*.

Case 2

A 63-year-old woman with rheumatoid arthritis, tobacco abuse, and coronary artery bypass 8 months earlier presents to the clinic complaining of fatigue, malaise, shortness of breath, and pleuritic chest pain.

Physical Examination: Her exam is notable for decreased breath sounds at both lung bases, but with clear lung fields anteriorly. Heart sounds are normal with no murmurs or gallops. Neck veins are not elevated and there is no peripheral edema. Chest radiography reveals bilateral pleural effusions. Given the systemic symptoms, a thoracentesis is done revealing turbid fluid. Centrifugation of the fluid yields a cloudy supernatant with the following cell count and differential: white blood cells 171 (62% segs, 26% lymphs, 11% monos). Other labs include glucose 1, protein 5.5, LDH 1830, and cholesterol 83 (crystals present). Gram's stain and bacterial culture are negative. The patient was diagnosed with a pseudochylothorax secondary to rheumatoid pleuritis. She was treated with corticosteroids as an outpatient and responded well.

Discussion: The diagnosis of rheumatoid pleuritis is usually made in the setting of long-term rheumatoid disease and pleural effusion. Pleural fluid analysis typically shows very low glucose and extremely high LDH. Additionally, the pleural fluid rheumatoid factor is high in rheumatoid pleuritis. By comparison, an empyema has a negative rheumatoid factor. Pseudochylothorax can be present in the setting of chronic effusions that result from long-standing inflammation. The turbid appearance is often confused with empyema, which must be ruled out by performing centrifugation. In empyema there is clearing of the supernatant, but the supernatant remains cloudy in chylothorax and pseudochylothorax. In addition, Gram's stain and cultures should be performed to rule out bacterial infection. Chylothorax contains chylomicrons and is caused by obstruction of the thoracic duct, is usually acute, and has a high triglyceride level (>110 mg/dL). Pseudochylothorax results from a long-standing inflammatory effusion that contains cholesterol crystals.

CLINICAL PEARL

The presence of turbid or milky fluid should prompt consideration of the following diagnoses: chylothorax, pseudochylothorax, and empyema. The supernatant of a centrifuged specimen will clear in an empyema, while remaining turbid in chylothorax and pseudochylothorax.

KEY CONCEPTS

① Clinically significant pleural effusions should be evaluated carefully in order to determine whether there is a systemic process (transudation) or a local process (exudate) that is responsible for the accumulation of pleural fluid. Once determined, the treatment of the underlying disease process can improve the pathophysiologic state that results from the presence of fluid in the pleural space.

② Fibrothorax and trapped lung are chronic pleural diseases that may cause severe derangements in respiratory physiology. Treatment should be reserved for those with severe disease who have relatively normal underlying lung function.

③ The presentation of pneumothorax is highly variable in that the presence of gas in the pleural space can potentially alter the physiology of the heart, lungs, and diaphragm.

STUDY QUESTIONS

11–1. A 21-year-old man presents to your office after he develops right-sided chest pain while watching TV. He denies shortness of breath, cough, or fever. He has a 5–pack-year history of tobacco use but denies any HIV risk factors. On examination he is 6 ft 2 in., 145 lb, RR 22 breaths/min, and heart rate 90 beats/min. There is no distress noted. Chest exam reveals hyperresonance to percussion and decreased breath sounds over the right hemithorax. A chest x-ray (CXR) shows a 40% right pneumothorax. What is the most appropriate management step?

    a. Obtain a high-resolution computed tomographic (HRCT) image of the chest.

    b. Administer 100% oxygen and repeat CXR in 4 hours.

    c. Refer the patient for video-assisted thoracoscopy and talc instillation.

    d. Insert a small-bore catheter via needle guidewire.

11–2. A 28-year-old HIV-positive woman presents to the emergency department with fever, shortness of breath, cough, and right-sided pleuritic chest pain. Last month her CD4+ count was 150 despite being treated with highly active antiretroviral therapy for the past 6 months. She is a 25–pack-year smoker and according to her clinic record she is compliant with oral PCP prophylaxis. On examination, her heart rate is 125 beats/min, respirations are 24 breaths/min, blood pressure is 110/70 mm Hg, and temperature is 102°F. The chest exam reveals dullness to percussion and decreased breath sounds at the base of her right lung. Chest x-ray reveals right lower lobe consolidation and a moderate-sized right pleural effusion that layers on lateral decubitus views. What is the most appropriate thing to do next?

a. *Empiric antibiotics alone*

b. *Thoracentesis alone*

c. *Four-drug therapy for tuberculosis*

d. *Bronchoscopy to look for PCP*

e. *a and b.*

SUGGESTED READING

Light RW. *Pleural Diseases.* 5th ed. Baltimore: Lippincott Williams & Wilkins; 2007.

Respiratory Abnormalities with Sleep Disorders

12

LaSandra Barton

OBJECTIVES

▶ *Identify sleep stages and their physiology in the normal subject.*
▶ *Describe the pathophysiology of obstructive and central sleep apneas.*
▶ *Understand the diagnostic, clinical, and management principles relating to sleep-related breathing disorders.*

GENERAL CONSIDERATIONS

It is well recognized that sleep disorders and respiratory functions are closely related. Sleep has a demonstrable effect on breathing patterns in individuals, producing a variety of specific clinical disorders such as obstructive sleep apnea (OSA) syndrome, or aggravating preexisting cardiopulmonary conditions such as chronic obstructive pulmonary disease (COPD) or congestive heart failure. This chapter will focus on this pathophysiologic relationship.

NORMAL SLEEP PHYSIOLOGY & DEFINITIONS

Sleep is divided into stages based on brain activity (as detected by the electroencephalograph [EEG]), eye movements (as detected by the electrooculogram [EOG]), and muscle activity (as detected by the electromyogram [EMG]). Additional parameters, including respiratory flow, oxygen saturation, and heart rate and rhythm, are simultaneously recorded during a polysomnogram (PSG) in order to diagnose sleep disorders (Figure 12–1).

Sleep is categorized in various ways. Based on eye movements, sleep is characterized as being without rapid eye movements (REM; non-REM sleep) or with

Acknowledgment: The authors acknowledge the use of some clinical material and images from Omidvari K. Sleep disorders. In: Ali J, Summer WR, Levitzky MG, eds. *Pulmonary Pathophysiology.* New York: McGraw-Hill; 1999 and Barton C. Sleep disorders. In: Ali J, Summer WR, Levitzky MG, eds. *Pulmonary Pathophysiology.* New York: McGraw-Hill; 2005.

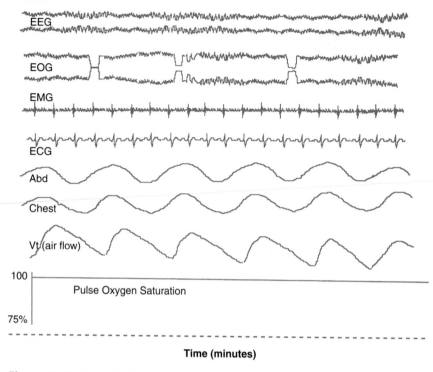

Figure 12–1. Normal polysomnogram

rapid eye movements (REM sleep). Non-REM (NREM) and REM sleep alternate throughout the night in roughly 90-minute cycles. During the night, the relative amounts of NREM and REM sleep vary, with more REM sleep occurring toward the end of the sleep period (Figure 12–2). *Stage 1* marks the transition from wakefulness to sleep and includes the state of drowsiness. During this stage, the EEG is characterized by mixed frequency low-voltage activity in addition to slow rolling eye movements. *Stage 2* is defined by the presence of two distinct waveform complexes on EEG: sleep spindles and K-complexes. During this stage, breathing can be irregular due to fluctuations in respiratory drive. Stages 1 and 2 are categorized as *light sleep*. *Stages 3* and *4* are called slow wave or delta sleep because they are defined by the amount of slow waves they contain, and are categorized as *deep sleep*. The EEG in REM sleep is composed of low-voltage mixed frequency activity with sawtooth waves. In normal subjects, almost all tonic muscle activity is suppressed, although phasic muscle twitches can occur. This is termed *muscle atonia*. Only extraocular and diaphragmatic muscle activity is preserved. Rapid eye movements are the hallmark of REM sleep. During this stage, intrinsic metabolic activity occurs that is not unlike that observed in the waking stage. Breathing is irregular. REM sleep generally occurs within 90–120 minutes of sleep onset and lasts 10–20 minutes. Episodes of REM sleep are of longer duration and occur more frequently toward the end of the sleep period (Table 12–1).

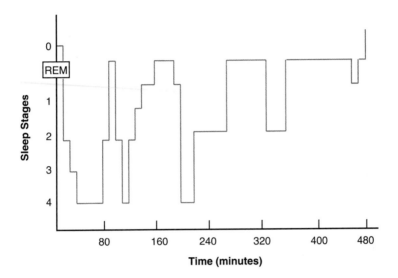

Figure 12–2. Depiction of "sleep architecture" in a typical 8-hour sleep period.

Table 12–1. Characteristics of sleep stages, normal sleep

Stage	EEG activity	EOM	EMG
1	Low-voltage mixed frequency	Slow, lateral, rolling movements	Present, but to a lesser degree than when awake
	Alpha activity slows, then becomes intermittent, then is replaced by theta waves POSTs Vertex waves[a]		
2	Sleep spindles[b] K-complexes[c] Occasional vertex and POSTs Delta waves (<20%) just before stage 3		Reduced
3	Delta waves (20%–50% of epoch)[d]		Low
4	Delta waves (>50% of epoch)[d]		Low
REM	Low-voltage mixed frequency sawtooth waves[e]	Fast lateral movements	Atonic, sometimes phasic twitches

Note: EEG, electroencephalogram; EOG, electrooculogram; EMG, electromyogram; POST, posterior occipital sharp transients; REM, rapid eye movement.

[a] Sharp, high amplitude transients, centrally located.
[b] Medium amplitude waveforms, 12–14 Hz frequency activity, centrally located.
[c] High amplitude, biphasic waves consisting of a sharp component followed by a slow wave whose duration is 1 to <4 Hz.
[d] High amplitude (>75 mV), long duration (≤2 Hz).
[e] Centrally located waveforms.

CLASSIFICATION OF SLEEP DISORDERS

The International Classification of Sleep Disorders categorizes sleep disorders into four groups (Table 12–2). *Dyssomnias* include disorders of initiating and maintaining sleep that produce excessive sleepiness, the patient's major complaint. *Parasomnias* include elements of undesirable phenomena or behavior such as rhythmic body movements or rocking that occur exclusively during sleep and are manifestations of nervous system activity. Excessive sleepiness is generally not the primary presenting complaint. *Medicopsychiatric sleep disorders* have features of disturbed sleep and wakefulness, although these are not generally the patient's primary complaint. This category includes psychiatric, neurologic, and other medical conditions such as infections, nocturnal cardiac ischemia, sleep-related asthma, gastroesophageal reflux disease (GERD), peptic ulcer disease, and fibromyalgia. The fourth category contains proposed sleep disorders for which there is insufficient evidence available to clearly define them, but include pregnancy-associated disorders and terrifying hypnagogic hallucinations.

Dyssomnia is further subdivided into three major groups: intrinsic, extrinsic, and circadian sleep disorders based on pathophysiologic mechanisms. *Intrinsic sleep disorders* arise from causes in the brain or body and include sleep-related breathing disorders (SRBDs), restless leg syndrome, and narcolepsy. *Extrinsic sleep disorders* are predominantly caused by disturbances of the environment. Some of these disorders depend on internal factors that initially cause a sleep disturbance, but continued sleep disturbance ultimately depends on external factors. When the external factors are removed, the sleep disorder disappears. This group includes stimulant-dependent sleep disorder and altitude insomnia. *Circadian sleep disorders,* although due to internal central nervous system

Table 12–2. The American Sleep Disorders Association International Classification of Sleep Disorders

---

Dyssomnias (disorders of initiating and maintaining sleep)
   Intrinsic sleep disorders
   Extrinsic sleep disorders
   Circadian sleep disorders
Parasomnias
   Disorders of arousal
   Sleep–wake transition disorders
   Parasomnias associated with REM sleep
   Other parasomnias
Medicopsychiatric sleep disorders
   Associated with affective disorders
   Associated with neurologic disorders
   Associated with other medical disorders
Proposed sleep disorders
   Not clearly defined

Note: REM, rapid eye movement.

(CNS) factors, are grouped separately because of their common chronobiologic basis. The patient's sleep pattern, which is internally generated, is out of synchrony with external societal demands, so the patient sleeps and wakes at times that are inappropriate and complains of insomnia or excessive sleepiness. Jet lag syndrome and shift-work sleep disorder are examples of these derangements.

RESPIRATORY PHYSIOLOGY DURING NORMAL SLEEP

In normal adults, tidal volume decreases by 15%–25% during sleep, with shallowest breathing occurring during REM sleep. Respiratory frequency can increase slightly during NREM sleep, but is irregular during REM and stages 1 and 2 of NREM sleep. Minute ventilation decreases by 0.5–1.5 L/min as a consequence of decreased tidal volume. Arterial carbon dioxide pressure ($Paco_2$) increases by 2–3 mm Hg while arterial oxygen pressure (Pao_2) decreases by 3–10 mm Hg such that the net result is a 0%–2% decrease in arterial oxygen saturation (Sao_2). Breathing during REM sleep becomes irregular due to changes in cortical activity associated with dreaming. Cyclical fluctuations in tidal volume, referred to as *periodic breathing,* are commonly observed during the transition from wakefulness to NREM sleep. This oscillatory breathing pattern results from fluctuations in respiratory center output in the brain. Alveolar ventilation is adjusted between the higher set point associated with wakefulness and the lower set point associated with sleep. At sea level, the fluctuations in alveolar O_2 tension are insufficient to produce noticeable changes in Sao_2. However, sleep at high altitudes potentiates periodic breathing and results in alterations in Sao_2. As sleep proceeds through slow wave sleep, ventilation becomes monotonously regular. Pauses in respiratory flow are frequently observed in normal patients. In normal subjects, they are generally short (<20 seconds in duration) and infrequent (<5 per hour of sleep). They can cause small decreases in Sao_2 and occur most commonly in REM and stage 1 and 2 sleep (NREM).

Age, male gender, use of alcohol or sedatives, obesity, and a history of hypertension, snoring, and upper airway muscle dysfunction are some of the risk factors for the occurrence of pathologic respiratory flow pauses called *apneas* and *hypopneas,* which are defined below.

Apneas and hypopneas can cause hypoxemia and hypercapnia. The amount of Sao_2 decrease is determined by the length of the pause, initial lung volume, ventilation-perfusion match, venous O_2 saturation, cardiac output, and factors affecting the oxyhemoglobin dissociation curve. Ventilatory responses to hypercapnia and hypoxia are blunted during sleep, most prominently in REM sleep. The decreased ventilatory response is due to increased airway resistance and decreased central ventilatory drive, among other factors. However, arousal from sleep occurs when the $Paco_2$ increases by 6–15 mm Hg. The arousal response to hypoxia is weaker than that to hypercapnia. Both of these may result in sleep stage transition and lighten sleep. However, most arousals are linked to airway obstruction and a secondary increase in the work of breathing.

HEMODYNAMIC CHANGES THAT OCCUR DURING NORMAL SLEEP

Changes in metabolic rate as well as parasympathetic and sympathetic tone in the nervous system cause a general decrease in systemic blood pressure and heart rate.

Systemic blood pressure reaches a nadir within several hours after sleep onset, followed by a gradual tendency to increase throughout the remainder of sleep. Mean arterial blood pressures decrease an average of 5%–9% during stages 1 and 2 and an average of 4%–8% during stages 3 and 4. During REM, blood pressure fluctuates widely, but is usually increased above NREM values. In contrast to significant changes in systemic blood pressure that can occur in sleep, pulmonary artery pressures remain in the physiologic range in normal individuals.

Heart rate decreases by 5%–8% during NREM sleep and increases to waking levels during REM sleep. Benign sinus arrhythmias with pauses up to 2 seconds in duration can be observed with type I second-degree atrioventricular block, which occurs in up to 6% of young adult males, but less often in young women and the elderly. In sleep, although there is a general reduction in ventricular ectopy, it can still be detected in 48%–73% of normal subjects, with the highest incidence of ectopy occurring during REM sleep. Ectopic rhythms can be complex (multifocal, repetitive, or both) in 15% of cases. Ventricular tachycardia is rare.

Sudden nocturnal death can occur in apparently healthy individuals, with the highest death rates occurring between 4 and 6 am, when REM sleep is most abundant. Prolonged sinus arrest and ventricular arrhythmias during REM sleep have both been proposed as possible mechanisms for sudden death. In those patients with known cardiac disease, cardiac monitoring demonstrates that the transition from ventricular tachycardia to ventricular fibrillation is the most common cause of sudden death. Lower heart rate as well as reduced stroke volume contributes to a decrease in cardiac output of about 10% during NREM sleep. Decreases in cardiac output parallel reductions of systemic blood pressure, resulting in little change in total peripheral resistance. Cardiac output is variable during REM sleep but can fall by as much as 26%.

PATHOPHYSIOLOGY OF SRBDs

SRBDs represent a spectrum of disorders that include OSA syndromes, central sleep apnea (CSA) syndromes, and hypoventilation syndromes. OSA is characterized by repetitive episodes of obstructive apneas and hypopneas that cause arousals and desaturations and result in a complaint of excessive daytime sleepiness. CSA is characterized by repetitive central apneas and hypopneas that also cause arousals and desaturations and result in complaints of insomnia, the inability to remain asleep with or without excessive daytime sleepiness.

Definition of Apnea

An apnea that occurs during sleep is defined by a significant decrease or complete absence of airflow for 10 seconds or longer. A hypopnea is defined as an incomplete absence of airflow resulting in an arousal from sleep or a decline in oxygen levels by 3% or 4% desaturation. Depending on the cause, apneas and hypopneas during sleep are divided into three types: central, obstructive, or mixed. *Central apnea* is defined as an apneic event characterized by cessation in oronasal air flow which coincides with the lack of effort detected in muscles of inspiration. It is due to the absence of CNS respiratory drive and is detected by chest wall monitors that remain silent during inspiration. *Obstructive apnea* occurs when respiratory flow is absent or significantly reduced despite the fact that activity in muscles of inspiration is detected by chest wall monitors. This signifies that although respiratory drive is normal, obstruction in the upper airway prevents respiratory inflow. *Mixed apnea* occurs when the initial respiratory effort is absent (central) but is then followed by a gradually increasing effort to draw in air against an occluded airway (obstructive) (Table 12–3). Regardless of their cause, apneas often terminate in arousal from sleep and are detected by changes in the EEG. An arousal detected by EEG is characterized by an abrupt increase in the frequencies of waveforms that last 3 seconds or longer.

The apnea–hypopnea index (AHI) or respiratory disturbance index (RDI) refers to the number of respiratory apneas/hypopneas that occur in 1 hour of sleep. Less than five apneas/hypopneas per hour are observed in normal young adults, and their frequency increases with age. In general, an AHI ranging from 5 to 15 indicates a mild condition, 15 to 30 is considered moderate, and one greater than 30 is considered severe. AHI alone does not reflect the severity of oxygen desaturations or sleep disturbance.

Pathophysiologic Changes During Apneic Events

In the absence of ventilation during apnea, the Pao_2 falls rapidly in contrast to the slow rise in the $Paco_2$. Significant desaturation does not begin until the Pao_2 falls below 60 mm Hg. Lung oxygen stores in the supine position at functional residual capacity are only 35% of what would exist at total lung capacity in the upright position. Obese patients with elevated abdominal pressures have marked reductions in expiratory reserve volume, causing them to essentially ventilate from residual lung volumes that may be as much as 25% lower than those of nonobese individuals with proportionate reductions in lung oxygen stores. These factors increase the rate of the fall in Sao_2. In contrast to the reduction in systemic blood pressure that occurs during sleep in normal persons, OSA patients demonstrate

Table 12–3. Types of apneas

Apnea types	Chest and abdominal wall monitors	Oronasal thermistor
Obstructive	Movement detected (effort)	Interruption of flow
Central	No movement detected (no effort)	Interruption of flow
Mixed	First phase: no movement (no effort) Second phase: movement detected (mounting effort)	Interruption of flow

substantial elevations in both systemic and pulmonary arterial blood pressures. The greatest increase in systemic and pulmonary pressures is related to the severity of the arterial hypoxemia that occurs during REM sleep, when oxyhemoglobin desaturation is most severe. The pressures increase until the apneic episode is terminated. Maximal pressure elevation is associated with the lowest Sao_2 level as recorded by oximetry, immediately following termination of the apnea. Although systemic pressures usually return to baseline between apneas, pulmonary artery pressures rise progressively and often fail to return to baseline values during the night. Whether pulmonary hypertension occurs during the day as a consequence of hypoxemia induced by nocturnal apneas is controversial, but it is likely that daytime pulmonary hypertension is due more to the effect of comorbid conditions such as concomitant lung disease and obesity. Carotid and aortic bodies are arterial chemoreceptors that respond to the low Pao_2, high $Paco_2$, and low arterial pH that accompany apnea. When activated, these chemoreceptors cause bradycardia, peripheral arteriolar vasoconstriction, and increased catecholamine release, factors that support systemic blood pressure elevations that are observed during an apneic event. When an arousal terminates apnea, tonic parasympathetic stimulation (vagal tone) is interrupted and the heart rate increases. Apnea also increases right and left ventricular afterload and decreases cardiac output due to increased sympathetic outflow, physiologic responses to hypoxia, and the generation of negative intrathoracic pressure during inspiration against an occluded airway. Large negative intrathoracic pressures generated in OSA increase venous return to the right ventricle, causing increased right ventricular end-diastolic filling. This shifts the septum to the left, impeding left ventricular filling and compliance. During systole, ventricular emptying is impeded as well. This increases the pressure gradient, causing an increase in both right and left ventricular afterload, thereby decreasing stroke volume and output. In addition, bradycardia decreases cardiac output. After an apnea ceases, cardiac output increases by 10%–15% in a compensatory fashion.

Obstructive Sleep Apnea

ETIOLOGY & PATHOGENESIS

This disorder is seen ~2 times more in males and has a prevalence of ~5%. Its prevalence increases with age but severity decreases. The majority of patients with OSA are overweight, but not all are morbidly obese. The true prevalence is likely underestimated in normal weight individuals because OSA is not considered in these individuals.

PATHOPHYSIOLOGY

The pharynx is the major site of upper airway obstruction in OSA. However, the exact sequence of events that cause closure of the upper airway in OSA remains incompletely understood. In general, it is known that there is an imbalance between pharynx dilation and closure. It has been suggested by imaging studies that those with OSA have narrower upper airways. In normal subjects airway closure or collapse occurs when airway pressures fall below -15 cm H_2O. However, patients with OSA fail to resist pressures lower than even -3 cm H_2O due to structural changes and altered pharyngeal muscle function. Neuromuscular control of pharyngeal muscles is coordinated by the CNS. During sleep, tonic and phasic activity of the pharyngeal dilator muscles, particularly the genioglossus, is reduced, especially during REM sleep, which facilitates the decreased tone (relaxation) of pharyngeal structures. In addition, supine position, inflammation of the upper airway, and neuromuscular damage can add to the effect of pharyngeal abnormalities and promote closure of the upper airway. With the airway closure, there is decreased ventilation and development of hypoxemia with continued ventilatory effort resulting in increased vagal tone. Hypoxemia, hypercarbia, and increased negative intrathoracic pressure are all possible stimuli resulting in arousal to establish a patent airway again.

Diagnostic & Clinical Considerations

Sleep-related symptoms are best obtained from a family member who observes the characteristic snoring pattern of the affected individual. The cardinal symptom of OSA is daytime hypersomnia. A questionnaire such as the Epworth Sleepiness Scale contains questions that are sensitive for the presence of excessive sleepiness and can be useful for detecting and scoring the patient's level of daytime sleepiness. Paradoxically, some patients may not perceive themselves as sleepy but will admit to napping during monotonous situations, such as while watching television or long distance driving. Other daytime symptoms include fatigue, awakening with dry mouth or headache, memory impairment, and impotence. Nocturnal symptoms include snoring with pauses and gasps, and restless sleep including periodic limb movements, nocturia, and nocturnal choking (Table 12–4). In contrast to the effect of napping in narcolepsy, which is restorative, sleepiness in OSA is only partially relieved by a nap. In severe cases, the effects of this disorder impair work performance and can lead to daytime sleepiness, fatigue, and motor vehicle accidents. Diagnostic testing using polysomnography (PSG) is the gold standard for evaluation of OSA and other sleep disorders. The variables that are measured in an overnight sleep study include sleep stages (EEG and EOG), respiratory effort (chest band monitors), airflow (nasal and oral thermistors), Sao_2 (pulse oximetry), body position (noted by a sleep technician), limb and chin movements (EMG), and cardiac rate and rhythm (ECG). The diagnostic portion of the study determines the number of apneic/hypopneic events (AHI) and severity of O_2 desaturations, which in turn permits grading of SRBD severity and its correction and reversal with the use of continuous positive airway pressure (CPAP) (Figure 12–5).

Management Principles

Positive airway pressure treatment is the preferred treatment for patients with OSA who are able to tolerate the treatment. Positive airway pressure is created by a fan-generated flow delivered through a mask to create a pneumatic splint to maintain airway patency. The most commonly used positive airway device is CPAP. CPAP produces a continuous 20–60 L/min flow using a fan at a set pressure which creates a 4–20 cm H_2O pressure that is delivered through a mask. The pressure is constant during inhalation and exhalation. This constant pressure prevents the collapse

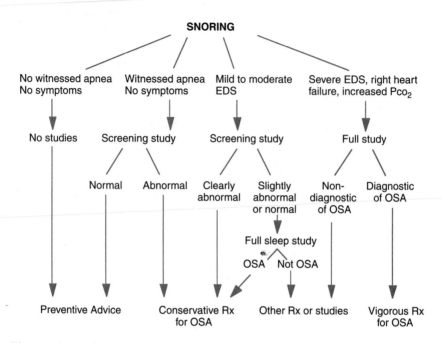

SNORING

No witnessed apnea
No symptoms → No studies

Witnessed apnea
No symptoms → Screening study → Normal / Abnormal

Mild to moderate
EDS → Screening study → Clearly abnormal / Slightly abnormal or normal

Severe EDS, right heart
failure, increased P_{CO_2} → Full study → Non-diagnostic of OSA / Diagnostic of OSA

Full sleep study → OSA / Not OSA

Preventive Advice

Conservative Rx
for OSA

Other Rx or studies

Vigorous Rx
for OSA

Figure 12–3. Algorithm for the work-up of patients with complaints of snoring. EDS, excessive daytime sleepiness; OSA, obstructive sleep apnea.

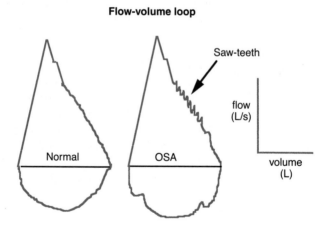

Flow-volume loop

Saw-teeth

flow
(L/s)

Normal

OSA

volume
(L)

Figure 12–4. Comparison of the typical flow-volume loop from a patient with OSA with that from a normal individual.

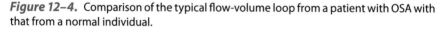

produced by inspiratory negative thoracic pressure. Weight loss of even 5%–10% is also a very effective treatment for this condition because it increases the lateral dimensions of the upper airway, decreases its collapsibility, and increases lung volume, and in doing so it produces a significant decrease in AHI. Body position

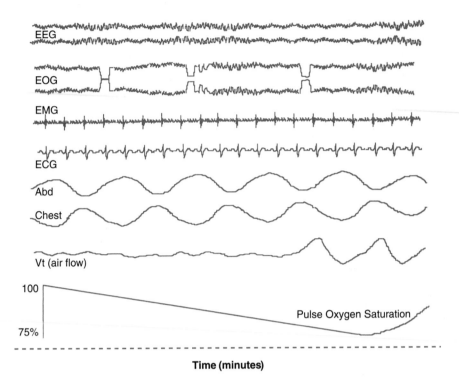

EEG

EOG

EMG

ECG

Abd

Chest

Vt (air flow)

100

Pulse Oxygen Saturation

75%

Time (minutes)

Figure 12–5. Polysomnogram of an individual with OSA. Note the presence of respiratory and abdominal muscle activity during apneic episodes.

also affects AHI. Sleeping in the supine position allows gravity to pull the tongue backward and narrows the upper airway. By maintaining sleep in the lateral decubitus position, position-dependent apneas can be almost completely eliminated if there is evidence of significant supine posture-related worsening of AHI. Likewise elevating the head of the bed 30° may also provide benefit. Oral appliances which function to open and dilate the upper airway by repositioning the mandible are also a treatment option. Tracheostomy is a definitive therapy for OSA and is indicated for patients who do not respond to CPAP therapy. Uvulopalatopharyngoplasty is useful for the treatment of severe snoring and in selected patients with OSA.

Central Sleep Apnea

ETIOLOGY & PATHOGENESIS

Central apneas and hypopneas are caused by cessation of the respiratory drive; they can trigger an episode of hyperpnea that restores oxygen levels. However, hyperventilation also decreases the $Paco_2$ level which can trigger a new apnea. When episodes of central apnea alternate with hyperpneas in a waxing and waning fashion, it is known as *Cheyne-Stokes respiration.* This scenario is more likely to occur in patients who have severe CHF with a severely depressed ejection fraction

Table 12–4. Symptoms associated with obstructive sleep apnea

Symptom	Incidence (%)
Loud snoring	95
Excessive daytime sleepiness	75
Restless sleep	99
Poor mentation	58
Personality changes	48
Impotence	40
Morning headaches	35
Nocturia	30
Enuresis	7
Waking up with dry mouth	?[a]

[a] Unknown incidence, but common.

Table 12–5. Conditions associated with obstructive apneas

Achondroplastic dwarfism
Acromegaly
Amyloidosis
Amyotrophic lateral sclerosis
Arnold-Chiari syndrome
Congestive heart failure
Chronic obstructive pulmonary disease
Down's syndrome
Hypothyroidism
Myotonic dystrophy
Polio and postpolio syndrome
Renal failure
Sickle cell disease
Structural abnormalities of the oropharynx (enlarged tonsils, adenoids, uvula, mandibular/maxillary hypoplasia)

(Table 12–7). Central apneic events generally occur in the transition from wakefulness to sleep in stages 1 and 2 and cause arousals such that these patients often complain of insomnia or inability to remain asleep, rather than or in addition to daytime sleepiness. Often CSA patients exhibit a combination of apnea types, central and mixed, although central apneas predominate. This syndrome is much less common than OSA and only affects about 15% of apnea patients. It is more likely to occur in women after menopause and obesity and snoring are much less common.

PATHOPHYSIOLOGY

The level of the partial pressure of carbon dioxide (P_{CO_2}) required to drive respiration (the apneic metabolic threshold) during wakefulness is lower

Table 12–6. Treatment of obstructive sleep apnea

Nonsurgical
Weight reduction
CPAP
Orthodontic devices
Miscellaneous
Nocturnal ventilation
Respiratory stimulants
Other drugs (naloxone, flutamide, dopamine antagonists, L-tryptophan)
Surgical
Tracheostomy
UPPP
Nasal and tonsillar-adenoid surgery
Inferior sagittal ostetomy with myotomy and suspension
Maxillomandibular and hyoid advancement
UPPP plus other surgical procedures

Note: CPAP, continuous positive airway pressure; UPPP, uvulopalatopharyngoplasty.

Table 12–7. Conditions that can cause central apneas

Conditions leading to daytime hypoventilation
Idiopathic central hypoventilation
Brain stem disease (eg, multiple sclerosis, stroke, tumor)
Neuromuscular weakness (eg, polio, postpolio syndrome, ALS)
Conditions that do not cause daytime hypoventilation
Cheyne-Stokes breathing due to:
Congestive heart failure or pulmonary congestion
Neurologic disease
During excessive CPAP titration
Idiopathic CSA
Pulmonary disease
Sleep at high altitude
Gastroesophageal reflux

Note: ALS, amyotrophic lateral sclerosis; CPAP, continuous positive airway pressure; CSA, central sleep apnea.

than that required during sleep because alertness provides an additional powerful stimulation for respiration. However, during the transition into sleep when alertness disappears, respiration depends more heavily on the level of P_{CO_2} to drive respiration, and it must rise to the critical level necessary to stimulate the next breath. In those moments, apneas or hypopneas can occur, even in normal patients. Patients who have cardiopulmonary abnormalities or live at high altitudes may experience relative daytime hypoxia. They may compensate with increased respirations that cause relative hypocapnia. As noted above, alertness compensates for hypocapnia, and the respiratory drive is maintained during wakefulness. However, when these patients fall asleep, the depressed Pco_2 level has further to go before it triggers respiration. Resulting central apneas can be prolonged and frequent. In addition, a patient with significant heart failure has circulation slowing such that the lag between the time of gas exchange in the lung bed and that detected by chemoreceptors in the brain stem and periphery is prolonged. This causes the system to exceed its metabolic set points, resulting in even wider cyclical swings in respiration. Another group of patients experience hypoventilation due to weakened respiratory muscles (neuromuscular disease), reduced respiratory drive (brain stem disease), or esophageal disease that reduces reflexes involved in triggering respiration and interrupts the feedback loop. For these patients, metabolic factors are less important in causing central apneas than are mechanical or structural abnormalities.

DIAGNOSTIC & CLINICAL CONSIDERATIONS

Symptoms associated with CSA include insomnia, recurrent nocturnal awakenings, morning fatigue, and headaches (Table 12–8). This condition occurs in association with hypoxia, metabolic derangements, heart disease, and CNS pathology. Most central apneas occur at sleep onset and are recurrent in nature, establishing a cycle of decreased or absent respiratory effort terminated by ongoing arousals, thereby causing periodic cyclical breathing that is usually observed by a bed partner. The differential diagnosis includes OSA; however, snoring is not a dominant feature. Daytime hypersomnolence resulting from sleep fragmentation is invariably present. Associated conditions, especially left ventricular dysfunction, should be evaluated. A polysomnographic study reveals the absence of respiratory and abdominal muscle activity during periods of apnea (Figure 12–6).

MANAGEMENT PRINCIPLES

Since CSA can be due to a heterogeneous group of factors, therapy must be tailored to the individual. For some patients, there is an association of cardiopulmonary disease and CSA. In these cases treating CSA can improve cardiac function. The beneficial effects of effective CPAP therapy on cardiac function include improved oxygenation, decreased afterload, and decreased sympathetic tone produced by frequent nocturnal arousals. In addition, the treatment of underlying cardiac dysfunction can improve CSA by improving metabolic and circulatory factors that contribute to apneas. Nasal CPAP is often effective. The addition of

Table 12–8. Symptoms associated with central sleep apnea

Insomnia
Recurrent nocturnal awakenings
Waking up with gasping sensation
Sleeping poorly
Morning headache
Excessive daytime sleepiness
Morning fatigue

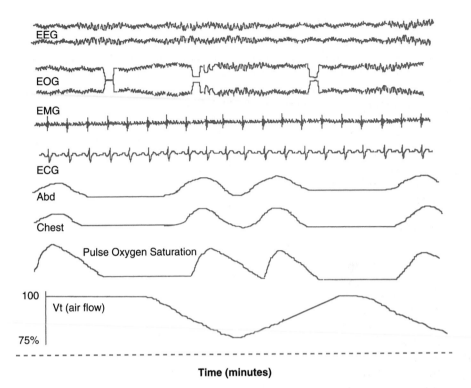

EEG

EOG

EMG

ECG

Abd

Chest

Pulse Oxygen Saturation

100

Vt (air flow)

75%

Time (minutes)

Figure 12–6. Polysomnogram of an individual with central sleep apnea (CSA). Note the absence of respiratory and abdominal muscle activity during apneic episodes.

oxygen may benefit selected patients, especially those with COPD who have persistent nocturnal hypoxemia. For patients with neuromuscular dysfunction, a full face mask with BiPAP is helpful to prevent nocturnal hypoventilation. During wakefulness, respiration may be maintained without the need for additional ventilation. Surgical therapy includes diaphragmatic pacing as well as tracheostomy to augment nocturnal ventilation with respiratory devices.

Obesity Hypoventilation Syndrome

ETIOLOGY & PATHOPHYSIOLOGY

Obesity hypoventilation syndrome is described by hypercapnic respiratory failure and the coexistence of obesity. The mechanism of this form of respiratory is not clear. A central origin with a defect in the respiratory controller has been proposed. In addition, fat deposit in the chest wall can change lung mechanics. Obesity can lead to decreased lung volume, chest wall and lung compliance, and inspiratory muscle strength. These changes lead to an increase in the work of breathing and increase dead space. There is a strong association between obesity hypoventilation syndrome (OHS) and OSA syndrome but not all patients with OHS have OSA syndrome.

Most patients have a body mass index (BMI) greater than 40 kg/m². Pulmonary function testing is not very useful in diagnosis which usually demonstrates a restrictive defect. This defect is likely more related to obesity since it has not been seen in pure OSAS matched for gender, BMI, and age. OHS leads to secondary pulmonary hypertension with increased total pulmonary vascular resistance due to prolonged periods of alveolar hypoxia. With normal lung function and ventilatory drive, apneas or hyponeas should only lead to an acute rise in CO_2 with no daytime hypercapnia. An impaired ventilatory drive or an impaired ventilatory function or both in a patient with OSAS can lead to persistent hypercapnia which is seen in OHS.

TREATMENT

The first line of treatment for OHS is weight loss. Weight loss can reverse the respiratory failure. NIMV treatment improves daytime symptoms and improves the respiratory failure. BiPAP improves tidal volume, respiratory muscles efficacy, and lung compliance. CPAP has been demonstrated to improve nocturnal apneic events but does not revert the respiratory failure.

CLINICAL SCENARIOS

Case 1

A 52-year-old man was referred to the clinic because "my wife can't stand my snoring." He did not report excessive daytime sleepiness, but his wife related that he had been involved in two automobile accidents in the past few months and often fell asleep watching TV. He had gained 60 pounds over the past few years and had a history of diabetes mellitus, high blood pressure, and coronary artery disease. He has a high score on the Epworth Sleepiness Scale.

Physical Examination: On examination, his BMI was found to be 39, neck circumference 18 in., BP 170/87 mm Hg, and HR 110/min. His exam also revealed a small anteroposterior oropharyngeal diameter. The PSG showed O_2 desaturation to 80% with an AHI of 22. The patient has moderately severe OSA with good reversibility with CPAP.

Discussion: Patients with OSA are often not aware of their own symptoms. A family member who observes the characteristic snoring pattern and notes symptoms that the patient may deny is very important to obtaining a complete history. In addition, a high score on the Epworth Sleepiness Scale will often correlate with the observed severity of OSA. Weight gain is causative in the development of OSA. Losing even 5%–10% of body weight will improve symptoms. Finally, conditions such as hypertension and heart failure can be improved by treating a patient's sleep apnea.

CLINICAL PEARL

When OSA is suspected in a patient, it is important to elicit a history of snoring and sleep disturbance from a family member.

Case 2

A 49-year-old man (smoker) is seen with severe GERD. He also has complaints of excessive daytime sleepiness and snoring.

Physical Examination: On examination he was found to be obese, with a BMI of 41 and BP of 159/72 mm Hg. The PSG reveals obstructive apneas during REM sleep (AHI = 34) in the supine position with the lowest Sao_2 of 83%. Titration with CPAP to a pressure of 10 cm H_2O suppressed the obstructive apneas. To completely suppress snoring, the pressure was increased, but central apneas occurred. The patient underwent cardiac and pulmonary evaluations. He was diagnosed with CHF and moderate COPD and treated accordingly for these conditions as well as for his GERD.

Discussion: The etiology of the patient's central apneas was multifactorial. In some cases, central apneas can be a consequence of aggressive titration with CPAP when pressures are too high and the patient is persistently aroused from sleep. In such cases the apneas are not pathologic since they are a by-product of first-time CPAP application. However, this patient had multiple preexisting conditions that cause central apneas, and most often they are related to unsuspected CHF. In this case, the patient also had severe GERD and moderate COPD. Treatment of underlying systemic conditions improved his sleep disorder. Further treatment of his sleep disorder with CPAP, weight loss, and smoking cessation improved his systemic conditions as well.

CLINICAL PEARL

As the cause of central apnea is multifactorial, treatment of associated comorbid conditions is key to improving the sleep disorder.

KEY CONCEPTS

Obstructive sleep apnea is recognized as one of the leading causes of daytime somnolence and fatigue and contributes to several cardiopulmonary derangements such as secondary pulmonary hypertension, right heart failure, cardiac arrhythmias, and strokes. It may also cause sudden death.

Central sleep apnea is generally multifactorial, causing mixed apnea patterns on the polysomnogram, and is often associated with cardiopulmonary disorders and metabolic derangements that trigger respiration.

When evaluating a patient with either OSA or CSA, it is often necessary to obtain history from a third party who can observe the patient while asleep; the diagnosis is confirmed when apneas are observed and measured during a PSG.

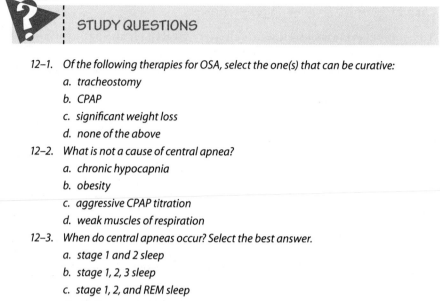

STUDY QUESTIONS

12–1. *Of the following therapies for OSA, select the one(s) that can be curative:*
   a. tracheostomy
   b. CPAP
   c. significant weight loss
   d. none of the above

12–2. *What is not a cause of central apnea?*
   a. chronic hypocapnia
   b. obesity
   c. aggressive CPAP titration
   d. weak muscles of respiration

12–3. *When do central apneas occur? Select the best answer.*
   a. stage 1 and 2 sleep
   b. stage 1, 2, 3 sleep
   c. stage 1, 2, and REM sleep
   d. all sleep stages

SUGGESTED READINGS

Chokroverty S, Daroff RB, eds. *Sleep Disorders Medicine: Basic Science, Technical Considerations and Clinical Aspects.* 2nd ed. Boston: Butterworth-Heinemann; 1999.

Kryger MH, Roth WT, Dement WC, eds. *Principles and Practices of Sleep Medicine.* 3rd ed. Philadelphia: WB Saunders; 2000.

Respiratory Failure

Jennifer Ramsey & Peter DeBlieux

OBJECTIVES

▶ Delineate and understand the symptoms and management of respiratory failure.

▶ Evaluate clinical presentations and coordinate appropriate mechanical ventilation therapies.

▶ Be familiar with the risks associated with instituting mechanical ventilation and complications that may result.

▶ Analyze and comprehend a clinical pathway for evaluating and treating a patient with respiratory failure with the help of clinical scenarios.

GENERAL CONSIDERATIONS

Respiratory failure, whether acute or chronic, remains one of the most common life-threatening medical problems encountered in critical care. It is estimated that 34% of patients in critical care in the United States receive mechanical ventilation. Short-term survival rates for patients with acute respiratory failure (ARF) that is not preceded by preexisting disease or associated multiorgan failure are more than 85%. Hospital mortality rates for acute exacerbations of chronic obstructive pulmonary disease (COPD) are less than 20%; however, quality of life and 1-year survival rates are generally poor. Outcomes of patients with ARF with preexisting disease depend primarily on the underlying conditions. Approximately 17% of patients placed on mechanical ventilation require support for more than 14 days.

Respiratory failure is a functional disorder caused by conditions that impair the ability of the respiratory system to remove carbon dioxide from and deliver oxygen to the pulmonary capillary bed. This inability to complete gas exchange results in abnormally low arterial oxygen tension with or without abnormally high arterial carbon dioxide tension.

The clinical manifestations of respiratory failure are linked to the patient's ability to adapt to hypoxemia and hypercapnia. The concept of *cardiopulmonary reserve* is vital to understanding a patient's ability to adapt. Cardiopulmonary

227

reserve refers to the interdependence of the heart, lungs, and oxygen-carrying capacity of any given patient. A patient with an impaired cardiac pump, preexisting pulmonary disease, or abnormalities in hemoglobin will have less "reserve" and will require a more urgent intervention for a respiratory event in comparison to a patient with normal physiology. Normal lungs, heart, and hemoglobin permit a degree of physiologic reserve that allows patients to compensate for an acute respiratory insult.

ETIOLOGY & PATHOGENESIS

Respiratory failure may be acute or chronic, depending on when the process develops, with varying pathogenic, physiologic, and therapeutic distinctions. Both acute and chronic respiratory failure can be classified into two main groups distinguishable by arterial blood gas analysis. The first category, hypoxic respiratory failure (HRF), is characterized by an abnormally low partial pressure of arterial oxygen (Pao_2) with a normal or low partial pressure of arterial carbon dioxide ($Paco_2$). The second category, hypercapnic-hypoxic respiratory failure (HHRF), is associated with an abnormally elevated $Paco_2$ coupled with an abnormally low Pao_2.

Acute Hypoxic Respiratory Failure

Hypoxic respiratory failure may be defined as any pulmonary condition resulting in severe arterial hypoxemia (Pao_2 <50 mm Hg) that cannot be corrected by increasing the fraction of inspired oxygen (Fio_2) to >50% (>0.5). Pathophysiologic causes of hypoxemia with an anatomic correlation are outlined in Table 13–1A and B

Table 13–1A. Causes of hypoxemia: Anatomic correlation with pathophysiological derangement

Anatomic	Pathophysiology
Airspace filling defect	V̇/Q̇ mismatch
Interstitial inflammation and fibrosis	Diffusion impairment
Vascular lesions/shunts	Shunt defects
Airway compromise or collapse	Hypoventilation

Table 13–1B. Clinical conditions associated with hypoxemia and relationship to arterial blood gas values (ABGs)

Clinical Diagnosis	ABGs
COPD, chronic asthma	Reduced Pao_2, increased Pco_2
Diffuse interstitial pulmonary disease	Reduced Pao_2, variable Pco_2
Congestive heart failure, pulmonary embolism	Reduced Pao_2, reduced Pco_2
UAO, OSA, morbid obesity, chest wall defects	Reduced Pao_2, increased Pco_2

Note: COPD, chronic obstructive pulmonary disease; UAO, upper airway obstruction; OSA, obstructive sleep apnea.

Acute respiratory failure limited to hypoxemia alone generally represents a disease process that involves only the lung, as it functions in gas exchange. Severity of ventilation-perfusion mismatching correlates well with the inability to increase Pao_2 despite subsequent increases in supplemental oxygen. Typically, the alveolar-arterial gradient increases with the addition of inspired oxygen, and the ratio of Pao_2:Fio_2 (PF ratio) becomes increasingly low.

Acute respiratory distress syndrome (ARDS) is the clinical correlate of a severe form of acute lung injury (ALI) that causes acute and persistent lung inflammation with increased capillary permeability. ARDS can occur without other organ damage as in severe inhalational injury or air embolism, and the early pathologic features are described as diffuse alveolar damage accompanied by the release of proinflammatory cytokines and toxic mediators, causing endothelial damage and acute lung injury (ALI). Alveolar and interstitial edema occurs due to protein and fluid shifts that overwhelm the capacity of the lymphatics. As a result, the air spaces fill with bloody, proteinaceous edema fluid and debris from degenerating cells with loss of surfactant and subsequent atelectasis. This in turn causes impaired gas exchange due to ventilation-perfusion abnormalities and severe right-to-left arteriovenous shunts with decreased compliance due to poorly aerated and stiff lungs. Further hypoxic vasoconstriction and vascular compression causes pulmonary hypertension. A chronic state may result in secondary erythrocytosis and increased blood viscosity leading to right ventricular strain and cor pulmonale (Figure 13–1). ARDS progresses through three relatively discrete pathologic stages. The initial "exudative" stage, characterized by diffuse alveolar damage, is followed by a "proliferative" stage, which is characterized by resolution of pulmonary edema and by proliferation of type II alveolar cells, squamous metaplasia,

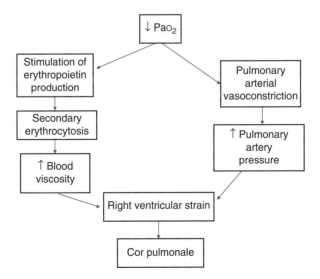

Figure 13–1. Consequences of chronic hypoxic respiratory failure.

and interstitial infiltration by myofibroblasts, and early deposition of collagen. Some patients progress to a third "fibrotic" stage, characterized by obliteration of normal lung architecture, diffuse fibrosis, and cyst formation.

Hypercapnic-Hypoxic Respiratory Failure

Hypercapnic-hypoxic respiratory failure is best defined as a ventilatory insufficiency resulting from a reduction in minute ventilation, or an increase in dead space ventilation that is associated with a direct reduction in alveolar ventilation.

A specific level of $Paco_2$ attributable to HHRF is difficult to assign without knowledge of the cause of the respiratory failure and the patient's previous condition. During hypoventilation, the carbon dioxide pressure ($Paco_2$) and Pao_2 levels change in opposite directions by nearly the same amount (Figure 13–2). HHRF is always associated with some degree of hypoxemia. Even with a severe degree of alveolar hypoventilation, resulting in a doubling of $Paco_2$, hypoxemia will not be a dominant feature in the normal lung due to a normal alveolar-arterial oxygen gradient. In contrast there is worsening hypoxemia in a diseased lung insulted with diminished alveolar ventilation. The primary etiology of HHRF is impaired gas exchange that results in increased dead space, ventilation-perfusion mismatches, and reductions in alveolar ventilation. The partial pressure of carbon dioxide within the alveoli ($Paco_2$) is increased and the Pao_2 is subsequently reduced.

In emphysema, the pathogenesis is thought to be secondary to destruction of the alveolar capillary interface. The mechanism is primarily a function of tobacco use, which causes excess oxygen stress with alveolar macrophage and neutrophilic inflammation damaging the alveolar septum. This results in loss of the vascular bed and lung recoil with marked overinflation, causing derangement of gas exchange and dead space ventilation. Bronchial asthma is the second most common cause of HHRF. There is increased large and small airway resistance secondary to mast cell and eosinophilic inflammation with edema,

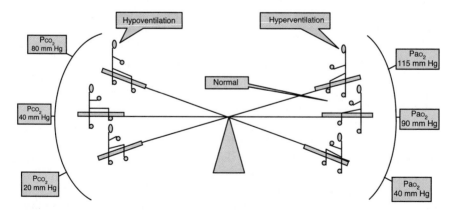

Figure 13–2. Relationship between Pao_2 and $Paco_2$: Illustrative examples.

airway remodeling, mucus hypersecretion, and muscle hypertrophy. HHRF may result from the failure of the structures that contribute to the ventilation of the lung, including central nervous system disorders, neuromuscular disorders, and fatigue. (See Chapter 6 for further discussion.) The primary mechanism for hypoxemia in HHRF secondary to COPD and asthma is the perfusion of poorly ventilated lung units or ventilation-perfusion mismatch. The clinical manifestations of respiratory failure are dictated by difficulties in gas transport and alveolar ventilation. The symptom complexes are linked to the patient's adaptability to changes in hypoxemia and hypercapnia. The degree of ventilatory response is more closely correlated with the capacity of the respiratory system to respond to hypoxemia than with its ability to respond to hypercapnia. As a direct result of hypoxemia, the sympathetic nervous system is activated, creating a direct outflow of catecholamines. The cardiovascular response to catecholamine stimulation is tachycardia, increased systemic vasoconstriction, and increased cardiac output. Arterial hypoxemia directly stimulates the carotid body chemoreceptors, leading to an increase in minute ventilation. In cases of severe hypoxemia the myocardium and central nervous system are at greatest risk of injury; tissue hypoxia is associated with impaired mental performance and myocardial dysfunction. Clinical manifestations of HHRF are compounded by the presence of hematologic or circulatory abnormalities. Acute hypercapnia causes central nervous system depression by lowering cerebrospinal fluid pH. The rapid decreases in serum pH, as opposed to absolute levels of serum $Paco_2$, best correlate with a depression in mental status. Hypercapnia does stimulate increases in minute ventilation in normal subjects, but this response is commonly blunted by the pathology that led to the episode of HHRF. This diminished response impairs effective improvement in alveolar ventilation.

DIAGNOSTIC & CLINICAL CONSIDERATIONS

Evaluation should initially focus on the events leading to the onset of respiratory distress, such as drug effect, infection, trauma, or neurologic events such as seizures, as well as any underlying disease such as asthma and COPD. Findings are dependent on the cause of respiratory failure and ARDS. These may include fever, hypotension, abdominal pain, or coma.

Common clinical causes of HRF are listed in Table 13–2 and include but are not limited to pneumonia, aspiration, sepsis, trauma, neurologic insults, and post-transplant lung injuries. Massive blood transfusions and leukoagglutinin reactions can cause severe acute lung injury, ARDS, and lead to respiratory failure.

In ARDS, respiratory distress usually follows 24–48 hours after some systemic insult, with rapidly worsening tachypnea, dyspnea, and hypoxemia requiring high concentrations of supplemental oxygen; dry cough and chest pain may also be present. The physical examination usually reveals cyanosis, tachycardia, tachypnea, and diffuse rales in the chest. Laboratory findings are nonspecific and may include increased white cell count, decreased platelets, evidence of disseminated intravascular coagulation (DIC), and metabolic acidosis or lactic acidosis. Arterial blood gases usually show an acute respiratory alkalosis, an elevated alveolar-arterial

Table 13–2. Causes of acute hypoxic respiratory failure (HRF)

Adult respiratory distress syndrome (ARDS)
Severe acute respiratory syndrome (SARS)
Aspiration
Atelectasis (lobar)
Cardiogenic pulmonary edema
Lung contusion or alveolar hemorrhage
Pneumonia
Pneumothorax
Pulmonary embolus
Transfusion-related acute lung injury

Table 13–3. Symptoms of hypoxemia and hypercapnia

Hypoxemia	Hypercapnia
Tachycardia	Somnolence
Tachypnea	Lethargy
Anxiety	Restlessness
Diaphoresis	Tremor
Altered mental status	Slurred speech
Confusion	Headache
Cyanosis	Asterixis
Hypertension	Papilledema
Hypotension	Coma
Bradycardia	
Seizures	
Lactic acidosis	

oxygen gradient and severe hypoxemia. A metabolic acidosis is often present in patients with sepsis and shock. The hypoxemic patient will appear agitated, and at times delirious (Table 13–3). As a direct result of hypoxemia, the sympathetic nervous system is activated, creating a direct outflow of catecholamines. The cardiovascular response to catecholamine stimulation is tachycardia, increased systemic vasoconstriction, and increased cardiac output. Arterial hypoxemia directly stimulates the carotid body chemoreceptors, leading to an increase in minute ventilation. In cases of severe hypoxemia the myocardium and central nervous system are at greatest risk of injury; tissue hypoxia is associated with impaired mental performance and myocardial dysfunction. It is important to identify the underlying cause (Table 13–4).

Although HHRF is always associated with some degree of hypoxemia, specific causes of HHRF are listed in Table 13–5. HHRF may result from the failure of the structures that contribute to the ventilation of the lung, including central nervous system disorders, neuromuscular disorders, and fatigue.

In patients with HHRF the chest radiograph often shows significant hyperinflation in asthma and COPD, or small lung volumes in neuromuscular disease and drug overdose.

Table 13–4. Causes of adult respiratory distress syndrome (ARDS)

Aspiration
  Fresh and salt water
  Gastric contents
  Hydrocarbons
Central nervous system
  Anoxia
  Increased intracranial pressure
  Seizures
  Trauma
Drug overdose or reactions
  Acetylsalicylic acid
  Cocaine
  Heroin and other opiates
  Paraquat
  Plaquenil
  Propoxyphene
Hematologic alterations
  Disseminated intravascular coagulation
  Massive blood transfusion
  Leukoagglutination reactions
Infections
  Pneumonia (bacterial, fungal, viral)
  Sepsis
  Tuberculosis
Inhalation injury
  Corrosive chemicals (NO_2, Cl_2, NH_3, phosgene)
  Oxygen
  Smoke
Metabolic disorders
  Pancreatitis
  Uremia
  Severe acute respiratory syndrome (SARS)
Shock
Trauma
  Cardiopulmonary bypass
  Fat emboli
  Lung contusion
  Multisystem nonthoracic trauma

The chest x-ray in ARDS or ALI typically shows diffuse air space disease with fluffy alveolar infiltrates in multiple lung zones with prominent air bronchograms (Figure 13–3). Similar changes can be seen in other processes such as diffuse pulmonary hemorrhage or congestive heart failure (CHF), with some subtle differences. Computed tomography (CT) demonstrates patchy ground-glass abnormalities with increased radiodensity in dependent lung zones. Oxygenation tends to improve somewhat over the first few days as pulmonary edema resolves, but most patients remain ventilator dependent due to continued hypoxemia, high minute ventilation requirements, and poor lung compliance. Radiographic

Table 13–5. Causes of hypercapnic hypoxic respiratory failure

Central nervous system
   Central hypoventilation
   Closed head injury
   Drugs, poisons, toxins
   Excess oxygen administration in a hypercapnic patient
   Intracranial mass effect
Neuromuscular diseases
   Acute polyneuritis
   Myasthenia gravis
   Polymyositis, dermatomyositis
   Spinal cord lesions
Metabolic derangement
   Hypokalemia
   Hypomagnesemia
   Hypophosphatemia
   Severe acidosis
   Severe alkalosis
Airway disease
   Upper (fixed, variable, sleep dependent)
   Lower (asthma, COPD)
Musculoskeletal
   Burns to chest wall
   Flail segment
   Kyphoscoliosis
Obesity hypoventilation
Myxedema coma

Note: COPD, chronic obstructive pulmonary disease.

densities become less opaque, reflecting resolution of pulmonary edema, while interstitial infiltrates remain. The development of interstitial emphysema and lung cysts may occur. Secondary events such as pneumothorax or pneumonia may complicate the radiographic presentations. At this point the clinical course may become dominated by complications such as volu-barotrauma, nosocomial infection, or the development of the multiple organ dysfunction syndrome (MODS). If the cause of the underlying process or complication is not clear, bronchoscopy with lavage may help identify the underlying process, such as occult aspiration, hemorrhage, or infection. Although transbronchial biopsy and open lung biopsy can be performed, their yield in this group of patients is usually disappointing, and does not aid in the diagnosis except in patients with disseminated cancer or diffuse pulmonary vasculitis.

MANAGEMENT PRINCIPLES

Management principles for HRF focus on oxygen supplementation and enhanced tissue oxygen delivery. Administration of oxygen via nasal cannula, Ventimask, and nonrebreather mask allows delivery of oxygen concentrations from 23% to approximately 70% FIO_2. Severity of ventilation-perfusion mismatching correlates

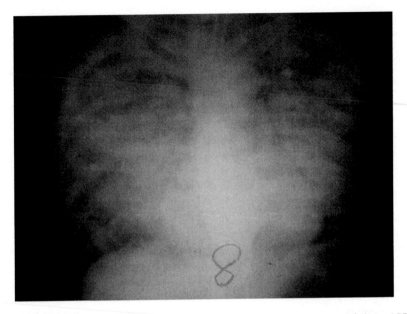

Figure 13–3. A patient with diffuse air space opacities and respiratory failure. ARDS, acute respiratory distress syndrome.

well with the inability to increase Pao_2 with subsequent increases in supplemental oxygen. Oxygen delivery with a semiclosed (noninvasive positive pressure ventilation [NIPPV]) or closed system (intermittent positive pressure ventilation [IPPV]) may be warranted to achieve adequate Pao_2 levels unobtainable with cannula and oxygen mask delivery. Benefits and limitations of these forms of mechanical ventilation are discussed later in this chapter. Positive pressure ventilation with increasing levels of positive end-expiratory pressure (PEEP) is usually required in patients with acute lung injury (ALI). The designation ALI covers a spectrum of pulmonary diseases, including early inflammatory conditions ranging in severity from pneumonitis to ARDS. The addition of PEEP to a ventilatory system must be undertaken in a careful fashion, by monitoring the patient's pulmonary compliance, cardiac output, and oxygenation to achieve a delicate balance between oxygenation, oxygen delivery, oxygen toxicity, and the risk of ventilator-induced lung injury (VILI). Early administration of antibiotics for presumed sepsis and early hemodynamic support for patients with shock are two examples of prompt supportive measures that affect HRF outcomes.

Management principles for HHRF are based on resolution of the ventilatory deficit, institution of appropriate oxygenation, and treatment of the active disease process. Often correction of the underlying cause for the reduced alveolar ventilation associated with HHRF will correct the abnormalities in Pco_2 and Pao_2. Choosing a means of correction in these patients is linked to cause, acuity, reversibility, and available technologies. Options include administration of bronchodilators and corticosteroids, invasive and noninvasive mechanical ventilation, reversal agents as naloxone and flumazenil, supportive care, and surgical airway management. Specific therapies and interventions are addressed below.

Oxygen Therapy

The role of oxygen therapy in the treatment of respiratory failure is disease-specific, ranging from patients with profound ventilation-perfusion mismatch to those with a pure alveolar hypoventilation hypoxia. Oxygen delivery systems can be grouped as either open or closed systems. Open systems, typically represented by nasal cannula, Ventimasks, and non-rebreather masks, limit the FIO_2 delivered due to entrainment of surrounding room air. Nasal cannula deliver a variable amount of oxygen (23–32%), based on flow rate and breathing pattern (nose versus mouth). The Ventimask system allows a more accurate estimate of FIO_2 (23–50%), due to mask delivery and improved control of entrained room air. The highest possible FIO_2 attainable with a 100% non-rebreather mask approaches 0.7.

A rough estimate of the FIO_2 is that each liter per minute of oxygen supplied by the nasal cannula increases the FIO_2 by 3–4%. However, the precise percentage of inspired oxygen cannot be determined as it is different in each patient based on how much room air is entrained via mouth breathing. Oxygen delivery via a nasal cannula is comfortable, minimally invasive, and allows people to eat and talk; however, even with humidified oxygen, the nasal cannula system will dry mucous membranes, causing them to become very irritated and bleed. Also, the amount of oxygen that can be delivered this way is limited by the increasing discomfort to the patient with increasing flow rates; 5 liters per minute is the usual limit of this delivery system. Nasal cannulas deliver a variable amount of oxygen (23–32%), based on flow rate and breathing pattern (nose versus mouth).

Masks can provide higher flow of oxygen in a way that is tolerable to the patient. Masks differ in the flow of O_2 and in the amount of exhaled air and room air inhaled with each breath. This administrative tactic is limited by a lack of seal between the mask and the patient's face and by the limit of 15 liters a minute, the maximum flow a wall unit is capable of delivering.

A patient in distress is capable of creating a minute volume of almost double that in liters per minute; the higher the minute volume the patient creates over the amount the wall unit can provide, the more the oxygen is diluted with room air, and the lower the FIO_2 the patient receives. High-flow oxygen is limited by discomfort the patient experiences and by the drying effect the high-flow oxygen creates. Comfort Flo™ is designed to deliver high-flow, heated, humidified oxygen through a nasal cannula. High-flow therapy allows spontaneously breathing patients to comfortably receive a wide range of flows (1–40 liters per minute).

A closed delivery system with endotracheal tube placement is indicated to attain an FIO_2 greater than 0.7. The oxygen concentration delivery available with an endotracheal tube varies from 0.21 to 1.0 FIO_2, and small changes in FIO_2 typically require approximately 3 to 5 minutes of equilibration time to be detected in patients via pulse oximetric studies or by blood gas analysis.

Risks & Complications of Oxygen Therapy

Risks associated with the administration of oxygen therapy can be categorized into two types: early and late complications. Early risks of oxygen therapy focus on the minority of COPD patients who have acute exacerbations of chronic lung disease and receive oxygen concentrations that are greater than their requirements to achieve an oxygen saturation >90%. These COPD patients are classified as oxygen sensitive. When high levels of oxygen are administered to these patients, the protective mechanism of hypoxic vasoconstriction in the pulmonary vascular bed is altered. This alteration results in a worsening ventilation-perfusion ratio, and increased dead space ventilation leading to an increase in $Paco_2$. Also, as hemoglobin becomes saturated with oxygen, carbon dioxide bound to the hemoglobin is pushed off. This dissolved form of CO_2 contributes to the pressure of carbon dioxide in the blood (the Haldane effect). Also, a primary mechanism initiating breathing in these patients is the "hypoxemic respiratory drive." As the hypercapnic respiratory drive has become blunted over time; and as the Pao_2 increases, this drive is lulled into a relaxed state, and neuronal firing to create breathing slows down. Progressive retention of CO_2 spirals into worsening respiratory acidosis and can lead to CO_2 narcosis (Figure 13–4).

Late complications of chronic oxygen therapy are primarily associated with the risk of developing oxygen toxicity and resultant fibroproliferative disease of the alveoli. The goal is to maintain Fio_2 requirements below 0.7 within the initial 24

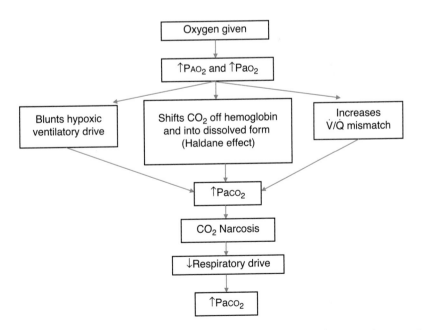

Figure 13–4. Baseline chronic hypercapnic respiratory failure plus acute hypoxemic respiratory failure.

to 48 hours and lower than 0.5 over a longer time span. The lung injury witnessed with hyperoxia involves cellular injury from toxic free radicals and oxidants that is exacerbated by elevated lung volumes, increased transpulmonary pressures, and inflammatory responses.

OBJECTIVES OF MECHANICAL VENTILATION

The primary objectives of mechanical ventilation are to ensure adequate gas exchange, relieve fatigued muscles of respiration, and guard against ventilator complications while allowing the underlying disease process to resolve. There are no specific parameters of respiratory rate, Pao_2, $Paco_2$, or pH that dictate the institution of mechanical ventilation. The decision is a clinical choice dependent on a number of variables that include those previously listed as well as respiratory muscle effort, mental status, reversibility of the precipitating event, comorbid conditions, and preexisting cardiopulmonary reserve.

 There are two distinct modes of mechanical ventilation, differentiated by the presence or absence of an endotracheal tube. IPPV is the standard form of mechanical ventilation utilizing an endotracheal tube and typically a volume- or pressure-controlled mechanical ventilator. NIPPV is characterized by the presence of a tight-fitting nasal or full-face mask to deliver pressurecontrolled mechanical ventilation. Both invasive and noninvasive forms of positive pressure ventilation have benefits and drawbacks, and both are associated with patient-ventilator complications.

NONINVASIVE POSITIVE PRESSURE VENTILATION (NIPPV)

There has been an increasing body of evidence to support the use of NIPPV in a number of clinical settings that were previously the realm of IPPV. NIPPV offers a number of theoretical advantages: avoidance of complications associated with endotracheal intubation, preservation of the cough reflex, enhanced comfort for the patient, improved communication by the patient through speech, and maintenance of the swallowing reflex. The two most popular forms of NIPPV are the continuous positive airway pressure (CPAP) mask and the bi-level positive airway pressure (BIPAP) mask. Clinical applications of NIPPV include post extubation respiratory failure in the intensive care unit and recovery room settings, acute exacerbations of COPD/asthma, reversible airway obstruction, hypoxemia, and cardiogenic pulmonary edema, as well as in patients refusing endotracheal intubation. See Table 13–6 for criteria for selecting patients for NIPPV. Oxygen delivery with a semi-closed (noninvasive positive pressure ventilation [NIPPV]) or closed system (intermittent positive pressure ventilation [IPPV]) may be warranted to achieve adequate Pao_2 levels unobtainable with cannula and oxygen mask delivery. NIPPV is characterized by the presence of a tight-fitting nasal or full-face mask to deliver pressure controlled mechanical ventilation.

INVASIVE POSITIVE PRESSURE VENTILATION (IPPV)

During spontaneous breathing, venous return is augmented during inspiration due to the negative pressure generated in the pleural space and increased abdominal pressure. This boost to venous return enhances right heart filling and right heart cardiac output. Conversely, positive pressure ventilation causes a positive intrathoracic pressure during inspiration and limits venous return, resulting in lower right heart cardiac output and a limited left ventricular preload. The addition of PEEP to positive pressure ventilation can further reduce cardiac output in particularly compliant lungs.

Hypotension following intubation and the institution of mechanical ventilation is commonplace and can be caused by hypovolemia, reduced preload, a decrease in sympathetic tone due to anesthetic agents, and possibly cardiac dysfunction. This hypotension is typically transient and responsive to fluid challenges, but may require the administration of vasopressors.

The physiologic effects of positive pressure can be beneficial in the setting of left heart failure. The decreased venous return as described above can help the heart clear the lungs of pulmonary edema Also, positive pressure and PEEP act in a ventricular assist method (Figure 13–5).

IPPV is the standard form of mechanical ventilation utilizing an endotracheal tube and typically a volume- or pressure-controlled mechanical ventilator. The

Table 13–6. Criteria for selection of patients for noninvasive positive pressure ventilation

Airway protection ensured
No impaired swallowing
Patient cough reflex intact
No excess secretions
Cardiovascular stability
Cooperative patient with intact mental status
No acute facial trauma
Proper equipment, tight-fitting facial mask (CPAP, BIPAP)

Note: BIPAP, bi-level positive airway pressure; CPAP, continuous positive airway pressure.

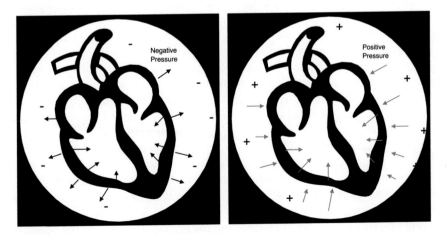

Figure 13–5. Effects of positive end expiratory pressure (PEEP) on ventricular "squeeze."

Table 13–7. Common findings leading to initiation of mechanical ventilation

Diminishing mental status
Pao_2 <70 mm Hg with Fio_2 >0.50
$Paco_2$ >50 mm Hg in a previously normocapnic patient
Respiratory rate >30 breaths/min despite therapy
Paradoxical respiratory efforts
Alveolar-arterial gradient >400 mm Hg on Fio_2 of 1.0
Maximum inspiratory force <–25 cm H_2O
Vital capacity <15 mL/kg body weight
Failure of noninvasive mechanical ventilation

oxygen concentration delivery available with an endotracheal tube varies from 0.21 to 1.0 torr Fio_2. The primary determinant dictating institution of mechanical ventilation is mental status. Patients who are alert and cooperative and who assist in their own therapy are given a trial of aggressive management with noninvasive ventilation regardless of their arterial blood gas test results. Efforts should be made to explain to the patient the goals and methodology of this trial to improve compliance and tolerance to NIPPV measures. Conversely patients requiring immediate ventilatory support for apnea, airway protection, excess secretions, and deteriorating mental status should not be given such a trial of conservative therapy despite the appearance of normal arterial blood gas values (Table 13–7).

Selection of a method of ventilation for acute respiratory failure most commonly results in the choice of volume-cycled mechanical ventilation. In volume-controlled ventilation, tidal volumes, flow rates, and flow profiles are predetermined by the clinician, and the resultant pressure generation is measured. Tidal volumes are typically based on ideal body mass and typically should be at the lower range of 6–8 mL/kg body weight. Higher tidal volumes can lead to dynamic hyperinflation and lung overdistention, resulting in ventilator-induced lung injury (VILI) or cardiovascular compromise, particularly in those patients with noncompliant lungs and elevated levels of PEEP. Lower tidal volumes in the range of 6 to 8 mL/kg ideal body weight are utilized in patients with severe reactive airway disease in order to reduce inspiratory time and increase expiratory time in an attempt to alleviate dynamic hyperinflation. In cases of ALI and ARDS, diminishing the tidal volume to 6 mL/kg ideal body weight has also been promoted as a method of avoiding further injury and improving patient outcome. The flow rate selected in volume-cycled ventilation can affect the patient's comfort and work of breathing. If the flow rate selected is less than the patient's demand, the patient's continued inspiratory effort during flow delivery increases the patient's work of breathing and leads to patient-ventilator dysynchrony. Inspiratory flow rates may range from 60 to 80 L/min in most cases, but may require even higher levels. Patients with exceedingly high ventilatory requirements may benefit from pressure-cycled mechanical ventilation, which can offer inspiratory flow rates in excess of 120 L/min. Causes of worsening hypoxemia during therapy for respiratory failure are outlined in Table 13–8.

The majority of volume-cycled mechanical ventilators allow for the selection of flow profile; square, sine, accelerating, and decelerating waveforms are the

Table 13–8. Causes of worsening hypoxemia during therapy for respiratory failure

Interventions
Bronchoscopy
Change in body position
Dialysis
Endotracheal intubation and mechanical ventilation
Thoracentesis
New medical problems
Anaphylaxis
Aspiration
Atelectasis
Bronchospasm
Cardiac output limitations
Fluid excess
Nosocomial pneumonia
Patent foramen ovale and other right-to-left shunts
Pneumothorax
Pulmonary embolus
Progression of primary disease
Acute lung injury
Asthma, chronic obstructive pulmonary disease
Cardiogenic pulmonary edema
Medications
β-blockers
Bronchodilators
Negative inotropic agents
Vasodilators

Table 13–9. Initial ventilator settings for respiratory failure utilizing volume-controlled ventilators

Mode: Assist control
Rate: 10–15 breaths/min
Tidal volume: 6 mL/kg idea/body weight (in ARDS)
F_{IO_2}: 1.0 initially with goal of <0.60 to be weighed against PEEP
Positive end-expiratory pressure: goal <10 cm H_2O but may need to increase >20 cm H_2O to maintain F_{IO_2} <0.80
Flow rate: >60 L/min
Plateau pressure: >30 cm H_2O measured at end inspiration

standard selections. Compared to the other profile choices, square wave profiles deliver the tidal volume with constant flow over the least inspiratory time. The other flow profiles require a higher flow rate or a longer inspiratory time to deliver the same tidal volume. There appears to be a modest benefit in terms of increased compliance, improved ventilation-perfusion matching, and reduced dead space percentage when utilizing decelerating flow profiles. Basic initial ventilator settings are outlined in Table 13–9.

RISKS & COMPLICATIONS OF MECHANICAL VENTILATION

Liberation from the ventilator as soon as clinically indicated should remain the goal from the outset. Early mobilization and "sedation holiday" play an important role in achieving this objective and to prevent VILI and ventilator associated infections. VILI is multifactorial and is a result of alveolar injury caused by excessive volumes, pressures, oxygen concentration, transalveolar pressure gradient, and pathologic insult. This injury may be manifested in alveolar rupture, scarring, or increased inflammation. A number of measures can be instituted to avoid the complications of volutrauma: reduction in tidal volumes, close monitoring for elevations in plateau pressures greater than 30 cm H_2O, measuring dynamic hyperinflation, and careful administration of PEEP to at-risk patients (Table 13–10).

Pneumothorax is a frequent and potentially lethal complication of positive pressure mechanical ventilation, occurring in 3% to 5% of patients. The primary mechanism for the development of pneumothorax in a mechanically ventilated patient is the dissection of air through the alveolus into the bronchovascular sheath, and from there tracking to the pleural space or to the mediastinum (Figure 13–6). Clinically a pneumothorax can present in a variety of ways: agitation on the part of the patient, hemodynamic compromise, hypoxia, decreases in lung compliance, and elevations in ventilator peak inspiratory pressures. Groups of patients at particular risk include those with COPD, asthma, ARDS, multilobar pneumonia, necrotizing pneumonia, and bleb or bullous disease. The clinical syndrome of tension pneumothorax is associated with diminished breath sounds on the involved side, a shift of the trachea away from the involved hemithorax, hypotension, tachycardia, jugular venous distention, and hyperresonance to percussion of the involved hemithorax. Immediate life-sustaining treatment is indicated: a 2-inch 18-gauge needle should be placed in the second intercostal space in the midclavicular line to permit rapid decompression of pressurized air. This emergent measure is immediately followed by the placement of a thoracostomy tube into the same hemithorax. Radiographic evidence of a pneumothorax can be subtle and can include increased radiolucency of the involved hemithorax, delineation of the epicardial fat pad, and the deep sulcus sign.

The deep sulcus sign is typically found in patients in a supine position and is denoted by a lucency that extends deep into the costophrenic sulcus of the hemidiaphragm. Repeating chest x-rays with the patient in the erect or decubitus position may assist in identifying the presence of a pneumothorax, but CT scanning of the

Table 13–10. Reducing the risk of ventilator-induced lung injury

Respiratory rate: <15 breaths/min
Tidal volumes: 6–8 mL/kg body weight
Consideration of permissive hypercapnia
Maintain low level of positive end-expiratory pressure: <10 cm H_2O
Utilize high inspiratory flow rate: 70–100 L/min
Maintain plateau pressures: <30 cm H_2O

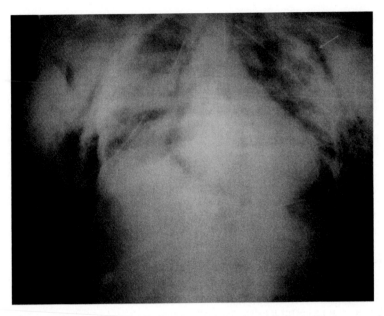

Figure 13-6. An intubated patient on mechanical ventilation. Chest x-ray shows pneumomediastinum.

Table 13-11. Diagnostic findings in patients with pneumothorax on mechanical ventilation

Bedside findings
Cardiovascular compromise (hypotension, tachycardia)
Sudden increases in peak inspiratory airway pressures
Chest x-ray findings
Deep sulcus sign
Mediastinal shift
Hyperexpansion of one hemithorax
Ventilator findings
ARDS and associated low compliance
Large tidal volumes: >12 mL/kg body weight
Plateau pressures: >30 cm H_2O
Respiratory rate: >30 breaths/min
Severe reactive airway disease

Note: ARDS, acute respiratory distress syndrome.

chest is the most sensitive and specific test for the diagnosis of pneumothorax (see Table 13–11 and refer to Chapter 11).

Ventilator complications have multiple causes (Table 13–12). Appropriate measures to take when ventilator alarms sound are highlighted in Table 13–13 It is essential to limit the harmful effects that mechanical ventilation may cause

Table 13–12. Ventilator-associated complications

ARDS
Aspiration
Bronchospasm
Cardiovascular collapse secondary to impaired venous return
Migration of endotracheal tube leading to extubation or right main stem intubation
Mucus plugging and atelectasis
Nosocomial pneumonia
Oxygen toxicity
Right-to-left shunt
Tracheobronchitis
Ventilator malfunction
Volutrauma

Note: ARDS, acute respiratory distress syndrome.

Table 13–13. Mechanical ventilation: What to do when the alarms sound

Disconnect patient from the mechanical ventilator
Bag-valve ventilation with 100% F_{IO_2}
Confirm endotracheal tube placement and patency
Rapid physical assessment (heart rate, blood pressure, breath sounds, oxygen saturation)
Review recent trends in ventilator parameters and patient's vital signs
Obtain chest x-ray and arterial blood gas analysis
Consider pain, withdrawal (alcohol, narcotics, benzodiazepines), patient-ventilator dysynchrony

the patient. Disconnecting the patient from mechanical ventilation and assuring patency of a properly positioned endotracheal tube are the hallmarks of primary assessment in such difficult cases. Patients should be ventilated via ambubag while the mechanical ventilator and patient are closely examined for problems and a chest x-ray is obtained.

CLINICAL SCENARIOS

Case 1

A 30-year-old man presents complaining of the most severe asthma attack he has ever experienced. Rapid administration of β-agonists, steroids, and oxygen fail to affect his respiratory distress. The patient becomes confused and unable to tolerate his oxygen mask. He is urgently sedated, and then intubated and placed on mechanical ventilation. His estimated body weight is 70 kg ideal body weight.

Discussion: A volume-cycled ventilator should be chosen and the ventilator mode set to assist control. The other settings should include tidal volume 6–7 mL/kg ideal body weight at 400–500 mL, respiratory rate 10 breaths/min, peak inspiratory flow rate 100 L/min, F_{IO_2} 100%, and PEEP 5 cm H_2O. Volume-cycled ventilators entail a reduced risk of dynamic hyperinflation compared to pressure-cycled ventilators. The ventilator settings would permit a prolonged expiratory time and diminish dynamic hyperinflation. Patients with asthma and reactive airway disease are at particular risk of VILI due to alveolar overdistention. Reduced tidal volumes and respiratory rates, coupled with an increased peak inspiratory flow, all function to relieve alveolar hyperinflation and minimize the risk of alveolar injury and hemodynamic compromise.

CLINICAL PEARLS

- Asthmatics are at increased risk for developing dynamic hyperinflation or auto-PEEP when placed on mechanical ventilation. These conditions can be life-threatening and are manifested by high plateau pressures and hypotension due to reduced venous return.
- Reducing the risk of dynamic hyperinflation is accomplished by prolonging the patient's expiratory time. Utilize low respiratory rates in the 8–12 breaths/min range, reduce tidal volumes to the 6–7 mL/kg ideal body weight range, and increase the inspiratory peak flow to the 80–120 L/min range.

Case 2

A 55-year-old man is in the recovery room following surgery for a ventral hernia. After he is extubated, he begins to have an increased respiratory rate and paradoxical respiratory efforts. An arterial blood gas analysis reveals a Pao_2 of 70 on 3 L of oxygen by nasal cannula and a Pco_2 of 55 mm. He is alert and cooperative, and requests not to be intubated.

Discussion: A BIPAP mask and machine are available. The settings should include an inspiratory pressure of 8–10 cm H_2O and an expiratory pressure of 3–5 cm H_2O, with an Fio_2 of 30%, utilizing a tight-fitting nasal or face mask. NIPPV is a viable option for patients with respiratory distress who can remain participatory and cooperative in their own care. Patients prematurely extubated within the intensive care unit or recovery room, and patients with acute reversible respiratory distress (eg, asthma, COPD, and congestive heart failure) may benefit from a trial of NIPPV. Failure to improve with NIPPV within the first hour is an indication to institute IPPV. Respiratory rate, accessory muscle use, symptom scores, and arterial blood gas values can be followed as indicators of the patient's response. For difficulties that are predominantly related to ventilation, 2- to 4-cm H_2O increments in the inspiratory component are indicated. For oxygenation difficulties, the Fio_2 and both the expiratory and inspiratory components should be increased in 2- to 4-cm H_2O increments.

CLINICAL PEARLS

- NIPPV should be considered as a viable option for treating those patients in respiratory distress who remain alert and cooperative. NIPPV may obviate the need to institute IPPV and result in reductions in morbidity, mortality, and costs.

• When instituting NIPPV, the lowest settings should be chosen, maintaining at least 5 cm H_2O difference between the inspiratory and the expiratory pressures. Close patient coaching and monitoring during initiation of this modality is associated with improved compliance, better tolerance by patient and increases the chance of success in avoiding intubation and IPPV.

KEY CONCEPTS

Respiratory failure is common, but the etiology is varied and may be multifactorial.

Management principles are centered on maintaining adequate oxygenation and ventilation while reducing the risks associated with treatment strategies.

Mechanical ventilation to treat respiratory failure may require endotracheal tube placement or noninvasive techniques such as a face mask with CPAP or BIPAP.

STUDY QUESTIONS

13–1. A 52-year-old man with a diagnosis of COPD secondary to chronic bronchitis is admitted with ARF and severe bronchospasm. His arterial blood gas analysis on room air reveals a $Paco_2$ of 76 mm Hg, Pao_2 of 42 mm Hg, and pH of 7.21. He is 5' 10" tall and weighs 90 kg. He is placed on a mechanical ventilator on the assist-control mode with the following settings: Fio_2 0.5, tidal volume 600 mL, inspiratory flow rate 100 L/min, and a respiratory rate of 12 breaths/min. Within 15 minutes of placement on the ventilator, he becomes hypotensive and tachycardic. What is the best option?

a. decrease the inspiratory flow rate

b. increase the tidal volume

c. decrease the tidal volume

d. remove the patient from the ventilator and place on 10 L/min oxygen

e. temporarily remove the patient from the ventilator and give a 500-mL fluid bolus

13–2. A 25-year-old man develops ARDS secondary to acute pancreatitis. He weighs 70 kg. He is placed on a mechanical ventilator with the following settings: tidal volume 500 mL, Fio_2 100%, inspiratory flow rate 90 L/min, respiratory rate 10 breaths/min, and PEEP 5 cm H_2O. After 24 hours he is slightly better clinically, with a blood pressure of 118/70 mm Hg and a good urine output. However, his arterial blood gas measurements on 100% Fio_2 and PEEP of 5 cm H_2O are Po_2 59 mm Hg, Pco_2 34 mm Hg, and pH 7.43. What should be done now?

a. *decrease the tidal volume*
b. *increase the tidal volume*
c. *increase the inspiratory flow rate*
d. *increase the PEEP to 12 cm H_2O*
e. *decrease the F_{IO_2}*

SUGGESTED READINGS

International Consensus Conferences in Intensive Care Medicine: Noninvasive positive pressure ventilation in acute respiratory failure. Am J Respir Crit Care Med 2001; 163:288.

Keith RL, Pierson DJ: Complications of mechanical ventilation: A bedside approach. Clin Chest Med 1996; 17:439.

Lee, WL and Slutsky, AS. Hypoxemic respiratory failure, including acute respiratory distress syndrome, pp 2352–2353. *Murray and Nadel's Textbook of Respiratory Medicine*, 4th ed. Philadelphia: Elsevier, 2005, pp. 2352–2353.

Pierson, DJ and Hill NS. Acute ventilatory failure. *Murray and Nadel's Textbook of Respiratory Medicine*, 4th ed. Philadelphia: Elsevier, 2005, pp. 2379–2382.

Sigillito R, DeBlieux P: Evaluation and initial management of the patient in respiratory distress. Emerg Med Clin North Am. 2003;21:239.

Lung Under Stress 14

Kendra J. McAnally & Stephen P. Kantrow

OBJECTIVES

- ▶ *Recognize lung injury caused by common therapeutic drugs and substance abuse.*
- ▶ *Identify the pulmonary complications that occur after lung and hematopoietic stem cell transplantation.*
- ▶ *Amplify on preoperative evaluation and understand the effects of operative procedures and anesthesia on lung function.*
- ▶ *Review changes in lung function that occur with aging.*

GENERAL CONSIDERATIONS

This chapter presents the clinical aspects of several stresses that can affect lung function. Therapeutic use of numerous drugs has been associated with significant lung dysfunction, and illicit drug use and cigarette smoking exact a tremendous toll on lung health in susceptible individuals. Lung transplantation exposes the donor lung to the remarkable stress of brain death, ischemia-reperfusion, and then recovery in a hostile immune environment. Hematopoietic cell transplantation offers an opportunity for cure of a number of diseases, but this therapy exposes the lung to a variety of noninfectious and infectious injuries. Surgical procedures and general anesthesia cause dysfunction in normal lungs and can represent a critical stress to patients with limited pulmonary reserve. Finally, aging is associated with alterations in pulmonary mechanics and host defense.

DRUG-INDUCED LUNG DISEASE

 Numerous therapeutic drugs have been reported to cause lung injury, with varied clinical and pathologic findings. This section discusses three well-documented causes of drug-induced lung disease: amiodarone,

Acknowledgment: The authors acknowledge the use of some clinical material and images from Dillon GS. Lung under stress. In: Ali J, Summer WR, Levitzky MG, eds. *Pulmonary Pathophysiology.* New York: McGraw-Hill; 1999.

bleomycin, and methotrexate. All of these compounds are in clinical use and can cause severe pulmonary disease (Table 14–1). In addition, several types of lung injury due to cigarette smoking and use of illicit drugs, including cocaine, heroin, and intravenously administered oral medications, are also reviewed.

Therapeutic Drugs

Amiodarone is used to treat a broad range of dysrhythmias, including life-threatening ventricular tachycardia and atrial fibrillation. While this drug has potent beneficial effects on electrical conduction in the heart, numerous adverse effects occur with amiodarone use, including hypothyroidism, liver dysfunction, and pulmonary injury. Higher daily doses of amiodarone (greater than 400 mg/d) are associated with a higher incidence of pulmonary toxicity (5%–15%), but toxicity also has been reported in patients on low-dose therapy (200 mg/d). Pathologic findings in pulmonary toxicity attributed to amiodarone include foamy, lipid filled macrophages (probably due to phospholipase inhibition and phospholipid accumulation), type II pneumocyte proliferation, and fibrosis. However, foamy macrophages occur in the absence of overt lung disease in individuals receiving amiodarone and thus are not specific for amiodarone pneumonitis. The pulmonary complications of amiodarone typically present with an insidious dyspnea and a radiographic pattern which may be asymmetrical or limited to the upper lobes. Less commonly, a syndrome of dyspnea, fever, and a focal infiltrate on chest x-ray has been described. Rarely, acute lung injury with respiratory failure can occur after cardiothoracic surgery or angiogram. The diagnosis of amiodarone toxicity is one of exclusion. Treatment consists of discontinuing the drug and patients may respond to corticosteroids for a treatment period of 2–6 months.

Table 14–1. Drug-induced lung disease

Therapeutic drugs	Lung involvement
Amiodarone	Interstitial lung disease, BOOP
Bleomycin	Interstitial lung disease
Methotrexate	Interstitial lung disease, eosinophilia
Nontherapeutic drugs	
Tobacco	Obstructive lung disease, cancer, interstitial lung disease
Cocaine	Barotrauma, hemorrhage, pulmonary edema
Intravenous injection of tablets	Nodular fibrosis, emphysema
Heroin	Pulmonary edema
Marijuana	Fungal contamination, obstructive lung disease?

Note: BOOP, bronchiolitis bliterans with organizing pneumonia.

Bleomycin is a cytotoxic antibiotic used to treat several types of cancer, including germ cell tumors and lymphomas. The pulmonary toxicity observed after bleomycin treatment can be rapidly or slowly progressive. Pathologically, epithelial and endothelial injury is prominent; fibroblasts are recruited and extensive fibrosis may occur. The combination of bleomycin, iron, and oxygen produces highly reactive oxygen intermediates that may contribute to the lung injury. Risk factors for bleomycin toxicity include the cumulative dose of the drug administered (usually >450 U), exposure to high concentrations of inspired oxygen, history of pulmonary disease, age over 70 years and thoracic radiation therapy.

Clinically, patients present with dyspnea and cough, inspiratory crackles on chest auscultation, and bilateral lower lobe infiltrates on chest x-ray. Mild deterioration of pulmonary function may improve after discontinuing bleomycin. More severe injury, with respiratory insufficiency, can improve after corticosteroid therapy, but mortality rates for this condition are high. Pulmonary function testing with frequent monitoring of diffusion capacity is recommended.

Methotrexate is a folate antagonist that has been used to treat malignant and inflammatory conditions. The incidence of clinical toxicity is less than 10% and occurs more frequently in patients receiving methotrexate for malignancy than in patients treated for inflammatory conditions. Pathologic studies usually demonstrate infiltration of lung parenchyma with mononuclear cells, including lymphocytes and plasma cells. Poorly formed granulomas are also commonly observed. Pulmonary toxicity presents with dyspnea, nonproductive cough, and fever. Chest x-ray often demonstrates bilateral reticular infiltrates, or less commonly, focal infiltrates. Hilar adenopathy and/or pleural effusion are seen in 10%–15%. Diffusion capacity tends to remain intact. Frequently patients also have blood eosinophilia, consistent with a hypersensitivity reaction. Rarely, methotrexate pulmonary toxicity occurs as noncardiogenic pulmonary edema after intrathecal administration or as an acute chest pain syndrome. Discontinuation of methotrexate and treatment with corticosteroids usually leads to clinical improvement. In some cases methotrexate can be reinstituted following resolution without triggering a subsequent reaction.

Cigarette Smoking

Lung disease is a common complication of substance abuse. A variety of pulmonary pathologic conditions can develop with years of cigarette smoking. Chronic obstructive pulmonary disease (COPD) develops in 10%–20% of heavy smokers. Nonsmokers can develop emphysema due to heritable α_1-antitrypsin deficiency, in which a single amino acid substitution leads to deficiency of this important antiprotease in serum, with aggregation of abnormal protein in liver endoplasmic reticulum. The onset of emphysema varies in susceptible populations: tobacco smokers become symptomatic at about 60–65 years of age, while nonsmokers with α_1-antitrypsin deficiency develop symptomatic disease 10–30 years earlier. Cigarette smokers with α_1-antitrypsin deficiency are highly susceptible to lung injury and emphysema and frequently become symptomatic in the third or fourth decade of life. Treatments include smoking cessation, antiprotease replacement therapy, and lung transplantation.

Pulmonary Langerhans cell granulomatosis (eosinophilic granuloma or pulmonary histiocytosis X) is a diffuse lung disease that develops almost exclusively (over 90% of cases) in cigarette smokers. Pathologically, Langerhans cells and eosinophils are prominent in lesions (but not in blood). Typically, patients become symptomatic in the third to sixth decade with cough, dyspnea, and chest pain. Chest x-rays demonstrate small (1-cm) stellate lesions, and later cystic enlargement of air spaces and honeycombing in mid- and upper lung fields. Pulmonary function testing reveals mild restriction and low diffusion capacity early in the course of the disease, and then increased total lung volume as cystic spaces develop. The prognosis overall is good, but some patients progress to respiratory failure. Treatments include smoking cessation, corticosteroids and/or cytotoxic therapy, and lung transplantation.

Respiratory bronchiolitis was previously considered an incidental finding in smoker's lung, but now appears to be part of a spectrum of disease that includes smoker's lung, respiratory bronchiolitis, and desquamative interstitial pneumonitis (DIP), in order of increasing severity. Pathologically, alveoli contain numerous brown-pigmented macrophages, and this disease is differentiated from others in the spectrum by extent of involvement (peribronchiolar, not diffuse). All patients with respiratory bronchiolitis smoke heavily, and cough and dyspnea are common. Chest x-rays may be normal or have an interstitial pattern, while high-resolution computed tomography (CT) scans may appear normal or demonstrate a ground-glass pattern. Pulmonary function studies demonstrate mild restriction and a low diffusion capacity. The prognosis is very good, and symptoms usually resolve with smoking cessation.

As with respiratory bronchiolitis, DIP occurs almost exclusively in cigarette smokers. Pathologically, DIP resembles respiratory bronchiolitis, but pigmented macrophages are present diffusely and some fibrosis may be seen in the interstitium. Symptoms develop in the third to fifth decade of life with cough and dyspnea. Chest x-rays often have an interstitial pattern and subpleural ground-glass opacities. One third of the reported cases progress to respiratory failure, while most others improve. Recommended therapies include smoking cessation and corticosteroids.

Smoking is the largest preventable cause of cancer and is responsible for approximately 30% of cancer deaths. Tobacco smoke contains many carcinogens and tumor promoters. It appears to be dose related and young smokers seem to be more susceptible to genetic alterations. Cancers most often associated with smoking include squamous cell of the head and neck and lung cancer. The lung cancers include adenocarcinoma, squamous cell, and small cell carcinoma. Risk decreases in ex-smokers in proportion to the length of time since smoking cessation, but never reaches that of a nonsmoker.

Illicit Drugs

Cocaine can be purified from coca leaves to an alkaloid or "free base," and in this form is heat stable and volatile at high temperature. Smoking the free-base preparation allows delivery of the drug rapidly to alveolar capillaries, where it is absorbed, mimicking the pharmacokinetics of intravenous injection. This type of substance abuse results in intense addiction with repetitive exposure of the lung to the drug and associated impurities contained in the drug or delivery system. Patients with "crack lung" from smoking cocaine typically present with chest pain and may have carbonaceous (black) sputum and hemoptysis. Chest x-rays are usually normal but may demonstrate focal infiltrates, diffuse acinar filling, or pneumomediastinum. Complications include noncardiac pulmonary edema, pneumomediastinum, alveolar hemorrhage, eosinophilic pneumonia, bronchiolitis obliterans (BO) organizing pneumonia, pulmonary infarction, and thermal airway injury. The cause of alveolar hemorrhage and hemoptysis after crack cocaine use is unknown, but pathologically hemorrhage, hemosiderin-laden macrophages, and fibrosis are common in autopsies of cocaine abusers. In crack users, deep inspiration during smoking, followed by application of additional positive airway pressure by accomplices (to enhance the drug delivery) may lead to pneumomediastinum, likely by dissection of air from ruptured alveoli along the bronchovascular sheath into the mediastinum.

Intravenous injection of oral drugs can also cause pulmonary disease. Two well-described examples are methadone and methylphenidate. Both are associated with panacinar emphysema and severe obstructive lung disease after years of intravenous injection, and methadone injection may cause upper lobe conglomeration and fibrosis that resembles the progressive massive fibrosis of silicosis. Although both methadone and methylphenidate contain talc (magnesium trisilicate) as filler, the damaging ingredient is unknown. Nearly all reported cases of lung disease occurred in cigarette smokers, and many of the patients developed symptoms at a very early age (ie, the third decade of life), suggesting a destructive interaction between cigarette smoke and intravenous drug abuse.

Sir William Osler (1880) first described narcotic-induced pulmonary edema after morphine poisoning. Pulmonary edema following heroin overdose is the modern version of this disease, and most cases resolve within 24–48 hours. The chest x-ray demonstrates bilateral perihilar edema, but unilateral edema has been described. Prolonged respiratory failure suggests complications such as aspiration or pneumonia, or an alternative diagnosis.

Marijuana contains more tar and carbon monoxide per inhalation than tobacco, and also delivers thousands of chemical species to the lung. However, a decline in the pulmonary function of long-term abusers has not been convincingly shown. Recent studies indicate obstructive lung disease risk may be increased in those who smoke both cigarettes and marijuana. Marijuana is often contaminated with *Aspergillus,* and may cause fungal pneumonia in immunosuppressed patients using the drug for recreational or therapeutic purposes. Marijuana smoking is also associated with bullous lung disease, pneumothorax and pneumomediastinum.

LUNG TRANSPLANTATION

The first human lung transplant was performed in 1963 at the University of Mississippi, and the patient survived for almost 3 weeks. Over the next 20 years, more than 40 lung transplants were performed, but results continued to be dismal. In the early 1980s, the introduction of cyclosporine, a potent inhibitor of immune cell activation, caused resurgence in organ transplantation. The availability of effective immunosuppressive regimens, improved surgical techniques, and advances in medical management has led to long-term survival in lung allograft recipients. Currently, approximately 2000 lung transplants are performed annually worldwide.

Indications & Contraindications for Transplantation

Common diagnoses for which lung transplantation is being performed include chronic obstructive lung disease, idiopathic pulmonary fibrosis, cystic fibrosis, alpha-1 antitrypsin deficiency and idiopathic pulmonary hypertension. Others include sarcoidosis, lymphangioleiomyomatosis, eosinophilic granuloma, and chronic rejection of a previous lung allograft. The number of lung transplants performed is limited by the availability of transplantable organs. About 10%–15% of patients deemed suitable candidates for lung transplantation die while on the waiting list. Generally, lung transplantation should be considered for patients with nonmalignant advanced lung disease that is unresponsive to medical therapy. In addition, the patient should be free of significant comorbidity. The major contraindications to lung transplantation are poor functional status, significant dysfunction of other major organs, active malignancy within 2 years, extrapulmonary infection, active substance abuse within 6 months (including cigarette smoking), hepatitis C with abnormal liver biopsy and psychosocial instability. Some relative contraindications include osteoporosis, mechanical ventilation and HIV infection.

Ideally, the transplantation should be done at a time when the patient is sufficiently ill to benefit from transplantation but is healthy enough to survive the procedure. Most centers recommend transplantation if the prognosis for survival is less than 2 years on maximal medical therapy. The prospect of improved quality of life is a strong motivation for transplantation, but to maximize the benefit of survival, prognosis and rapidity of clinical deterioration should determine the timing.

COPD is the most common indication for which lung transplantation has been performed. The presence of pulmonary hypertension, hypercarbia, and hypoxemia suggests poor prognosis and should be considered in determining when to proceed with transplantation. Selection guidelines include an FEV_1 less than 25% predicted and/or arterial Pco_2 greater than or equal to 55 mm Hg and/or increased pulmonary artery pressures.

Cystic fibrosis is a progressive obstructive and restrictive lung disease with chronic suppurative complications, including bronchiectasis. Poor prognostic signs in cystic fibrosis patients include a forced expiratory volume in the first second (FEV_1) of less than 30% of the predicted value on pulmonary function testing, hypercarbia, and hypoxemia. In general, patients with FEV_1 less than 30% of the predicted value should be considered for lung transplantation. A rapid decline in FEV_1, increased need for hospitalization, weight loss, and hemoptysis are associated with increased mortality rates and should lead to earlier consideration for transplantation. Cystic fibrosis has a set of problems unique to the disease, including colonization by highly resistant organisms, malnutrition, aminoglycoside-induced renal dysfunction, and pleural adhesions. Living donor lung transplant is an alternative for these patients because most recipients are children or young adults.

Idiopathic pulmonary fibrosis is a restrictive lung disease characterized by progressive decline in lung function despite optimal medical therapy. The rate of lung function deterioration is variable in patients with idiopathic pulmonary fibrosis, with a reported median survival of 2–5 years from the time of diagnosis. These patients should be referred for transplant evaluation when the restrictive abnormality is moderate (vital capacity or total lung capacity less than 65% of the predicted value), or when exercise-induced hypoxemia develops. In comparison to mortality rates for patients with other diagnoses, mortality rates for patients with pulmonary fibrosis are increased while on the waiting list for lung transplantation.

Idiopathic pulmonary hypertension is a disease that causes progressive vascular obstruction and manifests in the third or fourth decade of life as dyspnea and exercise intolerance. The median survival time after the diagnosis of pulmonary hypertension in untreated patients is 2–3 years. Signs of a poor prognosis include functional limitations consistent with advanced heart failure, elevated mean pulmonary artery pressure, elevated right atrial pressure, and decreased cardiac output. Recent advances in the medical management of pulmonary hypertension have decreased, but not eliminated, the need for transplantation for this disease.

Organ Procurement & Transplant Procedures

The United Network for Organ Sharing (UNOS) is a national nonprofit organization that facilitates procurement of donor organs and allocates them among various transplant centers. Previously, single lung transplant was more frequent than bilateral sequential lung transplant (BSLT.) However, in recent years, BSLT has been the most common procedure performed, currently just over half of the transplants. The advantages of this operation include increased lung reserve and slight improvement in long-term survival compared with single-lung allograft recipients. Mean survival for BSLT versus SLT is 5.9 and 4.4 years, respectively. Living related lobe transplantation has been developed to circumvent the scarcity of donor lungs and involves removal of a lung lobe from a related donor with immediate transplantation into the recipient, typically a child or small adult.

Heart-lung transplantation has been used for patients with Eisenmenger's complex, idiopathic pulmonary hypertension with right ventricular failure, and severe lung disease combined with heart disease. A major limitation is prolonged waiting time secondary to donor organ scarcity and an increased incidence of late complications.

Postoperative Care & Transplant Complications

The early postoperative care after transplantation includes ventilator management, hemodynamic support, immunosuppression, and infection prophylaxis. In general, patients are managed with ventilation strategies that limit airway and alveolar distending pressures, so low level positive end-expiratory pressure (PEEP) is used to prevent overinflation. In patients who are postoperative single lung transplant for emphysema, no PEEP is used secondary to the more compliant grafted lung and subsequent overinflation and volutrauma. All patients are susceptible to pulmonary edema, due in part to interrupted lymphatic drainage and to ischemia-reperfusion injury with alveolar epithelial and capillary leakage, so excessive vascular filling pressures are avoided (Table 14–2).

Immunosuppressive regimens for lung transplant recipients differ from center to center, but consist of corticosteroids, cyclosporine (or tacrolimus), azathioprine (or mycophenolate mofetil), and antilymphocytic therapy (eg, antithymocyte globulin) at the time of transplantation with typical maintenance immunosuppression with a three drug regimen consisting of prednisone and a calcineurin inhibitor (cyclosporine or tacrolimus), and an inhibitor of lymphocyte proliferation (azathioprine or myophenylate mofetil). Adjunctive therapies include interleukin-2–receptor antagonists and blockade of T-cell activation (costimulatory) pathways.

Because of the intensive immunosuppression required to limit rejection of the transplanted organ, host defense, particularly T-cell–mediated defense, is severely compromised. Prophylaxis against cytomegalovirus (CMV) and *Pneumocystis carinii (P. jirovecii)* is begun soon after transplantation, since these infections can cause significant rates of morbidity and mortality in this population of patients. Broad spectrum antibiotics are used in the perioperative period, until cultures from the grafted lung are obtained. The long-term management of lung transplant includes optimizing the immunosuppressive regimen and close clinical monitoring to identify and manage various pulmonary and extrapulmonary complications. Routine pulmonary function tests, and in some centers, surveillance bronchoscopy is performed to monitor for chronic rejection. In addition, blood tests are monitored for immunosuppressive drug levels and possible side effects from them.

Actuarial survival curves have shown that there is a bimodal pattern of increased mortality rates, with a peak during the first 3 months after transplantation and then another increase after 4–5 years. During the first month after transplantation, death is most commonly due to mechanical or hemodynamic complications and acute graft dysfunction. After the first month, infection is the most common cause of death during the first year. The reasons for increased incidence of infections include aggressive immunosuppression, depressed cough reflex, and

Table 14–2. Lung stress in transplantation

Lung transplantation
Ischemia-reperfusion injury
Acute rejection
Chronic rejection
Airway stenosis
Bacterial, viral, and fungal infection
Hematopoietic stem cell transplantation
Pulmonary edema
Alveolar hemorrhage
Interstitial pneumonitis
Bacterial, viral, and fungal infection

ineffective mucociliary clearance in denervated implanted lungs. Bacterial infections are common but usually easily treated. Viral and fungal infections occur less commonly but are associated with higher mortality rates.

Other postoperative complications include acute rejection, chronic rejection, and surgical airway complications. Acute rejection is a T-cell-mediated reaction that is manifested clinically as dyspnea, fever, cough, and worsening oxygenation. Radiographic findings can vary from normal to bilateral diffuse infiltrates and pleural effusions. Acute rejection is diagnosed using transbronchial lung biopsies, with bronchoalveolar lavage (BAL) to exclude infection. Perivascular mononuclear infiltrates and lymphocytic bronchiolitis characterize the histopathologic examination of lung biopsies from these patients. It is important that infection be ruled out when considering a diagnosis of acute rejection, since the treatment of rejection involves high-dose steroid therapy and more intense maintenance immunosuppression.

Chronic rejection is a persistent alloimmune reaction against donor antigens. It can present in two ways, chronic airway rejection and less commonly chronic vascular rejection. Chronic airway rejection, clinically presents as progressive dyspnea and worsening airflow obstruction. This problem is similar to obliterative bronchiolitis seen in the nontransplant population, with histopathologic findings of inflammation and fibrosis of the lamina propria and lumen of small airways. The late fibrotic lesion is probably preceded by lymphocytic infiltration, but the results of immunosuppressive therapy for established obliterative bronchiolitis have been disappointing. Lung function may stabilize in some patients, but progressive deterioration leads to graft loss and death if retransplantation is not an option. Chronic vascular rejection appears as atherosclerosis in the pulmonary vasculature. Recurrent, late and severe episodes of acute rejection is a risk factor for BO. Making the diagnosis of BO by transbronchial biopsy is difficult, so with clinically evident graft dysfunction without proven histology is called bronchiolitis obliterans syndrome (BOS). Gastroesophageal reflux may be a risk factor for BO, and in some transplant centers fundoplication is performed at the time of transplant.

Surgical airway complications occur in 10%–20% of patients undergoing lung transplantation. Stenosis is the most common airway complication and it usually occurs secondary to stricture or malacia. It is diagnosed bronchoscopically and is amenable to balloon dilatation or stent placement.

Retransplantations have been performed but have relatively poor outcomes when compared to primary transplantation. Retransplantation for chronic graft rejection has the best outcome compared to those done for acute primary graft dysfunction and airway dehiscense.

HEMATOPOIETIC STEM CELL TRANSPLANTATION

Over the past two decades, hematopoietic stem cell transplantation (HSCT) has emerged as a viable therapeutic option for several malignant and nonmalignant diseases, including leukemia, lymphoma, breast cancer, and aplastic anemia. Hematopoietic cell transplantation utilizes bone marrow, peripheral blood or umbilical cord blood as donor cell sources. Complications of HCT are caused by the radiation and chemotherapy used in pretransplant conditioning regimens, the profound immunosuppression that follows, and the immune response of the graft to the host (graft-versus-host disease [GVHD]). In addition, graft failure and/or relapse of malignancy are important causes of death in this population. Pulmonary complications are common in HSCT recipients and are responsible for substantial morbidity and mortality (Table 14–2).

Noninfectious Pulmonary Complications

Pulmonary edema is prevalent during the first month following HSCT. Patients usually complain of shortness of breath and cough. On examination, tachypnea, hypoxemia, cyanosis, and basilar crackles are common findings. Chest x-rays demonstrate bilateral lung infiltrates with basilar and perihilar predominance, and pleural effusions are common. The alveolar edema can be hydrostatic or nonhydrostatic in origin.

Hydrostatic pulmonary edema due to depressed cardiac function may occur when anthracyclines have been used in the conditioning regimen or prior chemotherapy. Hydrostatic pulmonary edema can also occur due to intravascular volume overload in the setting of hepatic venoocclusive disease, a cause of sodium and water retention that frequently complicates marrow transplantation. The diagnosis can be suggested by assessment of fluid balance, physical examination, and chest x-rays, but occasionally echocardiography and pulmonary artery catheterization may be needed to guide therapy. Nonhydrostatic pulmonary edema occurs when lung permeability increases and can have many causes, including sepsis, acute GVHD, chemotherapeutic agents (eg, cytosine arabinoside), and blood transfusion reactions. The management of both types of pulmonary edema consists of supportive care with careful manipulation of intravascular volume and treatment of the underlying disease process.

Diffuse alveolar hemorrhage clinically presents within weeks of HSCT as progressive dyspnea, hypoxemia, dry cough, and bilateral air space disease on chest x-ray. The diagnosis is confirmed by BAL in which successive aliquots become increasingly bloody, and alveolar macrophages obtained by BAL have increased hemosiderin content. Risk factors associated with alveolar hemorrhage in this population of patients include autologous HSCT, history of chest or whole-body irradiation, increased age, renal insufficiency, and transplantation for solid tumors. This complication of HSCT is associated with a high mortality rate, and the treatment is supportive, with high-dose steroids administered in most cases.

Interstitial pneumonitis without evidence of bacterial, viral, or fungal infection is seen in about 5%–15% of BMT recipients. The onset is within 3–4 months after HSCT, typically after engraftment of donor cells. This syndrome is referred to as idiopathic pneumonia syndrome and is diagnosed clinically if widespread alveolar injury is present without evidence of lower respiratory tract infection, even after invasive evaluation including BAL, and in some cases, transbronchial or open-lung biopsy.

The clinical presentation of idiopathic pneumonia is varied and ranges from asymptomatic radiographic infiltrates to acute respiratory distress requiring mechanical ventilation. The syndrome presents with dyspnea, hypoxemia, and cough, typically with widespread bilateral infiltrates on chest x-ray. The mortality rate associated with this process is high (approximately 60%–80%), with very few survivors if mechanical ventilation is required. Currently there is no effective therapy available, although high dose steroids are often given.

Infectious Pulmonary Complications

Bacterial pneumonia can occur any time after HSCT but is seen most frequently in the initial neutropenic period, when engraftment of the transplanted cells has not yet occurred. In addition to the marked immunosuppression, HSCT recipients are at high risk of pneumonia due to aspiration in the setting of mucositis and narcotic administration. Common organisms include *Pseudomonas aeruginosa*, Enterobacteriaceae, gram-positive organisms, and anaerobes. Clinically, bacterial pneumonia may not be typical, since some patients present without high fever, dyspnea, productive cough, or pleuritic chest pain. The diagnosis is based on a high index of suspicion, chest x-ray, appropriate cultures, and microscopic analysis of lung secretions.

Pneumocystis carinii (*P jirovecii*) pneumonia (PCP) is associated with a high mortality rate in this population of patients. The incidence of PCP has been decreased markedly by widespread use of effective chemoprophylaxis, most commonly trimethoprim-sulfamethoxazole, which can also further suppress bone marrow. In patients who do develop PCP, the onset is frequently acute, with tachypnea and hypoxemia. On chest x-rays, bilateral reticular infiltrates develop and may progress to dense bilateral consolidation. The diagnosis is confirmed by BAL fluid examination. Transbronchial lung biopsies increase the diagnostic yield, but carry the risk of bleeding and pneumothorax. Treatment consists of high-dose trimethoprim-sulfamethoxazole and corticosteroids, but it is often unsuccessful.

While morbidity and mortality rates associated with bacterial and *Pneumocystis* pneumonia have decreased, fungi have emerged as major pathogens in HSCT recipients. The two most common fungal pathogens are *Aspergillus* and *Candida* species. These infections typically occur during the first month after transplantation, when patients are neutropenic.

Invasive pulmonary aspergillosis occurs in about 5%–10% of HSCT patients and is fatal in the majority of cases. Although it usually occurs during neutropenia, it may occur later in patients who require corticosteroids for the management of GVHD. The lungs are portals of entry for spores of *Aspergillus,* and this fungus can invade vascular structures, resulting in thrombosis, infarction, hemoptysis, and systemic dissemination. Radiographically, vascular invasion is characterized by focal areas of consolidation. The presence of cavitation in an area of consolidation is characteristic of this fungal infection, but is usually a late finding. Flexible bronchoscopy with BAL and transbronchial lung biopsy can confirm, but not exclude, the diagnosis. Open-lung biopsy may be required to confirm the diagnosis.

Candidal infections are common in bone marrow recipients and, like *Aspergillus* infections, usually occur during prolonged neutropenia. Since effective prophylaxis and therapy are available, fatalities due to *Candida* infection are unusual. The common portals of entry for *Candida* are the gastrointestinal tract and intravascular catheters. *Candida* pneumonia is a rare cause of respiratory failure, and the clinical presentation is nonspecific. Chest x-rays may show patchy bilateral consolidation without cavitation. Because *Candida* is a frequent contaminant of respiratory isolates, open-lung biopsy may be required to confirm invasive infection. The diagnosis of systemic candidiasis is usually made by isolation of the organism from blood and evidence of invasion in other sites (eg, bladder or liver).

CMV pneumonitis usually occurs during the second and third months following allogenic HSCT. CMV-seropositive BMT recipients and CMV-seronegative patients who receive CMV-positive bone marrow or blood products are at risk of developing active infection following BMT. Because the pneumonitis develops during reconstitution of the immune system, an immunologic mechanism may contribute to the injury. Clinically, CMV pneumonitis presents with dry cough, fever, dyspnea, and hypoxemia. The radiographic findings are nonspecific and include a diffuse reticular pattern, a reticular and nodular pattern, or dense bilateral consolidation. The presence of coexisting infections often confuses the radiologic or clinical picture. Characteristic nuclear or cytoplasmic inclusion bodies in lung tissue confirm the diagnosis. However, positive BAL cultures for CMV or detection of CMV antigen in the appropriate clinical setting is usually sufficient to make the diagnosis and institute therapy.

The incidence and mortality rates associated with pneumonitis caused by other viruses, such as non-CMV herpes viruses, respiratory syncytial virus, and influenza and parainfluenza viruses, can be significant. Prophylaxis against some members of the herpes virus family is available (eg, herpes simplex), and treatment with acyclovir or ganciclovir can be administered. However, common respiratory viruses can cause epidemics in this immunocompromised population, and therapy for aggressive disease is frequently ineffective. Rapid diagnostic studies of respiratory secretions (eg, nasopharyngeal lavage or swab) are available.

OPERATIVE PROCEDURES & ANESTHESIA

Major surgical procedures place the lung under considerable stress, and pulmonary complications include hypoxemia, atelectasis, infection (pneumonia), and embolism. Preoperative pulmonary evaluation is undertaken to identify and minimize perioperative risk (Table 14–3). Identifying additional risk imposed by underlying pulmonary disease can modify the risk–benefit analysis of the therapeutic intervention. Several factors influence operative risk, including the planned procedure (eg, cardiothoracic versus peripheral) and the presence of comorbid conditions.

Influence of Operation & Anesthesia

 The incidence of pulmonary complications is highest with upper abdominal and thoracic procedures and lowest with peripheral procedures.

Table 14–3. Operative procedures and anesthesia

Complications
   Atelectasis
   Phrenic nerve injury
   Pulmonary embolism
   Bronchospasm
Evaluation for lung resection
   Step 1: If $FEV_1 < 2.0$ L for pneumonectomy (< 1.5 L for lobectomy), use quantitative perfusion scanning to estimate postoperative FEV_1 (ppoFEV_1)
   Step 2: If ppoFEV_1 and $D_{LCO} > 40\%$, proceed
   Step 3: If ppoFEV_1 or $D_{LCO} < 40\%$, use cardiopulmonary exercise testing to assess risk

Pulmonary dysfunction after upper abdominal procedures is typically manifested as persistently decreased lung volumes, atelectasis, and hypoxemia. The abdominal contribution to ventilation appears to be impaired, with limited diaphragm excursion and decreased cough. Almost half the patients undergoing abdominal procedures develop small ipsilateral pleural effusions that resolve spontaneously. Cardiac surgery is frequently complicated by atelectasis. Phrenic nerve injury is confirmed in less than 10% of patients after cardiac surgery and so is unlikely to be primarily responsible for atelectasis. Multiple causes have been proposed, including extended use of cardiopulmonary bypass and entry into the pleural space during the operation. Thoracic operations are also commonly complicated by atelectasis; diaphragmatic dysfunction, compression of the lung, decreased cough, and decreased respiratory excursion due to pain have been implicated. Operations performed on peripheral structures (eg, extremities) are infrequently complicated by prolonged respiratory compromise. However, the short-term (less than 24 hours) effects of anesthesia on lung function can be significant when there is underlying lung disease.

General anesthesia affects the shape and motion of the chest wall and diaphragm. There is a significant decrease in functional residual capacity secondary to a cephalad shift of the diaphragm. Also, loss of intercostal and diaphragmatic muscle tone appears to contribute to the development of atelectasis during general anesthesia. Because inhalational anesthetics inhibit hypoxic pulmonary vasoconstriction, gas exchange abnormalities due to shunting (from atelectasis or underlying pulmonary disease) may be exacerbated. However, the effects of general anesthesia are mild in the absence of significant cardiopulmonary disease. There is no strong evidence that regional anesthetic is safer than general anesthesia for patients at risk for pulmonary complications.

Patients are at increased risk for pulmonary embolism during the perioperative period, and patients with limited cardiac or pulmonary reserve have increased morbidity and mortality rates in the event of an embolism. Adequate prophylaxis against deep venous thrombosis is essential and varies with the operative procedure.

Underlying Pulmonary Disease

Specific pulmonary diseases do increase the risk for perioperative complications. Acute upper and lower respiratory tract infections increase the risk of atelectasis and pneumonia due to aspirated secretions, and elective surgery should be postponed until infection is controlled. Patients with asthma are susceptible to bronchospasm during the perioperative period. Endotracheal intubation may trigger an exacerbation and should be undertaken with caution. Drugs that release histamine should be avoided, while some inhalational anesthetics can prevent and reverse bronchospasm. Preparation of asthma patients for surgery includes use of bronchodilators and the addition of systemic steroids when asthma is severe.

Pulmonary complications of surgery occur commonly in patients with COPD. For individual patients, pulmonary function testing does not accurately predict postoperative hypoxemia or the need for prolonged mechanical ventilation. Generally, however, the risk of pulmonary complications is low for an FEV_1 greater than 2.0 L, moderate for an FEV_1 of 1.0–2.0 L, and high for an FEV_1 less than 1.0 L. Baseline hypoxemia and/or hypercarbia appear to be useful predictors of respiratory complications.

Patients with COPD should receive maximal outpatient therapy in preparation for surgery. Patients with chronic bronchitis may benefit from bronchodilator therapy, and antibiotics are frequently prescribed. Cigarette smokers (with or without COPD) undergoing surgery have an increased incidence of complications, including fever, cough, and abnormal chest x-rays. The adverse effects of smoking are particularly apparent in patients with limited pulmonary reserve. It seems reasonable to recommend 4–6 weeks of abstinence from smoking to minimize bronchial secretions, or 12–24 hours of abstinence to decrease the blood carboxyhemoglobin level and maximize blood oxygen-carrying capacity. In the postoperative period, patients are encouraged to use an incentive spirometer and to ambulate as early as tolerated.

Evaluation for Lung Resection

Resection of lung parenchyma may be recommended electively (eg, for carcinoma of the lung) or emergently (eg, for uncontrollable hemoptysis). Evaluation of candidates for lung resection is frequently challenging because patients who require this therapy often have impaired lung function and diminished pulmonary reserve. Some degree of COPD is found clinically or pathologically in most lung cancer patients, and the dysfunction is severe in 10%–20% of cases. Removal of a lobe (lobectomy) or a lung (pneumonectomy) decreases the remaining vital capacity, but generally to a lesser degree than predicted by the amount of lung tissue removed. Prediction of short-term survival time and long-term pulmonary function after lung resection is helpful in determining who should undergo these potentially life-saving procedures. Generally, a preoperative FEV_1 greater than 2 L is not a contraindication to pneumonectomy and patients with a preoperative FEV_1 greater than 1.5 L tolerate lobectomy. Patients with a lower FEV_1 are at higher risk for complications, including death or prolonged mechanical ventilation. However, common causes of death after lung cancer surgery include myocardial infarction, pulmonary embolism, and infection, and these diseases are not readily predicted by spirometric measures.

In order to select patients for whom recovery of independent ventilation and adequate pulmonary function can be expected, additional studies are useful.

Specifically, patients with a low FEV_1 (less than 2 L) or diffusion capacity (<80%) can be evaluated with a quantitative assessment of lung perfusion. An estimated postoperative $FEV_1 \geq 800$ mL or 40% of the predicted normal value is a widely used clinical guideline. Measurement of cardiopulmonary reserve with exercise testing also appears to be useful for operative risk stratification.

THE AGING LUNG

Age-related changes in pulmonary function do not typically contribute to limitation of routine activities. However, reserves available to meet additional stresses are compromised, and may contribute to worse outcomes during disease. Studies of lung parenchyma in older adults demonstrate a gradual loss of alveolo-capillary surface area, decreasing by approximately 15% by age 70. While enlargement of terminal air spaces is observed, there is uncertainty about whether destruction of alveolar septae analogous to that seen with smoking occurs with healthy aging. Changes in parenchymal lung tissue lead to decreased elastic recoil, which may contribute to the gradually increasing residual/closing volume during aging, which begins to encroach on tidal respiration first in the supine position and then while sitting (Table 14–4). Decreased elasticity of thoracic bone articulations appears to increase the work of breathing in older adults, and respiratory muscle strength decreases, although improved performance occurs with training.

An important difference in control of breathing appears to occur with aging, as older subjects have a markedly decreased ventilatory response to experimentally imposed hypercapnia and hypoxemia. Studies of pulmonary function testing in older adults are difficult to interpret because healthy subjects may represent an elite survivor population that differs at all ages from the control subjects. Given that caveat, total lung capacity appears to be preserved during aging. Residual volume increases, perhaps due to decreased expiratory effort and/or small airway closure, and carbon monoxide diffusion capacity decreases with age, consistent with loss of alveoli.

 Aging is also associated with an increased risk of pulmonary infection. This increased risk may be due to deficits in immune function. In addition, comorbid disease can increase the risk of pneumonia. For example, neurologic disease (eg, stroke) predisposes to aspiration, which presents a recurrent

Table 14–4. Changes in the aging lung

Pathology
Enlargement of terminal air spaces
Decreased alveolocapillary surface area
Pulmonary function
Increased residual volume
Decreased diffusion capacity
Respiratory drive
Decreased ventilatory response to hypercapnia and hypoxemia
Host defense
Increased frequency of bacterial infection

large volume infectious stress to the lung. Finally, elderly patients who require substantial nursing support in dedicated facilities are exposed to hospital-acquired pathogens. When elderly patients develop pneumonia, the usual signs and symptoms, including fever and dyspnea, may be absent. The diagnosis of pneumonia is associated with a higher mortality and longer hospital stays in older patients, and represents a dangerous stress on the aging lung and immune system.

CLINICAL SCENARIOS

Case 1

A 69-year-old man presents to the emergency room with progressive dyspnea and a nonproductive cough over the past month. He denies fever, chest pain, orthopnea, and paroxysmal nocturnal dyspnea. He was treated for congestive heart failure and ventricular arrhythmia 6 months ago, and since that time his medications include aspirin, a diuretic, a nitrate, an angiotensin-converting enzyme inhibitor, and amiodarone.

Physical Examination: On exam, he is mildly tachypneic with bibasilar crackles on auscultation. There is no elevation of the jugular venous pressure, and the cardiac exam is normal with the exception of tachycardia. Routine laboratory evaluation including complete blood count and basic metabolic profile is unremarkable. A chest radiograph demonstrates bilateral lower lung zone infiltrates without cardiomegaly or pleural effusions. An electrocardiogram shows sinus tachycardia with Q waves in the inferior leads, unchanged from previous studies. Arterial blood gas analysis without supplemental oxygen confirms a gas exchange problem: pH 7.44, P_{CO_2} 31, and P_{O_2} 65. Bronchoscopy with BAL is performed, and the recovered fluid contains foamy, lipid-laden macrophages. Special stains and cultures for various infectious agents are negative.

Discussion: The clinical scenario is very suggestive of amiodarone pulmonary toxicity. These findings occur in 5%–15% of patients receiving 400 mg/d of amiodarone and usually develop after 6 months of therapy. The symptoms, physical findings, radiographic abnormalities, and arterial blood gas analysis are all consistent with a progressive restrictive lung disease. The diagnosis can be further suggested by high-resolution CT scan, which may show areas of high attenuation. This increased attenuation is attributed to the radiopaque iodine content of the amiodarone, but the specificity of this finding is unknown. The presence of lipid-laden macrophages in BAL fluid does not confirm the diagnosis, as these cells can be seen in lavage from patients receiving amiodarone without pulmonary toxicity. The treatment consists of discontinuing amiodarone and administration of corticosteroids if the symptoms are severe. In spite of this, some patients develop progressive respiratory failure. Occasionally, amiodarone is the only drug that can control potentially lethal dysrhythmias in a given patient. In this situation, the patient may be placed on long-term corticosteroids along with the lowest effective dose of amiodarone. Angiotensin-converting enzyme inhibitors commonly cause a dry, nonproductive cough but are not causes of progressive interstitial lung disease.

Typical features of amiodarone toxicity in this case notwithstanding, drug-induced lung disease is very often a diagnosis of exclusion. Evaluation for other causes of lung dysfunction, especially congestive heart failure, that can cause the presenting signs and symptoms is necessary.

Case 2

A 63-year-old man is referred to a pulmonary clinic for evaluation of cough and dyspnea. He states that his symptoms started about 9 months ago and then gradually worsened to the point that he became dyspneic during minimal exertion. The patient is a retired teacher and quit smoking 4 years ago. He denies other medical problems, takes no medications, and is unaware of any environmental inhalational exposures. The patient is in mild respiratory distress.

Physical Examination: The vital signs are remarkable for a respiratory rate of 32 breaths/min. He has prominent bibasilar crackles on auscultation of the chest. The cardiac exam is normal. A chest radiograph shows bilateral lower lobe reticulonodular infiltrates. Pulmonary function tests demonstrate that the vital capacity is 65% and the diffusion capacity is 55% of the predicted value. The patient undergoes an open lung biopsy and is found to have usual interstitial pneumonitis. No evidence of asbestos or infection is identified. At this time he is prescribed prednisone (1 mg/kg) for interstitial pulmonary fibrosis (IPF).

Discussion: This patient has a gradually progressive clinical presentation consistent with a diagnosis of IPF. Confirmation of the disease and exclusion of infectious etiologies of interstitial lung disease will allow the physician to treat aggressively with immunosuppressive agents. The response to corticosteroids and cytotoxic therapies is variable and the majority of patients do not improve. This patient should be followed carefully for side effects of therapy and disease progression, with reassessment of pulmonary function within 6–12 weeks of initiation of therapy.

A progressive decline in lung volumes, increased need for oxygen supplementation, or worsening exercise tolerance should prompt early referral for lung transplantation evaluation. Patients with pulmonary fibrosis have the highest mortality of any primary lung disease group while on a waiting list for transplantation. In recognition of this fact, these patients are credited with additional days of waiting time when placed on the transplant list. Because patients with IPF tend to be older and often have a history of cigarette smoking, they should be carefully screened for other comorbid conditions (eg, malignancy or coronary artery disease).

Early referral for lung transplant evaluation is essential. Waiting time for organs may be as long as 2 years, and death while on the transplant list is common. A lung transplant specialist can assist in determining whether to proceed with transplant evaluation or to defer until the disease has progressed.

KEY CONCEPTS

 Therapeutic use of certain drugs, illicit drug use, and cigarette smoking can lead to a variety of lung injuries.

 Lung transplantation is performed for end-stage pulmonary disease and exposes the new lung to acute ischemic injury, chronic immunologic attack, and recurrent infections.

 Hematopoietic stem cell transplantation offers an opportunity for cure for many diseases, but introduces the potential for chemotherapy and radiation-induced injuries to the lung, as well as a chronically hostile immune environment and a risk for opportunistic infections.

 Operative procedures and anesthesia acutely affect pulmonary function and protective airway reflexes and can be associated with long-term loss of lung volume (resection) or loss of function (phrenic nerve injury).

 Age-related changes in pulmonary function decrease the reserve available to meet the stress of illness, and comorbid illness and deficits in pulmonary host defense increase the frequency and severity of lung infection.

 STUDY QUESTIONS

14–1. A 53-year-old woman who has undergone autologous hematopoietic stem cell transplantation for multiple myeloma 10 days earlier develops shortness of breath, dry cough, and hypoxemia. On examination, patient is afebrile with RR 28 breaths/min, HR 120 beats/min, and BP 110/70 mm Hg. Cardiac exam is unremarkable. Chest examination reveals bilateral crackles, and chest radiograph shows areas of patchy air space disease in lower lung zones bilaterally. A flexible bronchoscopy with bronchoalveolar lavage is performed. The lavage fluid shows gross blood and numerous hemosiderin-laden macrophages. Specific stains and immunoassays for various organisms are negative in the lavage fluid. The next step would be:

   a. Diuresis

   b. Intravenous amphotericin B

   c. Broad-spectrum intravenous antibiotics

   d. High dose methylprednisolone and platelet transfusion, if needed

   e. Comfort care only.

14–2. A 36-year-old man presents to the chest clinic complaining of increasing dyspnea and dry cough for 6 months. In the last 3 months he has received three courses of oral antibiotics, with azithromycin, amoxicillin, and ciprofloxacin, without any significant improvement in his symptoms. Patient has smoked one pack per day *for the past 20 years. Physical examination and routine laboratory results are unremarkable. Pulmonary function tests show a mild restrictive lung defect and a moderate decrease in diffusion capacity. A chest radiograph shows increased interstitial markings, and subpleural areas of ground-glass opacity are noted on high-resolution CT scan. The most likely diagnosis is*

a. Cystic fibrosis

b. Asthma

c. Desquamative interstitial pneumonitis

d. α_1-Antitrypsin deficiency

e. Atypical pneumonia.

SUGGESTED READINGS

Limper AH. Drug-induced pulmonary disease. In: Murray JF, Nadel JA, Mason RJ, Boushey HA, eds. *Murray and Nadel's Textbook of Respiratory Medicine.* 3rd ed. Philadelphia: WB Saunders; 2005:1888–1908.

Maurer JR, Zamel N. Lung transplantation. In: Murray JF, Nadel JA, Mason RJ, Boushey HA, eds. *Murray and Nadel's Textbook of Respiratory Medicine.* 4th ed. Philadelphia: WB Saunders; 2005:2433–2451.

List of Abbreviations

ABMA   antibasement membrane antibody
ACE   angiotensin-converting enzyme
ACS   acute coronary syndrome
AFB   acid-fast bacilli
AHI   apnea-hypopnea index
AIDS   acquired immunodeficiency syndrome
AIP   acute interstitial pneumonia
ALI   acute lung injury
AMS   acute mountain sickness
ANA   antinuclear antibody
ARDS   acute respiratory distress syndrome
ARF   acute respiratory failure
ATS   American Thoracic Society
AVM   arteriovenous malformation
BAE   bronchial artery embolization
BAL   bronchoalveolar lavage
BCG   bacille Calmette Guérin
BIPAP   bilevel positive airway pressure
BMI   body mass index
BMT   bone marrow transplantation
BNP   brain natriuretic peptide
BPD   bronchopulmonary dysplasia
CAD   coronary artery disease

cANCA   cytoplasmic antineutrophilic cytoplasmic antibody
CAP   community-acquired pneumonia
CF   cystic fibrosis
CFTR   cystic fibrosis transmembrane conductance regulator
CHF   congestive heart failure
CMV   cytomegalovirus
COP   cryptogenic organizing pneumonia
COPD   chronic obstructive pulmonary disease
CPAP   continuous positive airway pressure
CPEX   cardiopulmonary exercise
CSA   central sleep apnea
CT   computed tomography
CWP   coal worker's pneumoconiosis
CXR   chest x-ray
DAD   diffuse alveolar damage
DAH   diffuse alveolar hemorrhage
DIP   desquamative interstitial pneumonitis
D_{LCO} diffusion capacity
DOT   directly observed therapy
DPLD   diffuse parenchymal lung disease
ECG   electrocardiogram

EEG	electroencephalograph	LDH	lactate dehydrogenase
EOG	electrooculograph	LPS	lipopolysaccharide
ERV	expiratory reserve volume	LTBI	latent tuberculosis
ETH	ethambutol		infection
$FEF_{25\%-75\%}$	forced expiratory flow,	MBP	major basic protein
	midexpiratory phase	MDI	metered dose inhaler
FEV1	forced expiratory volume	MODS	multiple organ
	in the first second		dysfunction syndrome
F_{IO_2}	fraction of inspired oxygen	MOTT	mycobacteria other
FOB	fiber optic bronchoscopy		than *M tuberculosis*
FRC	functional residual	MRI	magnetic resonance
	capacity		imaging
FVC	forced vital capacity	Mtb, MTB	*Mycobacterium*
GER	gastroesophageal reflux		*tuberculosis*
GERD	gastroesophageal reflux	MVV	maximum voluntary
	disease		ventilation
GVHD	graft-versus-host disease	NAEPP	The National Asthma
HAP	hospital-acquired		Education and
	pneumonia		Prevention Program
HDI	hexamethylene	NIF	negative inspiratory
	diisocyanate		force
HEENT	head, eyes, ears, nose,	NIPPV	noninvasive positive
	and throat		pressure ventilation
Hgb	hemoglobin	NREM	non-REM sleep
HHRF	hypercapnic-hypoxic	NTM	nontuberculous
	respiratory failure		mycobacteria
HIV	human immunodeficiency	OSA	obstructive sleep apnea
	virus	P_2	component of second
HMD	hyaline membrane		heart sound that
	disease		represents closure of
HP	hypersensitivity		the pulmonic valve
	pneumonitis	PAC	pulmonary artery
HRCT	high-resolution		catheter
	computed tomography	Pa_{CO_2}	partial pressure of
HRF	hypoxic respiratory failure		arterial carbon dioxide
IgE	immunoglobulin E	pANCA	perinuclear
IgG	immunoglobulin G		antineutrophilic
INH	isoniazid		cytoplasmic antibody
IPF	interstitial pulmonary	$P_{AO_2} - Pa_{O_2}$	alveolar-arterial oxygen
	fibrosis or idiopathic		gradient
	pulmonary fibrosis	P_{AO_2}	partial pressure of
IPPV	intermittent positive		alveolar oxygen
	pressure ventilation	Pa_{O_2}	partial pressure of
IRV	inspiratory reserve volume		oxygen in systemic
LAM	lymphangioleiomyomatosis		arteries

Pco_2	Provocative concentration of methacholine at which 20% decline in FEV1 occurs	REM	rapid eye movement (sleep)
		RIF	rifampin
		RSV	respiratory syncytial virus
Pco_2	partial pressure of carbon dioxide		
		RV	residual volume
PCP	*Pneumocystis carinii* pneumonia	Sao_2	arterial oxyhemoglobin saturation
PEEP	positive end-expiratory pressure	SRBD	sleep-related breathing disorder
PEF	peak expiratory flow	TB	tuberculosis
PEFR	peak expiratory flow rate	TDI	toluene diisocyante
PFT	pulmonary function test	T/E Dis	thromboembolic disease
PLCH	pulmonary Langerhans cell histiocytosis	TLC	total lung capacity
		TNF	tumor necrosis factor
PMF	progressive massive fibrosis	TP	total protein
		TST	tuberculin skin test
PND	postnasal drip	TV	tidal volume
Po_2	partial pressure of oxygen	UIP	usual interstitial pneumonia
PPD	purified protein derivative (tuberculosis skin test)		
		UNOS	United Network for Organ Sharing
PPH	primary pulmonary hypertension	US LE	ultrasound lower extremity
PSG	polysomnogram	VATS	video-assisted thoracoscopic surgery
Pulse Ox	pulse oximetry		
PZA	pyrazinamide RDI respiratory disturbance index	VC	vital capacity
		VILI	ventilator-induced lung injury
QOL	quality of life	$\dot{V}/\dot{Q}$	ventilation-perfusion
RDS	respiratory distress syndrome	WBC	white blood cell count

Answers to Study Questions

SECTION 1

Chapter 1

1–1. d.   Airway obstruction is defined as a decrease in the FEV_1:FVC ratio of less than 70%. The degree of severity of obstruction is usually defined by comparing the change in the FEV_1 to the predicted value.

1–2. e.   All of the listed mechanisms are physiologic causes of dyspnea.

1–3. d.   All of the above are examples of airway obstruction that are associated with an equal decrease in the FVC and FEV_1 maintaining the FEV_1:FVC ratio above 70%.

Chapter 2

2–1. c.   In this patient, the accompanying symptoms of hoarseness, stridor, and shortness of breath indicate that the upper airway is the probable cause of the dry, hacking, nonproductive cough. All the other choices mentioned may cause increasing cough, but the absence of purulent sputum and symptoms of bronchitis and the paucity of findings suggestive of left ventricular failure or congestive heart failure make these diagnoses unlikely. Postintubation and/or posttracheotomy lesions generally are stenotic or due to tracheomalacia. Ulceration or scar formation involves the upper trachea or subglottic area. Endotracheal tube size, cuff pressure, tube design, and duration of intubation all determine the extent of injury. Cough involving a subglottic upper tracheal extrapulmonary lesion is due to stimulation of irritant receptors initiating the afferent loop of the cough reflex and is compounded by secretions. The flow volume loop shows the characteristic box pattern with obstruction in both the inspiratory and expiratory loops. Other than symptomatic treatment of the cough, avoidance of irritant exposure, mechanical and pharmacologic aids to facilitate clearance of secretions, and tracheal dilatation and placement of stents may be helpful in managing this condition.

2–2. c.   With a negative AFB smear and a normal chest x-ray and CT scan, it is unlikely that this patient has active TB. Latent TB, which this patient probably has based on her positive PPD, is generally asymptomatic.

All the other disorders listed could cause chronic cough in this clinical setting.

Chapter 3

3–1. c. Hemoptysis in a smoker may be due to many factors. Mild to moderate hemoptysis secondary to chronic bronchitis is the most common cause. In this instance, changes in the pulmonary arterial pressure gradient and development of precapillary bronchopulmonary anastomoses rupture superficial vessels, causing hemoptysis. Mucosal and submucosal edema occurs. Patients respond to treatment of chronic bronchitis, although hemoptysis may recur. Recurrence of TB is associated with other clinical symptoms, such as fever, generalized ill health, and increasing cough which are absent in this case, and recurrence can be confirmed by sputum bacteriologic studies. Rupture of an aneurysmal vessel in a cavitary TB focus generally causes massive hemoptysis. In case of old, inactive TB, bleeding and hemoptysis can occur due to underlying bronchiectasis, with or without purulent sputum. However, the chest x-ray is unlikely to be normal. In any patient with risk factors for carcinoma, hemoptysis may vary from mild to massive. The normal chest x-ray makes carcinoma also less likely in this case. However, if hemoptysis persists, a bronchoscopic evaluation would be needed to rule out an airway lesion or an endobronchial carcinoma.

3–2. d. This clinical scenario is classical for bronchiectasis with the pathogenesis described in the text. The chest x-ray findings suggest saccular or cystic bronchiectasis. It is not unusual to have hypoxemia and anemia with this degree of recurrent hemoptysis and repeated infections. Invasive pulmonary aspergillosis generally occurs in immunecompromised hosts recovering from neutropenia and *Candida* overgrowth is not uncommon in patients on frequent antibiotic therapy.

Chapter 4

4–1. b. Although the differential diagnosis is broad, this patient's history and physical examination are suggestive of an acute myocardial infarction. Therefore, an ECG should be promptly done to look for evidence of myocardial ischemia or infarction, while attempts are made to control the high blood pressure and to assess the need for urgent revascularization procedures. Because the murmur of aortic insufficiency also suggests the possibility of aortic dissection as a cause of this patient's chest pain, a chest x-ray should also be done immediately after obtaining an ECG. A chest x-ray will also reveal other possible causes for chest pain, such as a pneumothorax. If a widened mediastinum is seen on the x-ray, a transesophageal echocardiogram or a chest CT scan should be obtained to confirm aortic dissection. A serum lipase determination and a stool test for occult blood might be necessary later, if the results of the aforementioned tests are negative.

4–2. e. This patient's history of the sudden onset of pleuritic chest pain suggests an acute problem and in this case the findings indicate a tension pneumothorax. The appropriate first step would be to insert a small chest tube on the left to relieve tension. A chest x-ray would confirm the pneumothorax or, if he had a perforated gastric ulcer, the chest x-ray might show free air under the diaphragm. The other conditions listed as possible answers are in the differential but do not present with all the signs enumerated. Giving a β-adrenergic blocking drug might be appropriate to treat some tachyarrhythmias causing hypotension, although it would not be the first approach in this case. Giving a β-blocker to this patient could have disastrous results, since he is maintaining his blood pressure through his increased heart rate. A nasogastric tube to evaluate for blood in the stomach is not indicated in this patient. Hyperventilation during a panic attack and anxiety may be appropriately treated by having the patient rebreathe exhaled carbon dioxide from a paper bag. However, this patient is tachypneic because of respiratory and cardiovascular compromise and not because of anxiety.

4–3. d. The history and background information is strongly suggestive of GERD. Tests to confirm this such as pH monitoring are available and utilized in certain cases, but the best initial approach is to give a therapeutic trial of proton pump inhibitors and reduce acid reflux.

4–4. b. This history is suggestive of a hypercontracting esophagus, which includes the term "nutcracker esophagus" based on manometric studies. It has been shown that many patients with nutcracker esophagus also have a hypertensive or poorly relaxing lower esophageal sphincter suggesting an overlap between these hypercontractile motility abnormalities. However, not all patients with nutcracker esophagus have chest pain. Specific therapies have been difficult to define, since both the actual pathophysiology and the relationship of motility findings to symptoms remain obscure. However, use of calcium channel blockers significantly relieves chest pain. Although occasional uncontrolled observations have suggested that nitrates, phosphodiesterase inhibitors, anticholinergics, pneumatic dilatation, use of botulinunm toxin, or an extended myotomy may be beneficial, this is not universally accepted.

4–5. b. Coronary artery disease is foremost on the differential in this case. However, the symptoms are suggestive of pericarditis and the ECG will specifically show diffuse ST elevations. It is unlikely that these changes will be limited to the inferior leads as mentioned in C. Normal sinus rhythm and left ventricular hypertrophy will be nonspecific in this case.

4–6. d. This is one of those diagnoses that can be made by specific physical exam and reproducing symptoms in the absence of other competing diagnoses. In this case, the past history and workup has been negative and the location of the pain without a costal cartilage component or a neuropathic distribution is highly suggestive of lower rib pain syndrome.

4–7 c.   The clinical picture is highly suggestive of herpes zoster where the pain may be severe and often described as burning. Dermatomes may be involved and the presence of a rash increases the likelihood of this being the cause. There is no specific curative treatment but antivirals may reduce the duration of symptoms and prevent recurrences.

Chapter 5

5–1. c.   Both inspiratory and expiratory wheezing can be heard in severe asthma and chronic obstructive lung disease. However, wheezing exclusively in inspiration occurs typically in upper airway obstruction such as tracheal stenosis (see flow-volume loop in Chapter 1). Congestive heart failure typically causes crackles, and in some cases of pulmonary edema, expiratory wheezing is detected. This is thought to be due to peribronchial congestion, localized airway constriction, and decreased pulmonary elastance.

5–2. d.   Intensity of breath sounds may be decreased when there is decreased respiratory excursion due to muscle disease, restriction of chest wall, or pleural disease, or due to airflow limitation in obstructive lung disease. Pneumonia characteristically produces bronchial breath sounds due to increased transmission of sounds of central origin through a consolidated lobe.

5–3. c.   Pulmonary fibrosis due to any cause (in this case, asbestosis or idiopathic) produces mid- to late-inspiratory crackles. Pulmonary edema can cause crackles due to the opening and closing of airways at a peripheral air space/alveolar level. Bronchiectasis causes crackles that are described as leathery in nature and are said to originate from the terminal bronchioles. If significant, dependent lobar or segmental atelectasis caused by airway collapse typically results in decreased breath sounds and does not cause any adventitious sounds.

SECTION 2

Chapter 6

6–1. c.   Eosinophilic inflammation is commonly found in the airways of asthmatics and appears to be central to the pathogenesis of the disease. Interestingly, recent studies suggest that asthma management may be better when tailored to the sputum eosinophil count rather than symptoms. While eosinophils are not normally found in stable COPD patients, they are present during exacerbations. Histopathology in bronchiectasis does not include eosinophilic inflammation.

6–2. a. FEV$_1$ is predictive of mortality, 6-min walk distances, and QOL measures; however, the correlation is weak. Much stronger exercise and QOL associations have been found with IC, diffusing capacity, dyspnea, and activity of daily living questionnaires. This serves to emphasize the concept that while the mechanical *defect* in COPD is primarily airflow obstruction during expiration, the mechanical *consequences* restrict inspiration. The hyperinflation and air trapping denoted by a reduction in IC substantially increase the work of breathing. Diffusing capacity is a better estimate of the loss of alveolar surface area than is FEV$_1$. Activities of daily living and dyspnea are multidimensional constructs and cannot be reliably predicted by FEV$_1$, but correlate reasonably well with exercise capacity and QOL.

Chapter 7

7–1. c. Progressive pulmonary hypertension leading to cor pulmonale may occur as pulmonary fibrosis worsens. This is probably due to destruction and distortion of the pulmonary arterioles and capillaries; however, a primary vascular component has not been completely excluded. The progressive elevation of pulmonary vascular resistance leads to eventual right ventricular failure; this usually occurs in very late-stage disease.

7–2. c. The destruction of alveolar units in emphysema is not accompanied by fibrosis, but results in increased static lung compliance due to loss of elastic recoil. All of the other factors listed occur in the course of progressive fibrosis and contribute to loss of static lung compliance.

Chapter 8

8–1. a. This patient very likely had a pulmonary embolism and is a high risk for recurrent embolization, so observation would be risky. His lung scan is abnormal but is not diagnostic of pulmonary embolism because the ventilation-perfusion defects are matched. Warfarin should not be started until the diagnosis is confirmed. A D-dimer would not likely be helpful because it will probably be positive due to his recent trauma. Serial ultrasound exams are best utilized in patients with good cardiopulmonary reserve. This patient's borderline hypotension mandates a more urgent diagnostic approach. The CT angiogram should be positive in this patient with large defects on his ventilation-perfusion scan.

8–2. c. This patient has several clinical manifestations of severe pulmonary hypertension and right ventricular failure. All of the diseases listed may be causes of pulmonary hypertension; however, the presence of cyanosis should make one suspicious that a right-to-left shunt is present. Asthma is rarely associated with such severe pulmonary hypertension and the normal exam of the lungs makes severe asthma and left ventricular failure less likely. In severe asthma, diminished respiratory excursions and wheezing are often present. In left ventricular failure, crackles are often observed. Chronic pulmonary embolism and primary pulmonary hypertension are only associated with intracardiac shunts if a patent foramen ovale is present. Atrial septal defects are the most common congenital heart disease to present with pulmonary hypertension in adulthood. Atrial septal defects can escape detection in childhood because the murmurs are inconspicuous and the shunt is initially left to right.

8–3. b.   The acuteness of this patient's symptoms while stair climbing is very suggestive of heart disease. Pulmonary edema can result from left ventricular systolic, diastolic, or valvular dysfunction. A low plasma oncotic pressure is rarely the principal cause of pulmonary edema. Arterial blood gas analysis may be important in guiding therapy, but will not differentiate the possible causes of pulmonary edema. Pulmonary emboli occur in patients with heart failure, but rarely cause pulmonary edema. The pulmonary artery occlusion pressure is an approximation of the left atrial pressure. A high pulmonary artery occlusion pressure would suggest a cardiac cause of pulmonary edema (which we already suspect), but would not differentiate among the various diseases that elevate left atrial pressure. An echocardiogram would easily identify the suspected mitral stenosis in this patient.

8–4. a.   This patient has bronchiectasis, a chronic suppurative lung disease. Chronic inflammation in the lung leads to the development of large bronchial artery and intercostal artery anastomoses. These blood vessels are perfused at systemic pressures and are likely to bleed during acute exacerbations. Although patients can occasionally identify which lung is the source of bleeding, bronchial arteriography can usually best identify bleeding vessels. Once identified, embolization of the artery with synthetic materials can stop the bleeding. Blood is usually fully oxygenated by the time it is expectorated, regardless of whether the source of the bleeding is in the bronchial or the pulmonary circulation. Chest radiographs can sometimes suggest a likely lobe for the source of the bleeding, but when blood is aspirated into other lobes, the chest radiograph is less specific.

Chapter 9

9–1. c.   This man with silicosis is presenting as if he has an infectious disease with fever and a new cavity on his chest x-ray. The most likely diagnosis is tuberculosis, given the unique susceptibility of silicotics to tuberculosis and the new cavity on the chest x-ray. Diagnosis of infection would take priority over other treatments in such a patient. Silicosis causes interstitial fibrosis with decreased lung compliance and altered matching of ventilation to perfusion. Since bronchospasm is not a major feature of silicosis, bronchodilators would be of little value. The patient is hypoxemic with a widened alveolar-arterial difference, but his arterial oxygen saturation is greater than 90%. Administering supplemental oxygen to raise his arterial Po_2 would not significantly improve either the content of oxygen in the blood or the amount of oxygen delivered to the tissues. Although glucocorticoids are used to treat some inflammatory disorders of the lungs, they are contraindicated in most pulmonary infections because their immunosuppressive properties compromise host defenses against infection.

9–2. b. Near drowning when water reaches the alveolar space causes abnormalities of surfactant, leading to microatelectasis. This alveolar instability disrupts the normal matching of ventilation to perfusion. Hypoventilation is ruled out in this case, with a low arterial Pco_2. Heart failure is also unlikely, given the normal-sized heart on chest x-ray. Aspirated fresh water, as in this case, is rapidly cleared from the alveoli; thus, a diffusion defect should not be present.

9–3. c. Hypersensitivity pneumonitis results from immunologic sensitization to inhaled organic antigen, bird proteins in this case. Once a patient has become sensitized, they react to minute quantities of antigen. This makes respiratory protection with masks difficult. Breathholding is also unlikely to protect him from inhalation of antigen. Repetitive exposure to antigen in a sensitized host can only lead to disease progression. The only safe approach is cessation of exposure.

Chapter 10

10–1. b. BCG is an attenuated form of mycobacterium that has an extremely low risk of causing clinical disease. Its efficacy in preventing TB disease is variable at best, and due to this controversy it is not used routinely in the United States. It is felt that even though BCG vaccination may not prevent active pulmonary disease, it protects children from lifethreatening meningitis and miliary tuberculosis. Studies have shown that skin reactivity of BCG-vaccinated individuals wanes with time, and a positive skin test result 10 years after vaccination is more likely to be due to infection with tuberculosis than due to BCG. Therefore, immigrants from countries with a high prevalence of tuberculosis who received BCG vaccination as infants should be considered infected if their PPD test result is read as positive and should be evaluated and treated for clinical TB or offered chemoprophylaxis or treatment for latent TB if they do not have active disease.

10–2. e. Most often, bacterial pneumonias do respond to antibiotic therapy with gradual resolution of symptoms. Clinical response to the chosen empiric antibiotic regimen should be observed diligently so that patients who are responding slowly or not at all are identified promptly and further exploration may be undertaken. If a patient's condition is responding appropriately to therapy, improvement in clinical findings such as fever or leukocytosis is usually seen within

48–72 hours. Therefore, initial empiric therapy should not be changed until 72 hours have passed unless initial diagnostic studies identify a pathogen not covered by the original empiric therapy, a resistant pathogen is isolated from the blood or another sterile site (eg, pleural fluid), or there is clinical deterioration. Radiographic findings may lag considerably behind symptomatic resolution, and may in some cases initially worsen. Again, a change in empiric antibiotic coverage or an extensive diagnostic workup is not indicated unless there is a worsening of clinical status. When pneumonia fails to respond to initial therapy, probable explanations include inadequate empiric coverage, bacterial resistance to the chosen antibiotics, an uncommon pathogen, impaired host defense, a noninfectious condition, or a further complication. A diverse group of noninfectious diseases may masquerade as pneumonia and initially be misdiagnosed as infection. These diseases include acute respiratory distress syndrome, certain inflammatory lung diseases (eg, hypersensitivity pneumonitis, chronic eosinophilic pneumonia, Wegener granulomatosis, bronchiolitis obliterans organizing pneumonia, and pulmonary fibrosis), neoplastic processes (eg, bronchogenic carcinoma, pulmonary lymphangitic carcinomatosis, metastases), drug-induced lung disease, congestive heart failure, pulmonary embolism, and miscellaneous problems, such as an inhaled foreign body and lipoid pneumonia. Chest x-rays cannot differentiate these processes from infectious pneumonia; any of them can produce focal air space disease or diffuse infiltrates.

In this patient, a ventilation-perfusion scan is performed and shows little or no perfusion to the right lung and subsegmental perfusion defects in the left, unmatched with any ventilation defects. Antibiotics are discontinued, and anticoagulation with heparin is begun, followed closely by treatment with warfarin. His symptoms begin to improve, and he is discharged 6 days later on warfarin.

Chapter 11

11–1. d. This is a case of a primary spontaneous pneumothorax. HRCT of the chest to look for parenchymal lung disease is not indicated. Administration of 100% oxygen would be reasonable if the pneumothorax were less than 15%. An attempt at evacuation of the pneumothorax should be made with a small-bore catheter; if evacuation fails, consideration should be given to a more aggressive approach such as large-bore chest tube, pleurodesis, and possible thoracic surgery.

11–2. e. In the setting of suspected pneumonia, the presence of a significant pleural effusion (>10 mm on lateral decubitus film) is an indication for thoracentesis. The fluid should be evaluated for LDH, protein, pH, glucose and Gram's stain, as well as routine culture. Indications for chest thoracostomy include Gram's stain of pleural fluid positive for organisms; LDH >3 times the upper limit of normal for serum;

loculated pleural fluid; pleural fluid glucose <40 mg/dL; and pleural fluid pH <7.0.

Chapter 12

12–1. a. and c. Tracheostomy and significant weight loss can be curative. CPAP provides symptomatic treatment only.

12–2. b. Although obesity can affect patients with CSA, it is not causative.

12–3. c. Central apneas occur in the transition from wakefulness to sleep. To put it in a different way, central apneas are most likely to occur when it is easiest to arouse one from sleep: stages I, II, and REM.

Chapter 13

13–1. e. Hypotension with tachycardia seen soon after placement on a mechanical ventilator suggests gas trapping, decreased venous return, and reduced cardiac output. These effects are the results of reduced expiratory airflow due to dynamic hyperinflation and extreme airway resistance. Mechanical ventilation may not allow sufficient expiratory time for complete alveolar empty-ing. This incomplete emptying raises intrathoracic pressure and impedes venous return, increasing pulmonary artery resistance and reducing cardiac output. Immediately and temporarily removing the patient from the ventilator and thereby decreas-ing intrathoracic pressure can reverse this. Once infusing fluid restores volume, mechanical ventilation can be resumed with a lower tidal volume of 6–8 mL/kg ideal body weight.

13–2. d. Mechanical ventilation is initiated to achieve the following goals: improve oxygenation, optimize ventilation, and correct acid–base status. In this patient, mechanical ventilation was initiated successfully. However, in patients with ARDS, there is ALI, and a large number of alveolar units are either collapsed throughout the respiratory cycle or open only during inspiration. An ongoing continuum of injury ensues and oxygenation goals can be difficult to achieve. Recruiting alveoli for gas exchange can dramatically improve oxygenation. These collapsed alveoli can be recruited and maintained patent in a functional state with a small amount of PEEP. In patients with ARDS, PEEP at a level of 10–12 cm H_2O achieves this goal, prevents expiratory collapse, and allows a reduction in F_{IO_2}.

Chapter 14

14–1. d. The case scenario described is very suggestive of DAH. This patient is at increased risk for this complication because she has undergone autologous BMT for a solid malignancy. Even though DAH is associated with very high mortality, palliative care is premature at this time. There is no evidence of fluid overload or infection as a cause for the patient's symptoms. High-dose steroids and platelet transfusion support are the only therapeutic interventions available.

14–2. c.   Cystic fibrosis, asthma, and α_1-antitrypsin deficiency cause an obstructive lung defect. While atypical pneumonia can present with cough, dyspnea, and interstitial infiltrates, the duration of symptoms is usually days to several weeks. In addition, the patient has received adequate therapy for most causes of atypical pneumonia. The therapy for DIP includes smoking cessation and corticosteroids. The overall prognosis is good, with complete resolution of symptoms if the patient stops smoking.

Index

NOTE: A *t* following a page number indicates tabular material, and an *f* following a page number indicates a figure.

281